| DUE DATE | RETURN DATE | DUE DATE | RETURN DATE |
|----------|-------------|----------|-------------|
|          |             |          |             |

# ULTRASOUND ANNUAL 1983

# Ultrasound Annual
# 1983

## Editors

**Roger C. Sanders, M.D.**
*Associate Professor*
*The Russell H. Morgan Department*
*of Diagnostic Radiology*
*Department of Urology*
*Director of Abdominal Ultrasound*
*The Johns Hopkins Medical*
*Institutions*
*Baltimore, Maryland*

**Michael C. Hill, M.D.**
*Associate Professor of Radiology*
*Director of Diagnostic Ultrasound*
*The George Washington University*
*Medical Center*
*Washington, D.C.*

Raven Press ■ New York

Raven Press, 1140 Avenue of the Americas, New York, New York 10036

Made in the United States of America

International Standard Book Number 0-89004-954-8

The material contained in this volume was submitted as previously unpublished material, except in the instances in which credit has been given to the source from which some of the illustrative material was derived.

Great care has been taken to maintain the accuracy of the information contained in the volume. However, Raven Press cannot be held responsible for errors or for any consequences arising from the use of the information contained herein.

# Preface

The selection of topics for the second in this ultrasound series was not a difficult task. First, due to recent advances in real-time ultrasound, a chapter explaining the comparative merits of different types of real-time systems is included, along with a futuristic look at their development.

A second chapter focuses on the sonographic size of the normal common bile duct and the increasing role of ultrasound in this area. Sonography of the upper abdominal venous system was chosen as another topic of importance; problems involving the portal venous system, inferior vena cava, and hepatic veins are considered in one concise chapter. Due to the increasing use of small parts scanners, an update on scrotal sonography is included. The importance of sonography in patient management in this area is described in detail by Dr. Phillip. Transrectal prosthetic ultrasound using a linear array system has received scant attention within the United States until the recently published work of Rifkin and his group. The clinical efficacy of this modality and its use in guiding transperineal biopsies is discussed.

Although it may seem surprising to have a chapter on tropical diseases in a book on ultrasound, due to increasing world travel, it is not entirely improbable to be faced with a patient from a foreign country. A chapter discussing tropical diseases is included and deals with patients with amebiasis or hydatid disease of the liver.

Obstetrical ultrasound remains an area of rapid evolution. In this volume are two reviews of work in this area in which new information has emerged. Data on the use of doppler ultrasound in measuring fetal umbilical vein blood flow and how it is affected by some complications that occur in pregnancy is discussed. This ultrasonic method has been popularized and hopefully will prove useful in the early diagnosis of intrauterine growth retardation. With increasing use of *in vivo* and *in vitro* fertilization, ultrasound has assumed a critical role in monitoring ovarian follicular development in conjunction with serum estradiol levels. These developments are elucidated by Fleischer and his coworkers.

Finally, although ophthalmic ultrasound has been somewhat overshadowed by the development of computed tomography, it nevertheless is still useful in the diagnosis of certain ophthalmic disorders. Chang and his coworkers have presented in detail the current status of ophthalmic ultrasound.

Roger C. Sanders, M.D.
Michael C. Hill, M.D.

# Contents

# Contributors

**Henry J. Abrams**
*Department of Urology*
*State University of New York at*
*Stonybrook and*
*Long Island Jewish Hospital-Hillside*
*Medical Center*
*New Hyde Park, New York 11042*

**Albert L. Bundy**
*Department of Radiology and*
*Radiological Sciences*
*Ultrasound Section*
*Vanderbilt University Medical Center*
*Nashville, Tennessee 37232*

**Stanley Chang**
*Department of Ophthalmology*
*Cornell University Medical College*
*New York, New York 10021*

**J. L. Chezmar**
*Department of Radiology*
*The Johns Hopkins Medical*
*Institutions*
*Baltimore, Maryland 21205*

**D. Jackson Coleman**
*Department of Ophthalmology*
*Cornell University Medical College*
*New York, New York 10021*

**James F. Daniell**
*Department of Obstetrics and*
*Gynecology*
*Center for Fertility and Reproductive*
*Research*
*Vanderbilt University Medical Center*
*Nashville, Tennessee 37232*

**Arthur C. Fleischer**
*Department of Radiology and*
*Radiological Sciences*
*Ultrasound Section*
*Vanderbilt University Medical Center*
*Nashville, Tennessee 37232*

**D. Graham**
*Department of Obstetrics-*
*Gynecology and*
*The Russell H. Morgan Department*
*of Diagnostic Radiology*
*The Johns Hopkins Medical*
*Institutions*
*Baltimore, Maryland 21205*

**Michael C. Hill**
*Department of Radiology*
*The George Washington University*
*Medical Center*
*Washington, D.C. 20037*

**Yacov Itzchak**
*Tel-Aviv University School of*
*Medicine*
*Sheba Medical Center*
*Tel-Hashomer, Israel 52621*

**A. Everette James, Jr.**
*Department of Radiology and*
*Radiological Sciences*
*Ultrasound Section*
*Vanderbilt University Medical Center*
*Nashville, Tennessee 37232*

**P. Jouppila**
*Department of Obstetrics*
*University of Oulu*
*Oulu, Finland*

**P. Kirkinen**
*Department of Obstetrics*
*University of Oulu*
*Oulu, Finland*

**Shelia Kumari-Subaiya**
*Department of Radiology*
*State University of New York at*
*Stonybrook*
*Long Island Jewish Hospital-Hillside*
*Medical Center*
*New Hyde Park, New York 11042*

**Alfred B. Kurtz**
*Thomas Jefferson University*
*1015 Walnut Street*
*Philadelphia, Pennsylvania 19107*

**Frank P. Leo**
*Russell H. Morgan Department of*
*Radiology and Radiological*
*Science*
*Johns Hopkins Hospital*
*Baltimore, Maryland 21205*

**Wayne S. Maxson**
*Department of Obstetrics and*
*Gynecology*
*Center for Fertility and Reproductive*
*Research*
*Vanderbilt University Medical Center*
*Nashville, Tennessee 37232*

**Gail Phillips**
*Department of Radiology*
*State University of New York at*
*Stonybrook*
*Long Island Jewish Hospital-Hillside*
*Medical Center*
*New Hyde Park, New York 11042*

**Donald E. Pittaway**
*Department of Obstetrics and*
*Gynecology*
*Center for Fertility and Reproductive*
*Research*
*Vanderbilt University Medical Center*
*Nashville, Tennessee 37232*

**John E. Repp**
*Department of Obstetrics and*
*Gynecology*
*Center for Fertility and Reproductive*
*Research*
*Vanderbilt University Medical Center*
*Nashville, Tennessee 37232*

**Matthew D. Rifkin**
*Thomas Jefferson University*
*1015 Walnut Street*
*Philadelphia, Pennsylvania 19107*

**Zalman Rubinstein**
*Tel-Aviv University School of*
*Medicine*
*Sheba Medical Center*
*Tel-Hashomer, Israel 52621*

**R. C. Sanders**
*The Russell H. Morgan Department*
*of Diagnostic Radiology*
*The Johns Hopkins Medical*
*Institutions*
*Baltimore, Maryland 21205*

**E. Sauerbrei**
*Queen's University*
*Ultrasound Section*
*Department of Radiology*
*Kingston General Hospital*
*Kingston, Ontario*

**Ruth Shilo**
*Tel-Aviv University School of*
*Medicine*
*Sheba Medical Center*
*Tel-Hashomer, Israel 52621*

**Mary E. Smith**
*Department of Ophthalmology*
*Cornell University Medical College*
*New York, New York 10021*

**Gary A. Thieme**
*Department of Radiology and*
*Radiological Sciences*
*Ultrasound Section*
*Vanderbilt University Medical Center*
*Nashville, Tennessee 37232*

**Charles E. Torbit**
*Department of Obstetrics and*
*Gynecology*
*Center for Fertility and Reproductive*
*Research*
*Vanderbilt University Medical Center*
*Nashville, Tennessee 37232*

**Anne Colson Wentz**
*Department of Obstetrics and*
*Gynecology*
*Center for Fertility and Reproductive*
*Research*
*Vanderbilt University Medical Center*
*Nashville, Tennessee 37232*

Ultrasound Annual 1983, edited by R. C.
Sanders and M. Hill. Raven Press, New York
© 1983.

# Ultrasound of the Common Bile Duct

E. Sauerbrei

*Queen's University, Ultrasound Section, Department of Radiology, Kingston
General Hospital, Kingston, Ontario*

Until the past few years, intravenous cholangiography was the most common imaging test to evaluate the common bile duct. However, in a large minority of patients the duct was inadequately opacified for proper evaluation and the final interpretation was often in error (21). High resolution gray scale sonography, and especially real-time sonography, has replaced intravenous cholangiography as the primary imaging technique in evaluating the common bile duct both before and after cholecystectomy. Sonography is an accurate and reliable technique for evaluating the size of the common duct and intrahepatic ducts and for evaluating the neighboring soft tissue structures such as the liver, pancreas, and other structures of the porta hepatis. This chapter will discuss sonographic techniques, normal anatomy and anatomic variants, common duct size in various situations, obstructive and nonobstructive lesions affecting the duct, intraoperative bile duct scanning, and finally the role of ultrasound for the investigation of jaundice.

## NORMAL BILIARY TREE

### Normal Anatomy

The left and right hepatic ducts, which are intrahepatic, converge at the porta hepatis to form the common hepatic duct (CHD) which is extrahepatic. The cystic duct joins the CHD at a variable location to form the common bile duct (CBD) which then empties into the second portion of the duodenum (Fig. 1). Because the site of cystic duct insertion into the CHD is variable and because the cystic duct is uncommonly visualized in abdominal sonograms, the term common duct (CD) will be used to indicate the entire extrahepatic bile duct (13, 51, 55).

The CD is tethered cranially to the liver where the left and right hepatic ducts converge and caudally where it enters the posterior portion of the head of the pancreas. The remainder of the CD is relatively unfixed as it courses along the lateral edge of the hepatoduodenal ligament with the main portal vein and proper hepatic artery cranial to the pancreas. In the coronal plane,

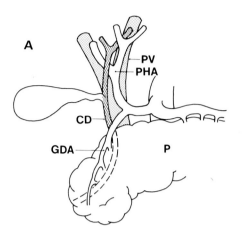

**FIG. 1A:** Normal anatomy. This drawing traces the course of the common duct (CD) from the porta hepatis caudally into the head of the pancreas (P). Note the position of the proximal common duct anterior to the right portal vein, and the position of the more distal common duct anterolateral to the portal vein (PV). The proper hepatic artery (PHA) courses medial to the common duct and anteromedial to the portal vein. Note the position of the gastroduodenal artery (GDA) on the anterior surface of the pancreas.

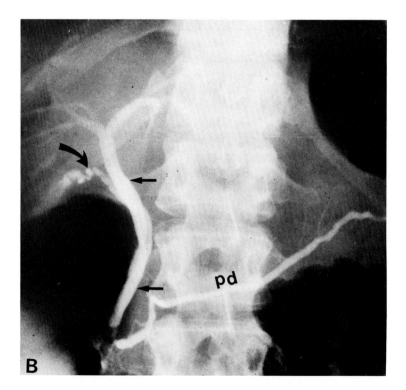

**FIG. 1B:** Normal anatomy. An AP radiograph taken from ERCP examination demonstrates excellent opacification of the pancreatic duct (PD), the common duct *(straight arrows),* and the cystic duct *(curved arrow).* This projection corresponds to **A.**

the CD, main portal vein, and proper hepatic artery course slightly obliquely from right to left as they course caudally in the hepatoduodenal ligament. In most people, the CD lies anterolateral to the portal vein, whereas the proper hepatic artery lies anteromedial to it (Fig. 1). This relationship holds true until the vessels exit the hepatoduodenal ligament just craniad to the pancreatic head, where the proper hepatic artery curves medially to form the common hepatic artery and the CD curves laterally to enter the second portion of the duodenum at the ampulla of Vater.

In a sagittal plane, the CD courses posteriorly as it travels caudally. The most anterior portion is usually the proximal CHD as it passes anterior to the right portal vein whereas the most posterior portion is the distal CBD as it courses through the posterior portion of the pancreatic head, immediately anterior to the inferior vena cava (Fig. 2).

### Sonographic Technique and Anatomy

Complete scans of the upper abdomen include a specific examination to define its course, diameter, lumen, wall, and surrounding tissues. The goal is to image the entire duct from the convergence of the left and right hepatic ducts to the ampulla of Vater, both in long and short axes. All sonographic techniques are tailored toward this end. In a retrospective study of 100 patients who had routine axial and sagittal scans of the liver with a static scanner (13), a portion of the CD was seen in only 39% whereas in a prospective study, in which the CD was examined specifically, the CD was seen in 87% of patients (87 of 100 patients) (13). Therefore, it is very important to search out the CD to obtain the appropriate images.

Several authors (3, 10, 13, 51) have shown that the CD or portions thereof can be demonstrated conveniently with the patient supine or in a right side-up anterior oblique position (ranging from 45° to 90°), the latter position allowing more frequent and easy demonstration of the CD. Static articulated-arm scanners and real-time scanners (sector format and linear array format) have both been used with success in evaluating the biliary tree but the highest success rates are obtained with real-time units. Cooperberg (10), using a real-time sector scanner, demonstrated the proximal CHD in 98 out of 100 consecutive adults without biliary tract disease, whereas Dewbury (13) demonstrated some portion of the CD in 87 of 100 consecutive patients in a prospective study using an articulated arm scanner.

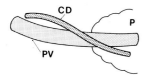

**FIG. 2.** Normal anatomy. This drawing depicts the course of the common duct (CD) in a parasagittal plane. In its proximal course, the common duct courses anterior to the portal vein (PV), while more distally, the common duct courses posteriorly and enters the posterior portion of the head of the pancreas (P).

In our laboratory, we use primarily real-time sector scanners and less frequently linear array units to examine the biliary tree. Scans are usually obtained with a 3.5-MHz medium-focus transducer although a 5-MHz transducer is available for thin patients. Patients are examined in a supine and right-side-up oblique position with the transducer placed on the skin in the right subcostal area, or more laterally in an intercostal space. The main portal vein is traced to its bifurcation where parasagittal scans demonstrate a small tubular structure (the proximal CHD) anterior to the right portal vein (Fig. 3). A small circle is usually identified between the CHD and right portal vein, corresponding to the right branch of the proper hepatic artery (see Fig. 12). This portion of the CD is visualized in virtually every patient, even those with previous biliary surgery. Then the transducer is rotated through 90° and the CD can be seen in cross section as a circle anterior to the right portal vein (Fig. 4A, B) and more caudally, anterolateral to the main portal vein (Fig. 4C). The distal CD is visualized less frequently than the proximal CD owing to the overlying gas in the duodenum and colon, but improved

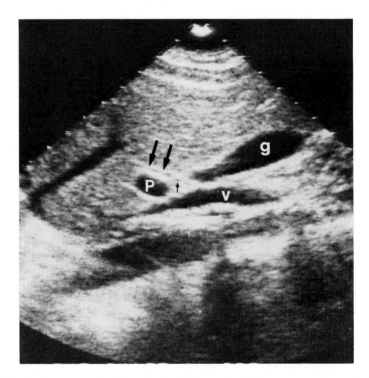

**FIG. 3.** Proximal common duct (longitudinal). A parasagittal sonogram demonstrates the proximal common duct *(large arrows)* coursing anterior to the right portal vein (P) and the right hepatic artery *(small arrow).* The inferior vena cava (v) and gallbladder (g) are also demonstrated. This portion of the common duct can be visualized in almost every patient.

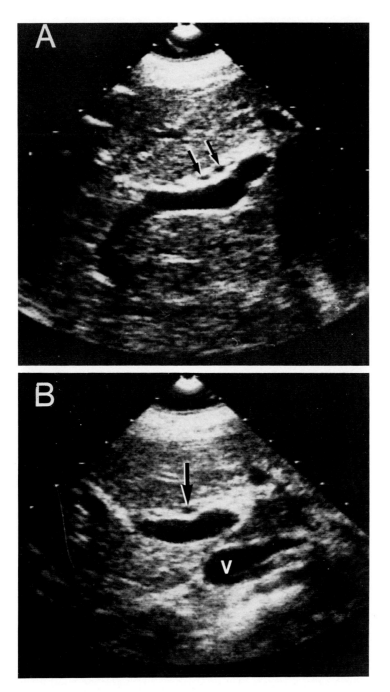

**FIG. 4. A:** Left and right hepatic ducts. A transverse oblique sonogram demonstrates the left and right hepatic ducts *(arrows)* anterior to the confluence of the right and left portal venous branches. The left and right hepatic ducts can be visualized in the majority of normal people. **B:** Proximal common duct (transverse). Transverse oblique sonogram caudad to **A** demonstrates the proximal common duct *(arrow)* anterior to the right portal vein at the confluence of the right and left portal venous branches which are anterior to the inferior vena cava (v).

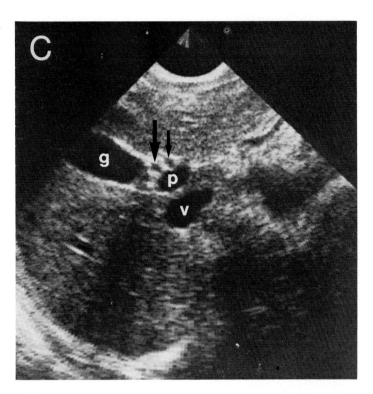

**FIG. 4C.** Mid-common duct (transverse). A transverse sonogram caudad to **B** demonstrates the common duct *(large arrow)* and proper hepatic artery *(small arrow)* anterior to the portal vein (p). This is the characteristic appearance of the triad of vessels in the hepatoduodenal ligament in a normal individual. The gallbladder (g) is situated lateral to the triad and the inferior vena cava (v) posterior.

visualization may result from filling the stomach and duodenum with water and temporarily paralyzing these structures with intravenous glucagon (53). The distal CBD may be visualized as it courses through the posterior aspect of the pancreatic head immediately anterior to the inferior vena cava (Fig. 5A, B).

### Anatomic Variants

Three common anatomic variants may cause confusion in scanning the CD: hepatic artery variants, the transverse common duct, and a redundant neck of the gallbladder.

The right hepatic artery courses anterior to the CD in about 15% of people studied sonographically (5, 56) (see Fig. 8A, C). Occasionally the hepatic artery is tortuous and the tomographic ultrasound sections may be confusing. Tracing the course of these structures to their origin often resolves the

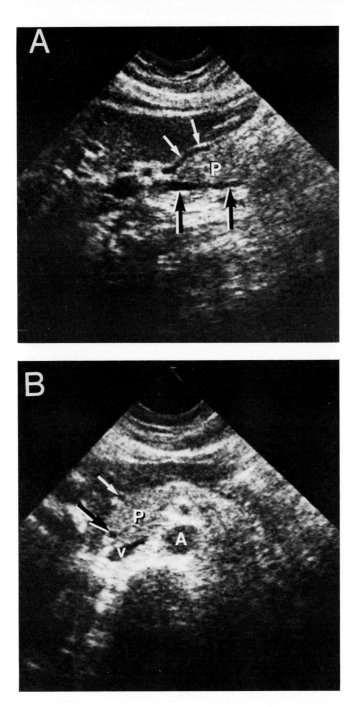

**FIG. 5. A:** Distal common duct (longitudinal). A parasagittal sonogram through the head of the pancreas (P) demonstrates the distal portion of a normal common duct *(large arrows)* coursing along the posterior aspect of the head of the pancreas and the gastroduodenal artery *(small arrows)* along the anterior aspect of the head of the pancreas. This portion of the common duct is visualized much less frequently than the proximal portion, as demonstrated in Fig. 3. **B:** Distal common duct (transverse). A transverse sonogram in the same person demonstrates the head of the pancreas (P) and body of the pancreas anterior to the inferior vena cava (v) and aorta (A). The distal common duct *(large arrow)* is seen along the posterolateral aspect of the head of the pancreas and the gastroduodenal artery *(small arrow)* along the anterior aspect.

problem although other signs (such as intrinsic pulsations and indentations of the artery into the more pliable CD and portal vein) and perhaps scanning with a duplex scanner (which is a combination of real-time imaging and pulsed doppler scanning) can clarify the anatomy (5).

The mid-portion of the CD may assume a transverse position in some patients. In a study of 118 intraoperative cholangiograms, Jacobson and Brodey (28) showed that about 6% of nonobstructed ducts will have a long transverse segment that may extend beyond the midline. In obstructed ducts, the proportion of patients with a transverse segment of the CD was significantly higher (18%) (Fig. 6). In these situations, a dilated transverse CD may be mistaken for the portal vein or splenic vein and a nondilated duct for the hepatic artery unless careful real-time scanning is performed to define the proximal and distal extents of the CD.

Another pitfall to avoid, especially on static scans, is mistaking a redundant neck of the gallbladder for the CD (32). Real-time scanning can eliminate this occasional problem by localizing the gallbladder and CD in their long and short axes.

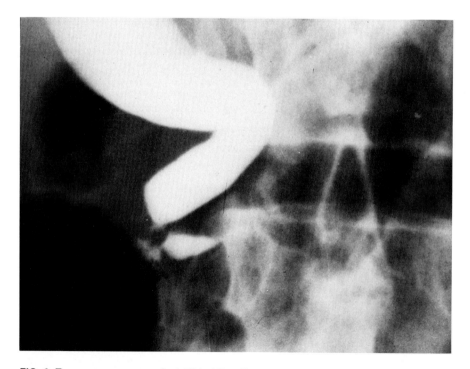

**FIG. 6.** Transverse common duct. This AP radiograph taken from a transhepatic cholangiogram demonstrates an unusually large common duct whose course is more tortuous than usual. The midportion of the common duct lies almost in a transverse plane, in contradistinction to most nondilated ducts which course in a longitudinal plane.

## Bile Duct Physiology

The primary function of the CD is the transport of bile from the liver to the duodenum. Bile will flow if the intraductal pressure (about 100 to 150 mm of water) is less than the hepatic secretory pressure. This pressure difference is affected by three mechanisms:

1. The activity of the sphincter at the distal end of the CD (the sphincter of Boyden).
2. Gallbladder filling and resorption of bile in the gallbladder.
3. Bile flow from the liver.

The contractility of the distal sphincter is probably the most important dynamic factor in affecting intraductal pressure. In normal people, there is a regular cycle of about 10 contractions and relaxations per minute, with each contraction causing an ejaculatory jet of bile into the duodenum (36). The CD has no motor role in bile flow because there is complete absence of smooth muscle fibers in the wall of the CD in the large majority of people (38). The wall is composed of elastic and fibrous tissue that can expand when the intraductal pressure increases and return to normal size when the pressure is reduced to normal. Contraction of the sphincter of Boyden will increase the intraductal pressure to 120 to 160 mm of water, at which point bile will flow into a normal gallbladder. During this contractile phase, however, bile still flows into the duodenum but at a reduced rate.

## COMMON DUCT SIZE IN NORMAL PEOPLE

### Gallbladder *In Situ*

In radiographic studies based on intravenous cholangiography, percutaneous cholangiography, and ERCP and early ultrasound studies (1, 6, 17, 35, 39, 57, 73), the upper limit of normal for the common bile duct diameter was between 8 and 11 mm in healthy adults with no apparent evidence of biliary obstruction. However, more recent studies, using real-time and static scanning in large numbers of people with the gallbladder *in situ* and with no evidence of biliary tract disease, portray a lower range of normal bile duct diameters.

In pediatric patients, the CD diameter gradually increases with age from 1 month to 16 years, but is less than or equal to 4 mm, as measured anterior to the right portal vein (40). The mean pediatric CD diameter is 2 mm. The normal range of CD diameters in adults has been less clearly established because recent ultrasound studies have produced conflicting results for the upper limit of CD diameters, ranging from 4 to 8 mm (3, 8, 10, 13, 49, 51, 59).

Table 1 lists five recent studies that examined the diameter of the CD in people with the gallbladder *in situ* and with no evidence of biliary obstruc-

TABLE 1.   *Bile duct diameter with the gallbladder* in situ

| Source | Number of people in study[a] | Upper limit of normal range (mm) | Number of ducts above normal range |
|---|---|---|---|
| Sample, 1978 (59) | 57[b] | 5 | 2 (4%) |
| Dewbury, 1980 (13) | 126[c] | 5 | 0 |
| Cooperberg, 1978 (10) | 98 | 4 | 0 |
| Bruneton, 1981 (8) | 750 | 4 | 40 (5%) |
| Niederau, 1983 (49) | 830 | 4 | 41 (5%) |

[a]All subjects were adults with no evidence of biliary obstruction.
[b]Fifty-seven patients with medical jaundice but no evidence of biliary obstruction. These patients had no previous biliary surgery.
[c]Author did not specify how many patients had gallbladder still *in situ*.

tion. In two series (13, 59) the upper limit of CD diameter (i.e. the internal lumen diameter) was found to be 5 mm, whereas three series (8, 10, 49) placed the upper limit at 4 mm. In the series by Bruneton et al. (8) (750 people) and the series by Niederau et al. (49) (830 patients), 95% of duct diameters were 4 mm or less. Five percent of normal people with the gallbladder *in situ* had a CD diameter greater than 4 mm but less than or equal to 7 mm (49). Given these statistics, the upper end of the normal range of CD diameters, most conveniently measured anterior to the right portal vein, is 4 mm. Diameters of 5 mm or more fall above the 95th percentile, and hence represent dilated ducts. In practice we consider CD diameters of 4 mm or less as normal, a diameter of 5 mm borderline enlarged, and a diameter of 6 mm enlarged.

### After Cholecystectomy

There is considerable confusion and debate regarding the size of the non-obstructed bile duct in people after cholecystectomy. Two major questions exist: What is the normal range of bile duct diameters in asymptomatic people after cholecystectomy? and, Does the bile duct dilate after a cholecystectomy? Ultrasound studies represent the optimal imaging technique to answer these questions because there is no inherent magnification in the system and because the normal biliary physiology and morphology are undisturbed during the examination. Several ultrasound studies have examined the range of bile duct diameters in normal post cholecystectomy patients (Table 2). Most authors measure the proximal duct diameter anterior to the right portal vein, or just caudal to this location in the hepatoduodenal ligament, because it is the easiest and most reliable location in which to image the bile duct (10, 22, 45, 49). In nondilated ducts, the diameter of the proximal portion is usually the same as the distal portion whereas in dilated systems, the proximal duct, on average, measures slightly less than the widest portion of the duct which is usually more caudal (49) (see Table 2).

According to the studies quoted in Table 2, there is no question that some normal people (i.e., people with no current bile duct obstruction) have a dilated bile duct after cholecystectomy. Mueller et al. (45) found that only 5% of 40 people had a dilated bile duct (greater than 5 mm was considered dilated), Graham et al. (22) found that 16% of 67 people had a dilated bile duct (greater than 4 mm was considered dilated) and Niederau et al. (49) found that 58% of 55 people had a dilated bile duct (greater than 4 mm was considered dilated). In the last two studies the percentages drop to 10% and 32%, respectively, if diameters greater than 5 mm are considered enlarged. To generalize, it appears that a majority of normal people postcholecystectomy have a normal caliber duct whereas a significant minority have a mildly dilated duct in the range of 5 to 10 mm. It is precisely the latter group that presents a difficult problem for the ultrasonographer because the pre-cholecystectomy status of the bile ducts is not usually known. If there is no clinical or laboratory evidence (i.e., raised bilirubin and alkaline phosphatase) of biliary obstruction, then further investigation is probably not warranted. Conversely, if there is some evidence of obstruction and the duct diameter is between 5 and 10 mm, then another test, such as percutaneous cholangiogram, ERCP, or CT scan, could be done to find the cause if the ultrasound scan cannot do so. The recently described technique of administering a fatty meal and observing any change in bile duct caliber can also be used to resolve the dilemma (67). This technique will be described in a later section (Common Duct Size in Biliary Obstruction). If the bile duct diameter is greater than 10 mm, the probability of bile duct obstruction is quite high.

Only two previous ultrasound studies have addressed the second question: does the bile duct dilate after a cholecystectomy in an otherwise normal person? (see Table 3) (22, 45). These studies indicate that very few bile ducts increase in size after cholecystectomy unless obstruction intervenes: in the range of 2.5 to 4.5% of patients. This suggests that most of the normal patients with mildly dilated bile ducts after cholecystectomy (ranging from 5 to 58% in different series) were dilated at the time of surgery and did not return to the normal range afterward. There is no evidence that the CD dilates merely in compensation for a missing gallbladder.

### Discrepancy Between Radiographic and Sonographic Bile Duct Measurements

Ultrasound studies indicate that the upper limit of normal for bile duct diameters before cholecystectomy is 4 or 5 mm (Table 1) whereas cholan-

TABLE 2. Bile duct diameter in asymptomatic people after cholecystectomy

| Source | Number in study | Upper limit of normal range (mm) | Mean diameter (mm) | Range of diameters (mm) | Percentage with enlarged caliber (%) |
|---|---|---|---|---|---|
| Niederau, 1983 (49)[a] | 55 | 4<br>5 | 5.2[b] | 1–11 | 58<br>32 |
| Bruneton, 1981 (8) | 77 | | 4.5 | | |
| Graham, 1980 (22)[a] | 67 | 4<br>5 | 3.7 | 2–10 | 16<br>10 |
| Mueller, 1981 (45)[a] | 40 | 5 | 3.5 | 2–7 | 5 |

[a]These authors measured the proximal portion of the common duct just caudal to the confluence of the left and right hepatic ducts.
[b]Niederau et al. (49) found the mean duct diameter increased to 6.2 cm when measured more caudally at the widest point of the duct.

TABLE 3. *Change in bile duct diameter after cholecystectomy*[a]

| Source | Number of people with scans pre and postcholecystectomy | Increased bile duct diameter (% of people) |
|---|---|---|
| Graham, 1980 (22) | 67 | 4.5 (3 of 67) |
| Mueller, 1981 (45) | 40 | 2.5 (1 of 40) |

[a]In these studies, the bile ducts were scanned preoperatively and several months post-operatively. In all cases, there was no evidence of biliary obstruction.

giographic studies indicate 9 or 10 mm (17). There are several factors responsible for this discrepancy (60):

1. Radiographic techniques will overestimate the BD diameter by a factor of approximately 1.3 because of radiographic magnification.

2. Ultrasound scans slightly underestimate the luminal diameter because ultrasound portrays a falsely thickened duct wall that will encroach on the luminal measurement by 1 or 2 mm.

3. A choleretic effect causes mild distension of the duct in about 30% of people having intravenous cholangiography, while direct injection of contrast material under pressure can certainly cause transient dilatation in some cases (46).

4. In cholangiograms one usually measures the maximum transverse diameter of the CD, whereas in sonograms one usually measures the sagittal diameter of the proximal CD. In dilated systems, the average proximal CD is slightly smaller than the distal CBD (49).

## COMMON DUCT SIZE IN BILIARY OBSTRUCTION

### Gallbladder *In Situ*

Although intrahepatic duct dilation can occur with CD obstruction (Fig. 7A), dilatation of the CD itself is a more sensitive indicator for the presence of obstruction (59, 74) (Figs. 7B–E). In a series of 170 patients (some with gallbladder *in situ* and some postcholecystectomy), Cooperberg et al. (11) used 4 mm as the upper limit of normal CHD diameter to obtain a sensitivity of 99% in detecting obstruction.

Sensitivity = true positives/(true positives + false negatives)

This reflects very few false negative examinations. The specificity was 84%, thus reflecting a false positive rate of 16%.

Specificity = true negatives/(true negatives + false positives)

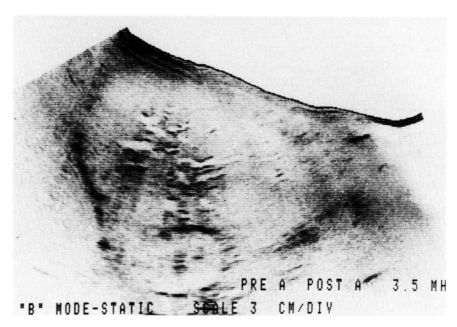

**FIG. 7A.** Dilated intrahepatic ducts. A parasagittal sonogram in the right lobe of the liver demonstrates multiple fluid-filled tubes stacked one on top of another within the parenchyma of the liver. This "too many tubes" sign is characteristic of dilated intrahepatic ducts. Note the accentuated through transmission behind the dilated ducts.

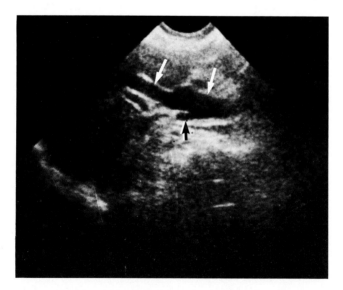

**FIG. 7B.** Dilated common duct (longitudinal). A parasagittal sonogram in the right upper quadrant demonstrates a dilated common duct *(white arrows)*. The proximal common duct is anterior to the oval cross-section of the right portal vein and the distal common duct courses toward the head of the pancreas. Occasionally, one may see a fluid-filled cystic duct remnant *(black arrow)* attached to the distal common duct, as this postcholecystectomy patient demonstrates.

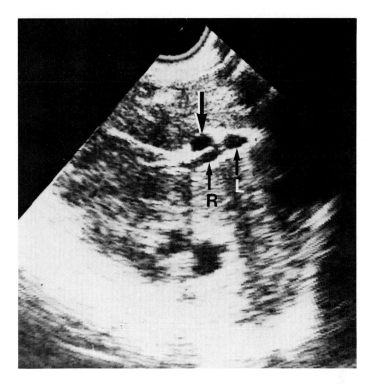

**FIG. 7C.** Dilated proximal common duct (transverse). A transverse oblique sonogram in another patient with bile duct obstruction demonstrates a dilated proximal common duct *(large arrow)* anterior to the right portal vein (R) and lateral to the left portal vein (L).

Using 5 mm as the upper limit of normal, CHD diameter decreased the sensitivity to 94% without improving the specificity. It appears, therefore, that using only the CD diameter one detects most cases of biliary obstruction but this also falsely indicates obstruction in a small but significant minority with mild ductal dilatation (5 to 10 mm). Most of these patients are postcholecystectomy (11).

### After Cholecystectomy

If one considers only postcholecystectomy patients, a CHD diameter greater than 4 mm will give a sensitivity of 88% for detecting obstruction and a specificity of 57% (false positive rate of 43%) (23). The decreased sensitivity usually reflects the presence of partially obstructing stones in a nondilated duct (see Fig. 11). The rather low specificity, which actually reflects the presence of a mildly dilated duct but without obstruction, may be tolerable for a screening test for right upper quadrant pain postcholecystectomy. These patients may be subjected to further imaging tests to include or ex-

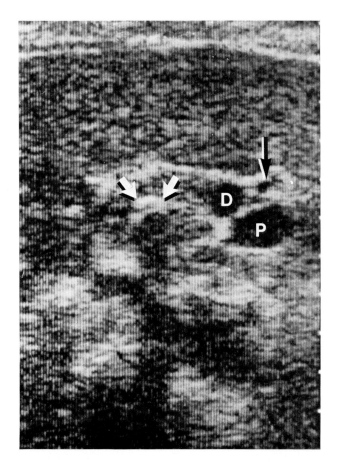

**FIG. 7D.** Dilated mid-common duct (transverse). A transverse sonogram taken more distally through the mid-portion of the common duct in a patient with biliary obstruction. Note the dilated common duct (D) anterolateral to the main portal vein (P) and lateral to the proper hepatic artery *(arrow)*. This is the characteristic appearance of a dilated common duct in its midportion in the hepatoduodenal ligament. Note the calculus *(small arrows)* within a contracted gallbladder, lateral to the triad of vessels.

clude biliary obstruction especially if the serum alkaline phosphatase or bilirubin is raised. As pointed out by Weinstein and Weinstein (72), dilatation of the CD does not occur as a simple consequence of cholecystectomy. The problem arises owing to the common occurrence of persistent dilatation from prior obstruction because prolonged and/or severe obstruction may destroy the elasticity of the CD wall. This impairs the duct's ability to retract to normal caliber. For this reason, it is almost impossible to define an exact value for the upper limit of normal duct diameter in the postcholecystectomy patient.

To further investigate postcholecystectomy patients with a mildly dilated

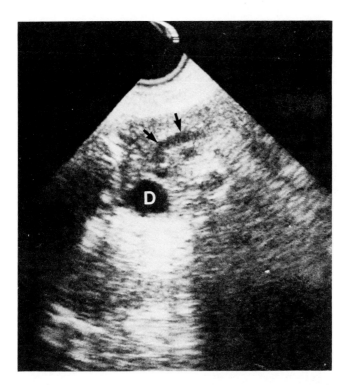

**FIG. 7E.** Dilated distal common duct (transverse). Transverse sonogram taken through the head of the pancreas in another patient with obstruction at the ampulla of Vater. The distal common bile duct (D) is markedly dilated and the pancreatic ducts *(arrows)* in the head and neck of the pancreas is also dilated due to the obstruction at the ampulla.

CD (5 to 10 mm) biliary sonography can be performed 45 minutes after a standard fatty meal (67). After cholecystectomy, a mildly dilated but non-obstructed CD will decrease to 5 mm or less (67). We have also found that larger ducts (10 mm) also decrease in diameter after a fatty meal when there is no obstruction present (Figs. 8, 9). After cholecystectomy, an abnormal response to a fatty meal occurs when a mildly dilated duct remains the same or increases in size after the fatty meal. This indicates biliary pathology, and further investigation is warranted. When fat enters the duodenum, the duodenal mucosa secretes cholecystokinin, which has three major effects: relaxation of the sphincter of Boyden, contraction of the gallbladder, and increased bile flow from the liver. Therefore, in a nonobstructed duct with a normal sphincter, a fatty meal will relax the sphincter, allow more drainage of bile into the duodenum, and theoretically decrease the diameter. Others, however, feel that the nonobstructed postcholecystectomy CD does not al-

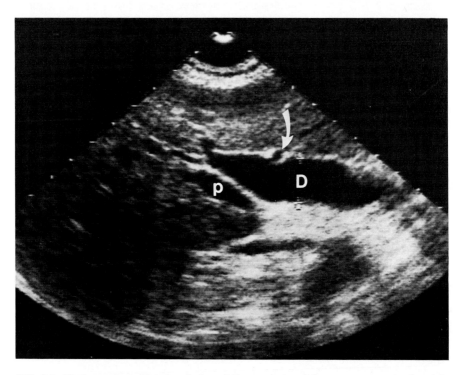

**FIG. 8A.** Common duct dilatation before fatty meal. An oblique sonogram in the right upper quadrant demonstrates a markedly dilated common duct (D) whose maximal diameter measured 16 mm. The proximal common duct is anterior to the right portal vein whereas the right hepatic artery *(arrow)* lies anterior to the common duct.

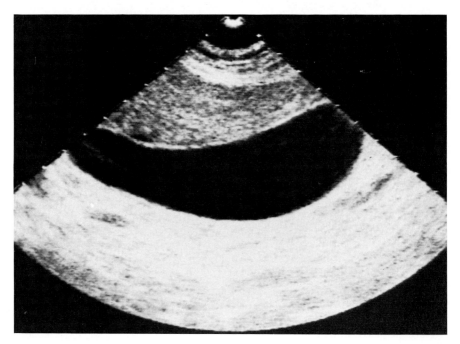

**FIG. 8B.** Distended gallbladder before fatty meal. A parasagittal sonogram in the right upper quadrant of the same patient demonstrates a fluid-filled gallbladder whose maximum AP diameter measured about 3.3 cm.

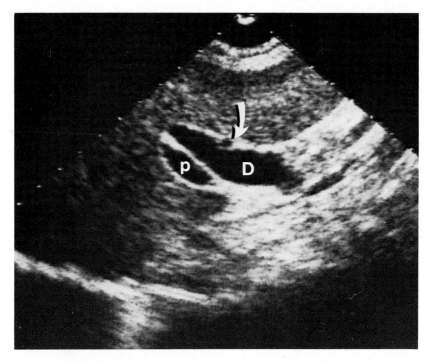

**FIG. 8C.** Common duct after fatty meal. Forty minutes after a fatty meal, the common duct (D) had decreased in diameter to 12 mm.

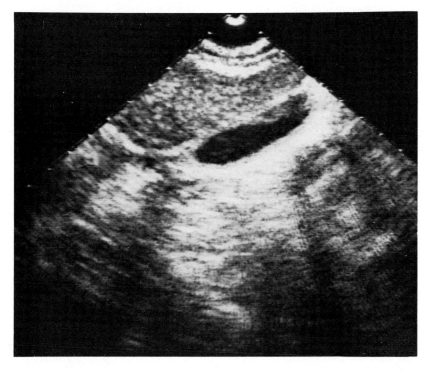

**FIG. 8D.** Gallbladder after fatty meal. A parasagittal scan through the gallbladder demonstrates marked decrease in volume of the gallbladder after the fatty meal. There was no clinical or biochemical evidence of biliary obstruction in this patient.

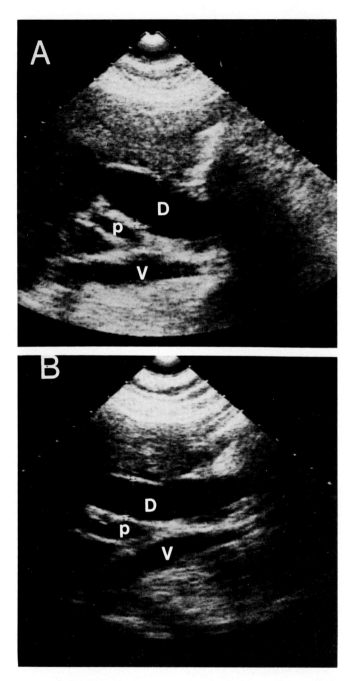

**FIG. 9. A.:** Dilated common duct (previous cholecystectomy). A parasagittal sonogram demonstrates a markedly dilated common duct (D) whose maximum diameter measured 20 mm. The right portal vein (p) and inferior vena cava (V) are small in comparison. **B:** Common duct after fatty meal. Forty-five minutes after administration of an oral fatty meal, common duct (D) measured 14 mm in diameter. This patient has been followed for 2 years with repeat sonograms and clinical evaluation and there is no evidence of biliary obstruction.

ways decrease in size following a fatty meal (*personal communication:* Dr. Michael Hill).

A fatty meal can also be used with the gallbladder *in situ* in a patient with a slightly dilated duct. If the duct is of normal caliber or slightly dilated before the fatty meal, but increases in diameter after the fatty meal, then a biliary lesion is probably present and further tests should be performed unless ultrasound can define the specific abnormality.

The fatty meal may thus resolve the problem in many patients with a dilated duct after cholecystectomy. This would reduce the number of false positive exams (given as 43% by Graham et al.) (23) by isolating those patients with significant functional obstruction causing their dilated duct. A more difficult problem is the group of patients with an obstructing lesion associated with a normal caliber duct. The sonologist or sonographer must examine the entire length of CD, if possible, even when the CD is normal caliber, in order to diagnose stones or tumors causing partial or intermittent obstruction (Figs. 10, 11).

## DYNAMICS OF BILE DUCT DILATATION

### Human Studies

The CD is actually a passive tube whose wall contains elastic tissue (38) which permits rapid distension of the duct when the intraductal pressure increases. When the pressure decreases, the elastic recoil causes a corresponding decrease in the luminal diameter if the elastic properties of the wall have not been altered. Severe distension, prolonged distension, and inflam-

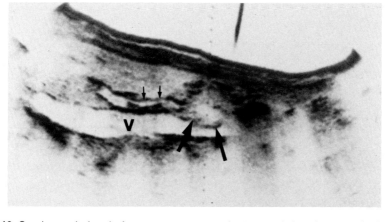

**FIG. 10.** Carcinoma in head of pancreas, common duct normal size. A parasagittal sonogram through the length of the inferior vena cava (v) demonstrates a 3 cm solid mass (*large arrows*) arising in the head of the pancreas. This was a carcinoma which failed to obstruct the common duct (*small arrows*).

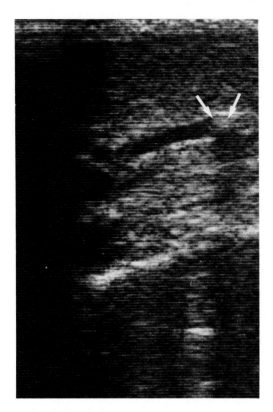

**FIG. 11.** Stone in nondilated duct. A parasagittal sonogram through the distal common duct in the head of the pancreas demonstrates a faintly shadowing calculus *(arrows)* within the distal portion of the common duct, which was not dilated. The common duct measures 4 mm in its internal caliber. This patient had abdominal lymphoma but had no clinical nor biochemical evidence of biliary obstruction.

mation in the wall may all decrease the elasticity of the wall and hence impair the duct's ability to revert to normal caliber after the pressure is relieved (18).

In patients, one may observe caliber changes from one minute to the next (18) or over a period of hours or days (20, 44, 50, 61). The cause for the increasing or decreasing intraductal pressure (and corresponding increasing or decreasing ductal diameter) may be due to physiologic changes (18, 50, 67), iatrogenic pressure changes such as direct injection of contrast medium (44, 60), or pathological lesions (20, 44, 61).

Spontaneous relaxation and contraction of the sphincter of Boyden can cause rapid changes in the pressure and diameter of the duct (Fig. 12). Similarly if a fatty meal is administered, this may cause a significant increase in duct diameter when obstruction is present, or decrease in diameter when obstruction is absent (67) (Figs. 8, 9). When contrast is injected or withdrawn directly in the CD, then instantaneous changes in the bile duct diameter can be observed (46). This phenomenon may explain some of the discrepancies between sonographic diameters and cholangiographic diameters. In a similar fashion, the passage of a stone or resolution of an obstruct-

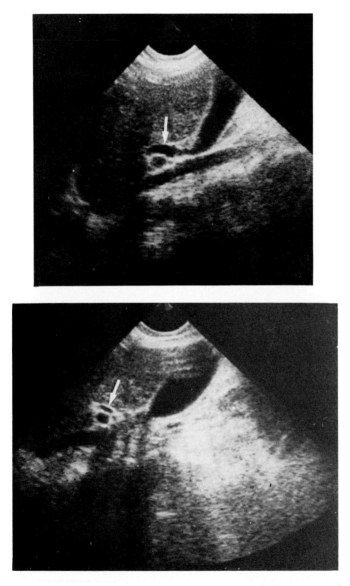

**FIG. 12. A:** Spontaneous change in bile duct size. A parasagittal sonogram in the right upper quadrant of an individual with no clinical or biochemical evidence of biliary pathology demonstrates a mildly dilated common duct *(arrow)* anterior to the right portal vein. The internal diameter of the common duct measures 7 mm. **B:** A parasagittal sonogram in the same individual 2 min later demonstrates the same common duct *(arrow)* anterior to the right portal vein. Now the internal diameter of the common duct measures 3 mm and is within normal limits. This represents a spontaneous rapid change in bile duct diameter in an individual with no clinical or biochemical evidence of biliary obstruction.

ing mass can allow rapid return of the duct toward the normal range (20, 44, 61) (Fig. 16).

### Obstruction Without Dilatation

A very recent obstruction may cause little if any dilation immediately but will cause dilatation hours or days later (44, 47, 61). This probably explains some cases where an early or intermittent obstruction fails to cause distension of the CD (see Fig. 11). In patients with a normal duct caliber, but strong clinical suspicion of biliary pathology, it is worthwhile repeating the sonogram a few days later to reevaluate the system.

### Dilatation Without Jaundice

Despite these pitfalls in using ductal diameter as an indicator of ductal pathology, BD dilatation is an early and reliable sign of obstruction and may precede the rise in serum bilirubin and even alkaline phosphatase, although the latter is usually elevated in patients with dilated bile ducts (72, 75). Weinstein et al. (72) described 33 patients with dilated bile ducts but normal serum bilirubin, all of whom had obstructing lesions related to the biliary tree; 77% had a raised serum alkaline phosphatase. Therefore in anicteric patients with a dilated CD, if the obstructing lesion is not demonstrated, further investigation of the biliary tree is warranted.

### Animal Experiments

Animal studies have examined the temporal and spatial patterns of ductal dilatation after complete occlusion of the distal CD and these confirm early CD dilatation before serum bilirubin elevation (65, 76). Zeman et al. (76) occluded the distal CD in 3 dogs after cholecystectomy and Shawker et al. (65) occluded the distal CD in 7 rhesus monkeys with the gallbladder still in place. The CD became dilated by 4 hr in the dogs and by 24 hr in the monkeys, before the serum bilirubin became elevated. Shawker et al. (65) concluded that dilatation of the CD is the earliest reliable sign of obstruction. It appeared that the bile duct expanded centrifugally from the point of obstruction, involving first the distal CD, then the proximal CD, and finally the intrahepatic ducts. After relief of obstruction the process reversed itself and the intrahepatic ducts returned to normal before the CD (Fig. 13). There was a long delay (30 to 50 days) before the CD of the monkeys returned to normal but this is probably because complete obstruction was present for 1 to 2 weeks, during which time the elasticity of the walls probably altered.

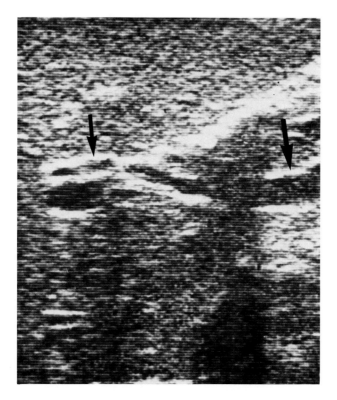

**FIG. 13.** Variation in bile duct diameter. A parasagittal sonogram in a patient with a previous cholecystectomy, but now asymptomatic, demonstrates a normal size proximal common duct *(small arrow)*, whereas the distal common duct *(large arrow)* is slightly dilated, measuring 10 mm in internal caliber.

## OBSTRUCTIVE LESIONS

### The Presence, Level and Cause of Obstruction: Ultrasound Accuracy

Several authors have examined the usefulness of ultrasound in distinguishing obstructive jaundice from nonobstructive jaundice and in assessing the level and cause of obstruction (2, 19, 26, 31, 58, 71) (see Tables 4 and 5). Using varying upper limits of normal CD diameter (6 to 8 mm), the sensitivity in selecting out those patients with obstructive jaundice varied between 87 and 97% while the specificity varied between 85 and 100% depending on the study. The level of obstruction could be determined in 60 to 94% of cases and the actual cause of obstruction in 39 to 81% of cases (Table 5). Our experience is similar to that of Baron et al. (2) in that the exact level of obstruction can be determined in approximately 60% of patients and the actual cause in about 40%. Difficulties usually arise because of bowel gas

TABLE 4. *The presence, level, and cause of obstruction: ultrasound accuracy*

| Source | Number in study | Upper limit of normal CD diameter (mm) | Presence of obstruction | | Level of obstruction accuracy (%) | Cause of obstruction accuracy (%) |
| | | | Sensitivity (%) | Specificity (%) | | |
|---|---|---|---|---|---|---|
| Baron, 1982 (2) | 92 | 6 | 87 | 89 | 60 (24/40) | 39 (18/47) |
| Haubek, 1981 (26) | 84 | 8 | 97 | 85 | 95 (35/37) | 68 (25/37) |
| Goldberg, 1978 (19) | 23 | 7 | 89 | 100 | — | — |
| Salem, 1981 (58) | 105 | 6 to 7 | 89 | 100 | 79 (52/66) | — |
| Koenigsberg, 1979 (31) | 32 | 8 | — | — | 94 (30/32) | 81 (26/32) |
| Vas, 1981 (71) | 50 | 6 to 7 | — | — | 86 (43/50) | 52 (26/50) |

TABLE 5.  Specific causes of biliary obstruction

| Source | Number with obstruction | Stones (%) | Pancreatic carcinoma (%) | Portal masses (%) | Bile duct carcinoma (%) | Pancreatitis (%) | Other[a] (%) |
|---|---|---|---|---|---|---|---|
| Baron, 1982 (2) | 47 | 19 | 26 | 26 | 4 | 4 | 21 |
| Haubek, 1981 (26) | 44 | 27 | 32 | 18 | 7 | 7 | 9 |
| Salem, 1981 (58) | 66 | 42 | 29 | 11 | 9 | 3 | 6 |
| Koenigsberg, 1979 (31) | 32 | 25 | 47 | 6 | 6 | 9 | 7 |

[a]Other includes: GB carcinoma, liver tumor, and duodenal tumor.

obscuring the detail around the distal CBD. However, the sensitivity in isolating those with obstructive jaundice is increased if one uses 4 or 5 mm as the upper limit of normal CD diameter as opposed to 6 to 8 mm.

Careful CT scanning with 5 mm slices after intravenous and oral contrast enhancement is probably more accurate in detecting the level and cause for biliary obstruction. Baron et al. (2) correctly predicted the level of obstruction in 88% of patients (35 of 40) and the cause in 70% (33 of 47) with careful CT scanning. Percutaneous transhepatic cholangiography is also more accurate in predicting the level and cause of biliary obstruction. Vas and Salem (71) correctly predicted the level of obstruction in 100% of patients (50 of 50) and the cause in 86% (43 of 50) with percutaneous transhepatic cholangiography. These tests can be used if sonography fails to delineate the level and cause of obstruction (see section on The Role of Ultrasound for the Investigation of Jaundice).

## Specific Causes of Obstruction

### *Choledocholithiasis*

Although many causes of biliary obstruction exist, the majority of lesions consist of CD stones and pancreatic carcinoma (Table 5). Stones in the CD account for between 19 and 42% of bile duct obstruction (Table 5). Choledocholithiasis may coexist with stones in the gallbladder or may be diagnosed after cholecystectomy, either because a stone has been retained in the CD or because new stones have formed months to years later (Fig. 14). The CD caliber may range from normal to severely dilated depending on the degree of functional obstruction present. Demonstrated calculi may vary greatly in size and they may be nonobstructive (Fig. 11), intermittently obstructive (Fig. 15), or impacted in the distal CD causing severe obstruction (Fig. 16). Care must be taken not to mistake echogenic bile or debris for calculi, nor to mistake indentations from the neighboring hepatic artery for intraductal stones. Occasionally a false positive diagnosis can be made when a surgical clip is present adjacent to the CD, or when there is gas in the CD (43), but these problems can be resolved by reviewing the plain radiographs in patients undergoing ultrasonography.

Three recent articles have shown that sonography is quite limited in diagnosing choledocholithiasis (2, 12, 24, 33, 71). The overall sensitivity ranged from 11% (12) to 29% (33), although Laing and Jeffrey (33) stated that the sensitivity rose to 55% in the last part of the study because more reliance was placed on real-time scanning and greater expertise was developed to scan the distal common bile duct which is the probable site for a stone to lodge. The reasons for the low sensitivity included gas in the duodenum and colon, obscuring the distal common bile duct which is usually the site of

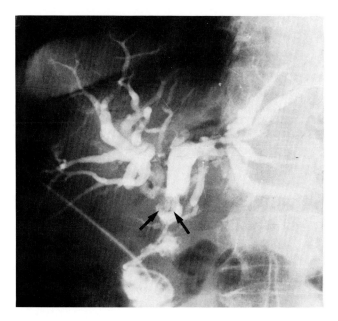

**FIG. 14A.** Growing common duct stone, postcholecystectomy. A T-tube cholangiogram several weeks after surgery for biliary-enteric anastomosis demonstrates a filling defect *(arrows)* within the distal portion of the dilated bile duct remnant just proximal to the biliary-enteric anastomosis.

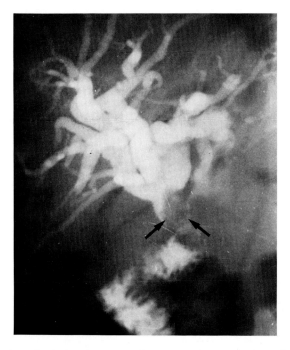

**FIG. 14B.** A transhepatic cholangiogram on the same patient several months after Fig. 14A demonstrates growth in the filling defect *(arrows)* within the distal portion of the dilated bile duct remnant. However, there was passage of contrast material from the dilated biliary tree into the bowel lumen, as demonstrated.

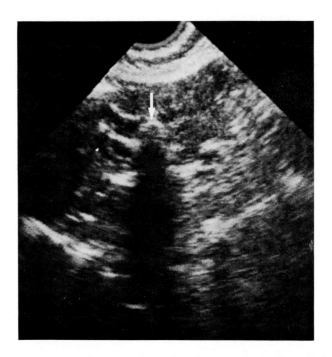

**FIG. 14C.** A parasagittal sonogram performed on the same day as Fig. 14B demonstrates a definite calculus *(arrow)* with distal shadowing in the distal portion of the dilated bile duct. This is excellent evidence that the filling defect is a calculus and not a tumor.

obstruction and the common occurrence of stones in a nondilated bile duct. In one series, 31 of 87 patients (36%) (12) with choledocholithiasis had a normal size duct whereas in another, 10 of 33 patients (30%) (33) had a normal size duct. The lack of fluid surrounding an obstructing stone in a normal or even dilated bile duct makes the diagnosis difficult. A non-obstructing stone might be seen in the proximal CD whereas the obstructing stone in the distal end could be missed. In the 31 patients with stones in a normal size bile duct (12), 27 of 31 (87%) had elevated serum alkaline phosphatase and bilirubin values. In this group, transhepatic cholangiography or endoscopic retrograde cholangiopancreatography would demonstrate the calculus.

### Pancreatic and Portal Masses

Tumors arising in the head of the pancreas account for 26 to 47% of patients with biliary obstruction (Table 5) and this lesion is probably the single most common pathology causing obstruction (Figs. 17, 18). Sonography is more successful in detecting a pancreatic mass than choledocholithiasis. Over 50% of tumors can be diagnosed with ultrasound. Baron et al. (2)

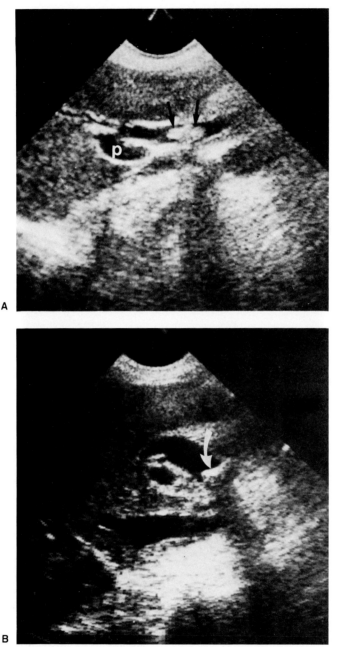

**FIG. 15. A:** Nonimpacted stone in common duct. A parasagittal sonogram demonstrates a mildly dilated proximal common duct anterior to the right portal vein (p). The midportion of the common duct contains a fairly large calculus *(arrows)* which was mobile and did not appear to cause obstruction at this point in time. **B:** Calculus impacted in mid-common duct. A parasagittal sonogram demonstrates a dilated common duct with a fairly large calculus *(arrow)* impacted in the midportion causing obstruction.

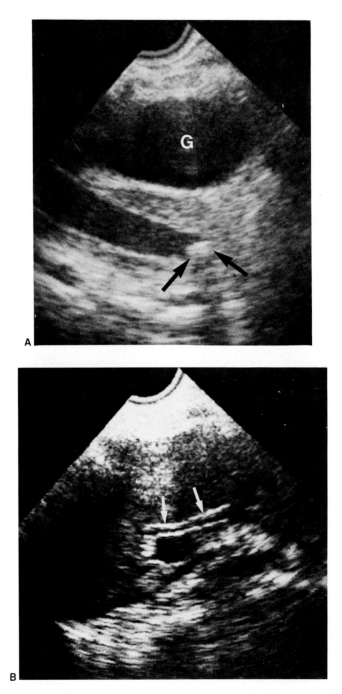

**FIG. 16. A:** Calculus impacted in distal common duct. A parasagittal sonogram demonstrates a dilated distal common duct within the head of the pancreas. There is a calculus *(arrows)* impacted in the distal end of the duct causing acute obstruction. Note the shadowing behind the calculus and note the distended gallbladder (G). **B:** Decrease in duct size after stone removal. Several days after removal of the impacted calculus, a repeat sonogram demonstrates a dramatic decrease in diameter of the common duct *(arrows)* which is now within normal limits, measuring only 2 or 3 mm.

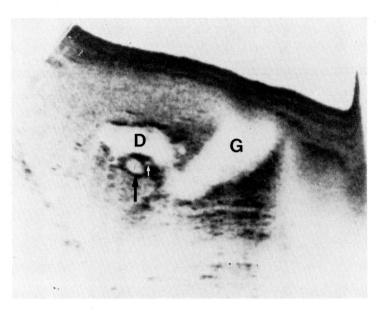

**FIG. 17.** Courvoisier gallbladder. A parasagittal sonogram demonstrates a markedly distended common duct (D) anterior to the right portal vein *(black arrow)*. Right hepatic artery *(white arrow)*. Dilated gallbladder (G). This patient had a small tumor in the head of the pancreas.

correctly diagnosed 8 of 12 patients while Vas and Salem (71) diagnosed 15 of 22 patients. Smaller masses in the head of the pancreas (less than 3 cm diameter) and carcinoma of the ampulla of Vater are typically the masses that go undetected even with excellent sonographic technique. Portal masses are a less common cause of biliary obstruction (6 to 26% of patients) but the majority of these may also be diagnosed with ultrasound (Fig. 19). Although most masses in the porta hepatis represent lymphoma or lymph node metastases, other uncommon lesions such as polycystic liver disease (14) and aortic aneurysm (69) have been implicated.

When a pancreatic mass or a mass in the porta hepatis is evident, one may easily perform a transcutaneous thin needle (usually 22 gauge) aspiration biopsy under ultrasound control. Cytological analysis of the specimen can then allow a tissue diagnosis of malignancy and thus obviate the need for any further diagnostic tests to determine the diagnosis.

### Other Causes

Less common causes of biliary obstruction which can be more difficult to diagnose with ultrasound include bile duct carcinoma, pancreatitis, bile duct stricture (Fig. 20), hepatic tumors, parasitic and mycotic lesions such as

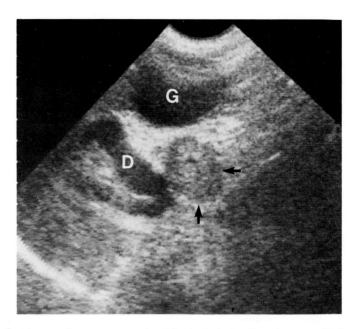

**FIG. 18.** Carcinoma of pancreas causing bile duct obstruction. A parasagittal sonogram demonstrates a solid mass *(arrows)* arising in the head of the pancreas and causing obstruction and dilatation of the common duct (D). G = gallbladder.

ascariasis, sclerosing cholangitis, and recurrent oriental pyogenic cholangitis and aortic aneurysm. These various lesions account for about 10% of cases seen in North American populations (Table 5).

Cholangiocarcinoma is usually not detected by ultrasound because it is often an infiltrating lesion that causes slight thickening of the wall and narrowing of the lumen. On occasion, however, it is possible to clearly outline the lesion itself and the proximal ductal dilatation (Fig. 21). Uncommonly a cholangiocarcinoma may present as a focal intraductal mass. The mass will appear as a solid lesion usually with midlevel echoes within the bile duct lumen (62). The lack of distal shadowing allows discrimination from an intraductal calculus. Identical appearances have been described in a benign bile duct polyp (7) and extension of tumor into the bile duct from a hepatoma (37) and a gallbladder carcinoma (62). Sclerosing cholangitis is another uncommon disease that may cause biliary obstruction; this is rarely diagnosed with ultrasound although Caroll and Oppenheimer (9) have described a patient with sclerosing cholangitis in whom there was diffuse thickening of the intrahepatic and extrahepatic bile duct walls.

Recurrent pyogenic cholangitis (Oriental Cholangiohepatitis) is occasionally encountered in North America in immigrants from Southeast Asia (15, 54). Typically the patients are 30 to 40 years of age with a history of recur-

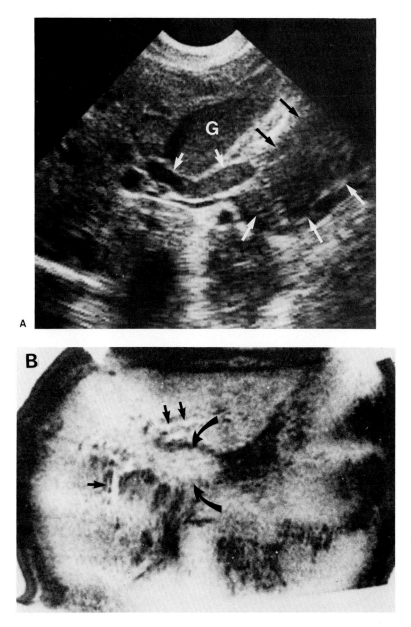

**FIG. 19. A:** Lymphoma in the peripancreatic nodes. An oblique sonogram of the right upper quadrant demonstrates a dilated common duct *(short arrows)* proximal to a solid mass *(long arrows)*. Note the echo-free fluid in the proximal common duct and the echogenic bile within the distal portion of the common duct. This echogenic bile is related to stasis and has the same appearance as the echogenic bile in the gallbladder (G). **B:** Metastatic mass in the porta hepatis. A transverse sonogram demonstrates a mass in the porta hepatis *(curved arrows)* due to metastasis from a carcinoma of the stomach. The common duct could not be visualized but there was dilatation of the intrahepatic ducts *(small arrows)* in the left and right lobes of the liver.

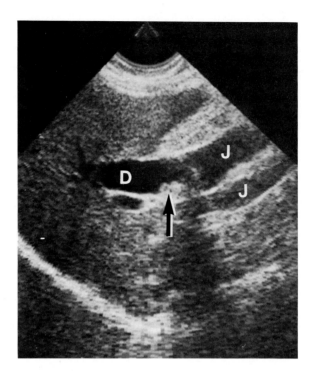

**FIG. 20.** Stricture at the site of biliary-enteric anastomosis. A parasagittal sonogram demonstrates a dilated common duct (D) down to its junction with the fluid-filled loop of jejunum (J). Note the low level echoes within the jejunal fluid which did not reflux into the duct during the real time examination. There was a small amount of mobile echogenic bile or sludge *(arrow)* within the duct.

rent right upper quadrant pain, fever, and jaundice. Pathologically the disease is characterized by pericholangitis, fibrotic changes, and polymorphonuclear infiltrates in the wall, often associated with soft calcium bilirubinate stones and massive dilation of the CD. Sonography can demonstrate marked CD dilatation and intrahepatic duct dilation associated with calculi, which can mimic soft tissue masses without much posterior shadowing.

Biliary ascariasis is another unusual cause of obstruction, the sonographic signs of which include intraductal echogenic material, which does not shadow, and bile duct dilatation (63, 64). The worms may appear as featureless fragments, coils, single strips, or multiple strips within the CD and gallbladder. Ascaris lumbricoides is a round worm that is a very common infestation in Africa, the USSR, the Far East, and Latin America but much less common in the United States and Canada. The adult worm resides commonly in the jejunum but can extend into the CD and thence into the gallbladder. Intraductal worms can cause biliary colic, raised liver enzymes, and occasionally a raised serum bilirubin but clinical jaundice is uncommon.

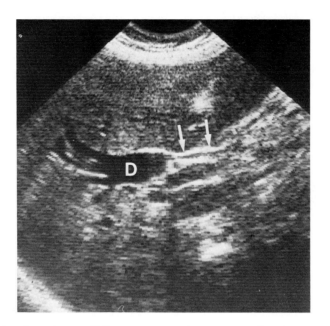

**FIG. 21.** Cholangiocarcinoma. Oblique sonogram demonstrates dilated intrahepatic ducts proximal to the malignant stricture *(arrows)* of the common hepatic duct anterior to the right hepatic artery *(small circle)*. (This case was contributed by Dr. Peter Cooperberg, Director of Division of Ultrasound, Vancouver General Hospital, Vancouver, Canada.)

Sonography after medical therapy can verify expulsion of the worms and a return of the CD to normal size (63).

## OTHER BILE DUCT ABNORMALITIES

### Biliary Gas

After biliary-enteric anastomosis, there is usually reflux of bowel content, including gas, into the CD and intrahepatic ducts. Sonography can easily demonstrate gas in the nondependent branches of the intrahepatic bile ducts and in the CD itself. Gas within intrahepatic ducts appears as thin echogenic lines which usually do not shadow nor cause "ring down" artifacts (Fig. 22A). This must be distinguished from portal venous gas, which usually appears as echogenic lines in the peripheral portions of the liver parenchyma (Fig. 22B) (52), whereas biliary gas tends to occupy more central portions of the liver.

Gas in the CD must be distinguished from a calculus. When "ring down" or reverberation echos (68) are present behind an echogenic focus inside the bile duct, intraductal gas is diagnosed (Fig. 22C). A well-defined shadow

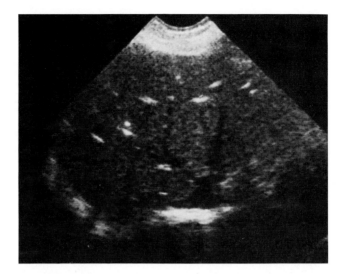

**FIG. 22A.** Biliary gas. A transverse sonogram through the right and left lobes of the liver demonstrate multiple linear echogenic foci within the parenchyma without posterior shadowing. This is the characteristic appearance of gas within the intrahepatic bile ducts. The cause for the biliary gas in this patient was a previous biliary enteric anastomosis.

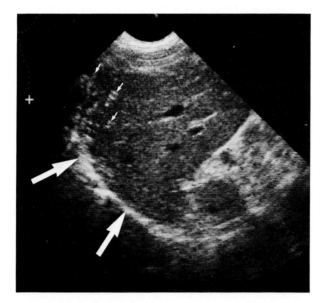

**FIG. 22B.** Portal venous gas. A parasagittal sonogram through the right lobe of the liver demonstrates multiple linear echogenic foci in the peripheral portion of the liver parenchyma near the right hemidiaphragm *(large arrows)*. This represents an example of portal venous gas in a patient who had necrosis in the sigmoid colon. Characteristically, the distribution of intrahepatic portal venous gas is peripheral compared to intrabiliary gas which is usually in the more central portions of the liver parenchyma.

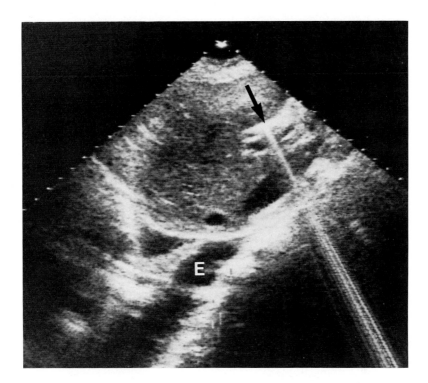

**FIG. 22C.** Gas in the common duct. A parasagittal sonogram through the right lobe of the liver demonstrates a densely echogenic collection within the common duct *(arrow)* associated with a very dense ringdown (or reverberation) echo posterior to the echogenic focus. This is characteristic of gas within the common duct. The gas in this patient is due to a previous biliary enteric anastomosis. Incidentally note moderate sized effusion (E) within the right chest.

may be present behind a focus of gas in the bile duct and thus can be mistaken for a stone. However, with real time examination, one can readily observe the flow of gas and fluid within the duct.

Without a previous history of biliary surgery, gas in the bile ducts can arise owing to a pathological biliary-enteric anastomosis. Common causes include gallstone ileus (erosion of calculus through the gallbladder wall into bowel lumen), malignant tumors, and inflammatory conditions of the bowel. Gas-containing intrahepatic abscesses and cholangitis may also be associated with intraductal gas.

### Cystic Lesions

Choledochal cysts are uncommon congenital lesions of the common duct, which can be classified into three main categories: cystic dilatation of the CD (the most common type) with or without intrahepatic biliary dilatation,

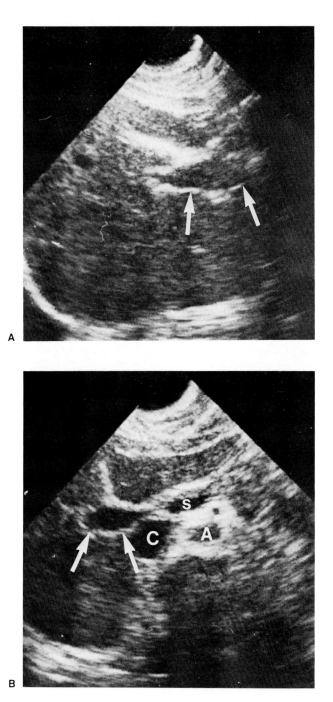

**FIG. 23. A:** Choledochal cyst (longitudinal). A parasagittal sonogram demonstrates a bulbous dilatation of the common duct *(arrows).* The proximal portion of the duct tapers into a more normal sized duct in this 8-year-old patient. **B:** Choledochal cyst (transverse). A transverse scan through the distal duct in the same patient demonstrates focal enlargement of the duct *(arrows)* anterolateral to the inferior vena cava (C). The splenic vein (s) and aorta (A) are also visualized.

diverticulum of the CD with or without intrahepatic biliary dilatation, and a choledochocele (30). The incidence of intrahepatic biliary dilatation associated with a choledochal cyst was 45.9% of 41 patients reported by Todani et al. (70). Choledochal cysts are usually diagnosed in the first 10 years of life, and symptoms may range from none to the triad of right upper quadrant pain, palpable mass, and jaundice, the triad occurring in only 20 to 25% of patients (29). Sonographic findings include a cystic mass of varying size in the porta hepatis. Real-time scanning can demonstrate the confluence of the bile ducts with the cyst (Fig. 23) and the separation between the cyst and the gallbladder (16, 25, 29, 42). Preoperative imaging with high resolution real-time ultrasound and $^{99m}$Tc IDA cholescintigraphy should be diagnostic and should eliminate the need for invasive procedures in most patients (25).

Caroli's disease is another congenital cystic biliary lesion that affects the intrahepatic ducts but usually does not directly involve the CD. Symptoms typically begin between 20 and 30 years of age and are related to bile stasis, stone formation, and cholangitis. Ultrasound and CT scanning will demonstrate intrahepatic cysts of varying size, usually in association with a normal CD unless it is altered due to the presence of a stone or cholangitis (27, 41, 48). A specific diagnosis can be made when $^{99m}$Tc IDA scanning (27, 41) or CT cholangiography (48) demonstrates a communication between the observed cysts and the biliary tree.

## INTRAOPERATIVE BILE DUCT SCANNING

Using a small parts real-time scanner with a 7.5-MHz or 10-MHz probe, it is possible to scan the CD directly with the probe placed into the abdominal wound during the surgical procedure. The diameter of the CD can be accurately measured but, more importantly, the presence or absence of calculi can be ascertained with an accuracy equivalent to that of operative cholangiography (34, 66). In a study of 100 patients, ultrasound had a sensitivity of 96% and a specificity of 93% for detecting calculi in 31 patients in whom the duct was explored (34). Operative cholangiography had a sensitivity of 96% and a specificity of 96%. In 12 of 100 patients the operative cholangiogram was a failure for technical reasons, but sonography was able to evaluate the ducts in these cases. Additional positive features of operative ultrasonography include its speed of diagnosis (3 to 5 min), the noninvasive nature of the study, and the safety of the procedure. In contrast, operative cholangiography was slower (10 to 15 min) and invasive. If a high resolution small parts scanner is available in the operating room and if the involved personnel can operate the probe and interpret the images in a competent way, then operative choledochosonography may eclipse operative cholangiography for evaluating the CD during surgery.

## THE ROLE OF ULTRASOUND FOR THE
## INVESTIGATION OF JAUNDICE

The initial imaging technique in the evaluation of jaundice is sonography (Fig. 24) (4). As previously described, sonography of the intrahepatic ducts and the extrahepatic duct can accurately differentiate between those with biliary obstruction (i.e. enlarged caliber) and those with no obstruction (i.e. normal caliber). In patients without duct dilatation, the jaundice is almost always caused by cholestasis associated with hepatocellular disease. If the CD is dilated and the cause is determined at ultrasound, then definitive therapy is indicated. If a mass is seen to cause the obstruction, a percutaneous needle aspiration biopsy is very useful for cytological confirmation of malignancy.

When duct dilation is present but the cause is not determined, a further imaging test is required. The least invasive alternative is a closely monitored CT scan that not only can diagnose the cause in many cases, but also give

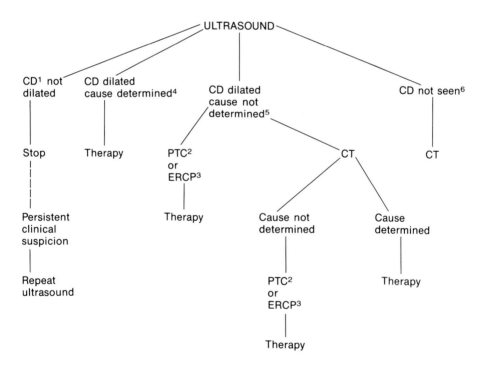

**FIG. 24.** Investigation of jaundice. 1—Common duct. 2—Percutaneous cholangiogram. 3—Endoscopic retrograde cholangiopancreatography. 4—Thin needle aspiration biopsy may be used to establish malignancy in a visualized mass. 5—A fatty meal can help distinguish between obstructive and nonobstructive bile duct dilatation, (see section entitled Common Duct Size in Biliary Obstruction). 6—The CD is occasionally not seen owing to overlying intestinal gas or surgical dressings.

useful ancillary information. For example, in pancreatic carcinoma, CT will demonstrate the local extent of the tumor and delineate nodal and liver metastases. If choledocholithiasis is suspected, percutaneous cholangiography is a safe and accurate method for diagnosing intraductal calculi as well as other obstructing lesions (46). If one wishes to evaluate the pancreatic duct or if one contemplates a sphincterotomy, then ERCP offers these additional advantages in addition to excellent imaging of the bile ducts and related pathology. Occasionally ultrasound will be unable to visualize the CD owing to either extreme obesity or extensive intestinal gas or surgical dressings in the right upper quadrant. In these patients, a CT scan of the upper abdomen is a reasonable next step in evaluating the CD and surrounding tissues.

## ACKNOWLEDGMENTS

The author would like to thank Mrs. Heather Impola for her patience and skill in preparing the manuscript, and also Dr. Peter Cooperberg for contributing Fig. 21.

## REFERENCES

1. Ariyama, J., Shirakabe, H., Ohashi, K., et al. Experience with percutaneous transhepatic cholangiography using the Japanese needle. *Gastrointest. Radiol.*, 2: 359–365, 1978.
2. Baron, R. L., Stanley, R. J., Lee, J. K. T., Koehler, R. E., Melson, G. L., Balfe, D. M., and Weyman, P. J. A prospective comparison of the evaluation of biliary obstruction using computed tomography and ultrasonography. *Radiology*, 145: 91–98, 1982.
3. Behan, M., and Kazam, E. Sonography of the common bile duct: value of right anterior oblique view. *Am. J. Roentgenol.*, 130: 701–709, 1978.
4. Berk, R. N., Cooperberg, P. L., Gold, R. P., Rohrmann, C. A., and Ferrucci, J. T. Jr. Radiography of the bile ducts: A symposium on the use of new modalities for diagnosis and treatment. *Radiology*, 145: 1–9, 1982.
5. Berland, L. L., Lawson, T. L., and Foley W. D. Porta hepatis: sonographic discrimination of bile ducts from arteries with pulsed doppler with new anatomic criteria. *Am. J. Roentgenol.*, 138: 833–840, 1982.
6. Bolandi, L., Gandolfi, L., Ross, A., Caletti, G. C., Fontana, G., and Labo, G. Ultrasound in the diagnosis of cholestatic jaundice. *Am. J. Gastroenterol.*, 71: 168–176, 1979.
7. Bondestam, S., Kivilaakso, E. O., Standertskjöld-Nordenstam, C. M., Holmström, T., and Hästbacka, J. Sonographic diagnosis of bile duct polyp. *Am. J. Roentgenol.*, 135: 610–611, 1980.
8. Bruneton, J. N., Roux, P., Fenart, D., Caramella, E., and Occelli, J. P. Ultrasound evaluation of common bile duct size in normal adult patients and following cholecystectomy. A report of 750 cases. *Eur. J. Radiol.*, 1 (2): 171–172, 1981.
9. Carroll, B. A., and Oppenheimer, D. A. Sclerosing cholangitis: sonographic demonstration of bile duct wall thickening. *Am. J. Roentgenol.*, 139: 1016–1018, 1982.
10. Cooperberg, P. L. High-resolution real-time ultrasound in the evaluation of the normal and obstructed biliary tract. *Radiology*, 129: 477–480, 1978.
11. Cooperberg, P. L., Li, D., Wong, P., Cohen, M. M., and Burhenne, H. J. Accuracy of common hepatic duct size in the evaluation of extrahepatic biliary obstruction. *Radiology*, 135: 141–144, 1980.
12. Cronan, J. J., Meuller, P. R., Simeone, J. F., O'Connell, R. S., van Sonnenberg, E., Wittenberg, J., and Ferrucci, J. T. Jr. Prospective diagnosis of choledocholithiasis. *Radiology*, 146: 467–469, 1982.

13. Dewbury, K. C. Visualization of normal biliary ducts with ultrasound. *Br. J. Radiol.*, 53: 774–780, 1980.
14. Ergun, H., Wolf, B. H., and Hissong, S. L. Obstructive jaundice caused by polycystic liver disease. *Radiology*, 136: 435–436, 1980.
15. Federle, M. P., Cello, J. P., Laing, F. C., and Jeffrey, R. B. Jr. Recurrent pyogenic cholangitis in Asian immigrants. *Radiology*, 143: 151–156, 1982.
16. Filly, R. A., and Carlsen, E. N. Choledochal cyst: report of a case with specific ultrasonographic findings. *J. Clin. Ultrasound*, 4: 7–10, 1976.
17. Fromhold, W., and Fromhold, M. Roentgenology of the biliary tract. In: *Alimentary Tract Roentgenology*, edited by A. R. Margulis and H. J. Burhenne, p. 1264. Mosby, St. Louis, 1973.
18. Glazer, G. M., Filly, R. A., and Laing, F. C. Rapid change in caliber of the nonobstructed common duct. *Radiology*, 140: 161–162, 1981.
19. Goldberg, H. I., Filly, R. A., Korobkin, M., Moss, A. A., Kressel, H. Y., and Callen, P. W. Capability of CT body scanning to demonstrate the status of the biliary ductal system in patients with jaundice. *Radiology*, 129: 731–737, 1978.
20. Gooding, G. A. W. Acute bile duct dilatation with resolution in 43 hours: an ultrasonic demonstration. *J. Clin. Ultrasound*, 9: 201–202, 1981.
21. Goodman, M. W., Ansel, H. J., Vennes, J. A., Lasser, R. B., and Silvis, S. E. Is intravenous cholangiography still useful? *Gastroenterology*, 79: 642–645, 1980.
22. Graham, M. F., Cooperberg, P. L., Cohen, M. M., and Burhenne, H. J. The size of the normal common hepatic duct following cholecystectomy: an ultrasonographic study. *Radiology*, 135: 137–139, 1980.
23. Graham, M. F., Cooperberg, P. L., Cohen, M. M., and Burhenne, H. J. Ultrasonographic screening of the common hepatic duct in symptomatic patients after cholecystectomy. *Radiology*, 138: 137–139, 1981.
24. Gross, B. H., Harler, L. P., Gore, R. M., Callen, P. W., Filly, R. A., Shapiro, H. A., and Goldberg, H. I. Ultrasonic evaluation of common bile duct stones: prospective comparison with endoscopic retrograde cholangiopancreatography. *Radiology*, 146: 471–474, 1983.
25. Han, B. K., Babcock, D. S., and Gelfand, M. H. Choledochal cyst with bile duct dilatation: sonography and [99mTc] IDA cholescintigraphy. *Am. J. Roentgenol.*, 136: 1075–1079, 1981.
26. Haubek, A., Pedersen, J. H., Burcharth, E., Gammelgaard, J., Hancke, S., and Willumsen, L. Dynamic sonography in the evaluation of jaundice. *Am. J. Roentgenol.*, 136: 1071–1074, 1981.
27. Imai, Y., Watanabe, T., Kondo, Y., and Nakanishi, F. Caroli's disease: its diagnosis with non-invasive methods. *Br. J. Radiol.*, 54: 526–528, 1981.
28. Jacobson, J. B., and Brodey, P. A. The transverse common duct. *Am. J. Roentgenol.*, 136: 91–95, 1981.
29. Kangarloo, H., Sarti, D. A., Sample, W. F., and Amundsen, G. Ultrasonographic spectrum of choledochal cysts in children. *Pediatr. Radiol.*, 9: 15–18, 1980.
30. Kimura, K., Ohto, M., Ono, T., Tsuchiya, Y., Saisho, H., Kawamura, K., Yogi, Y., Karasawa, E., and Okuda, K. Congenital cystic dilatation of the common bile duct: relation to anomalous pancreaticoduodenal ductal union. *Am. J. Roentgenol.*, 128: 571–577, 1977.
31. Koenisberg, M., Wiener, S. N., and Walzer, A. The accuracy of sonography in the differential diagnosis of obstructive jaundice: a comparison with cholangiography. *Radiology*, 133: 157–165, 1979.
32. Laing, F. C., and Jeffrey, R. B. Jr. The pseudodilated common bile duct: ultrasonographic appearance created by the gallbladder neck. *Radiology*, 135: 405–407, 1980.
33. Laing, F. C., and Jeffrey, R. B. Jr. Choledocholithiasis and cystic duct obstruction: difficult ultrasonographic diagnosis. *Radiology*, 146: 475–479, 1983.
34. Lane, R. J., and Coupland, G. A. E. Ultrasonic indications to explore the common bile duct. *Surgery*, 91: 268–274, 1982.
35. Lasser, R. B., Silvis, S. E., and Vennes, J. A. The normal cholangiogram. *Am. J. Dig. Dis.*, 23: 586–590, 1978.
36. Lynn, J. A. Physiology of the extrahepatic biliary tree. In: *Liver and Biliary Disease:*

*Pathophysiology, Diagnosis, Management,* edited by R. Wright et al., pp. 228–232, Saunders, London, Philadelphia, 1979.

37. Maffessanti, M. M., Bazzochi, M., and Melato, M. Sonographic diagnosis of intraductal hepatoma. *J. Clin. Ultrasound,* 10: 397–399, 1982.
38. Mahour, G. H., Wakim, K. G., and Soule, E. H. Structure of the common bile duct in man: presence or absence of smooth muscle. *Ann. Surg.,* 166: 91–94, 1967.
39. Malini, S., and Sabel, J. Ultrasonography in obstructive jaundice. *Radiology,* 123: 429–433, 1977.
40. McGahan, J. P., and Phillips, H. E., and Cox, K. L. Sonography of the normal pediatric gallbladder and biliary tract. *Radiology* 144: 873–875, 1982.
41. Mittelstaedt, C. A., Volberg, F. M., Fischer, G. J., and McCartney, W. H. Caroli's disease: sonographic findings. *Am. J. Roentgenol.,* 134: 585–587, 1980.
42. Morgan, C. L., Trought, W. S., Oddson, T. A., and Thompson, W. M. Type II choledochal cyst: ultrasonographic appearance. *Radiology,* 132: 130, 1979.
43. Mueller, P. R., Cronan, J. J., Simeone, J. F., van Sonnenberg, E., and Hall, D. A. Choledocholithiasis: ultrasonographic caveats. *J. Ultrasound Med.,* 2: 13–16, 1983.
44. Mueller, P. R., Ferrucci, J. T. Jr., Simeone, J. F., van Sonnenberg, E., Hall, D. A., and Wittenberg, J. Observations on the distensibility of the common bile duct. *Radiology,* 142: 467–472, 1982.
45. Mueller, P. R., Ferrucci, J. T. Jr., Simeone, J. F., Wittenberg, J., van Sonnenberg, E., Polansky, A., and Isler, R. J. Postcholecystectomy bile duct dilatation: myth or reality? *Am. J. Roentgenol.,* 136: 355–358, 1981.
46. Mueller, P. R., Harbin, W. P., Ferrucci, J. T. Jr., Wittenberg, J., and van Sonnenberg, E. Fine needle transhepatic cholangiography: reflections after 450 cases. *Am. J. Roentgenol.,* 136: 85–90, 1981.
47. Muhletaler, C. A., Gerlock, A. J. Jr., Fleischer, A. C., and James, A. E. Jr. Diagnosis of obstructive jaundice with nondilated bile ducts. *Am. J. Roentgenol.,* 134: 1149–1152, 1980.
48. Musante, F., Derchi, L. E., and Bonati, P. CT cholangiography in suspected Caroli's disease. *Journal of Computer Assisted Tomography,* 6 (3): 482–485, 1982.
49. Niederau, C., Müller, J., Sonnenberg, A., Scholten, T., Erckenbrecht, J., Fritsch, W. P., Bruster, T., and Strohmeyer, G. Extrahepatic bile ducts in healthy subjects, in patients with cholelithiasis, and in postcholecystectomy patients: a prospective ultrasonic study. *J. Clin. Ultrasound,* 11: 23–27, 1983.
50. Oppenheimer, D. A., and Carroll, B. A. Spontaneous resolution of hyperlimentation-induced biliary dilatation: ultrasonic description. *J. Ultrasound Med.,* 1: 213–214, 1982.
51. Parulekar, S. G. Ultrasound evaluation of common bile duct size. *Radiology,* 133: 703–707, 1979.
52. Pearse, B. F., and Sauerbrei, E. E. The ultrasound and CT diagnosis of gas in the mesenteric-portal venous system. *J. Can. Assoc. Radiol.,* 1982.
53. Pon, M. S., and Cooperberg, P. L. Oral water and intravenous glucagon—to aid ultrasonic visualization of the common bile duct. *J. Can. Assoc. Radiol.,* 30: 173–174, 1979.
54. Ralls, P. W., Colletti, P. M., Quinn, M. F., Lapin, S. A., Morris, U. L. and Halls, J. Sonography in recurrent pyogenic cholangitis. *Am. J. Roentgenol.,* 136: 1010–1012, 1981.
55. Ralls, P. W., Quinn, M. F., and Halls, J. Biliary sonography: ventral bowing of the dilated common duct. *Am. J. Roentgenol.,* 137: 1127–1129, 1981.
56. Ralls, P. W., Quinn, M. F., Rogers, W., and Halls, J. Sonographic anatomy of the hepatic artery. *Am. J. Roentgenol.,* 136: 1059–1063, 1981.
57. Sabel, J., Graham, D. Y., Davis, R. E., and Marini, S. The value of grey scale ultrasound in the differential diagnosis of surgical and nonsurgical jaundice. *Am. J. Gastroenterol.,* 69: 149–153, 1978.
58. Salem, S., and Vas, W. Ultrasonography in evaluation of the jaundiced patient. *J. Can. Assoc. Radiol.,* 31: 30–34, 1981.
59. Sample, W. F., Sarti, D. A., Goldstein, L. I., Weiner, M., and Kadell, B. M. Gray-scale ultrasonography of the jaundiced patient. *Radiology,* 128: 719–725, 1978.
60. Sauerbrei, E. E., Cooperberg, P. L., Gordon, P., Li, D., Cohen, M. M., and Burhenne, H. J. The discrepancy between radiographic and sonographic bile-duct measurements. *Radiology,* 137: 751–755, 1980.

61. Scheske, G. A., Cooperberg, P. L., Cohen, M. M., and Burhenne, H. J. Dynamic changes in the caliber of the major bile ducts, related to obstruction. *Radiology*, 135: 215–216, 1980.
62. Schnur, M. J., Hoffman, J. C., and Koenigsberg, M. Ultrasonic demonstration of intraductal biliary neoplasms. *J. Clin. Ultrasound*, 10: 246–248, 1982.
63. Schulman, A., Loxton, A. J., Heydenrych, J. J., and Abdurahman, K. E. Sonographic diagnosis of biliary ascariasis. *Am. J. Roentgenol.*, 139: 485–489, 1982.
64. Schulman, A., Roman, T., Dalrymple, R., Fataar, S., and Morton, P. Sonography of biliary worms (Ascariasis). *J. Clin. Ultrasound*, 10: 77–78, 1982.
65. Shawker, T. H., Jones, B. L., and Girton, M. E. Distal bile duct obstruction: an experimental study in monkeys. *J. Clin. Ultrasound*, 9: 77–82, 1981.
66. Sigel, B., Coelho, J. C. U., Spigos, D. G., Donahue, P. E., Wood, D. K., and Nyhus, L. M. Ultrasonic imaging during biliary and pancreatic surgery. *Am. J. Surg.*, 141: 84–89, 1981.
67. Simeone, J. F., Mueller, P. R., Ferrucci, J. T. Jr., van Sonnenberg, E., Hall, D. A., Wittenberg, J., Neff, C. C., and O'Connell, R. C. Sonography of the bile ducts after a fatty meal: an aid in the detection of obstruction. *Radiology*, 143: 211–215, 1982.
68. Sommer, F. G., and Taylor, K. J. W. Differentation of acoustic shadowing due to calculi and gas collections. *Radiology*, 135: 399–403, 1980.
69. Spinelli, G. D., Kleinclaus, D. H., Wenger, J. J., Christmann, D. J. L., Matter, D. F., and Warter, P. C. Obstructive jaundice and abdominal aortic aneurysm: an ultrasonographic study. *Radiology*, 144: 872, 1982.
70. Todani, T., Narusue, M., Watanabe, Y., Tabuchi, K., and Okajima, K. Management of congenital choledochal cyst with intrahepatic involvement. *Ann. Surg.*, 187: 272–280, 1978.
71. Vas, W., and Salem, S. Accuracy of sonography and transhepatic cholangiography in obstructive jaundice. *J. Can. Assoc. Radiol.*, 32: 111–113, 1981.
72. Weinstein, B. J., and Weinstein, D. P. Biliary tract dilatation in the nonjaundiced patient. *Am. J. Roentgenol.*, 134: 899–906, 1980.
73. Whiteside, C. G. Radiology of the biliary tract. In: *Surgery of the Gallbladder and Bile Ducts*, edited by R. Smith and S. Sherlock, pp. 99–100, Butterworth, London, 1964.
74. Zeman, R. K., Dorfman, G. S., Burrell, M. I., Stein, S., Berg, G. R., and Gold, J. A. Disparate dilatation of the intrahepatic and extrahepatic bile ducts in surgical jaundice. *Radiology*, 138: 129–136, 1981.
75. Zeman, R. K., Taylor, K. J. W., Burrell, M. I., and Gold, J. Ultrasound demonstration of anicteric dilatation of the biliary tree. *Radiology*, 34: 689–692, 1980.
76. Zeman, R. K., Taylor, K. J. W., Rosenfield, A. T., Schwartz, A., and Gold, J. A. Acute experimental biliary obstruction in the dog: sonographic findings and clinical implications. *Am. J. Roentgenol.*, 136: 965–967, 1981.

Ultrasound Annual 1983, edited by R. C. Sanders and M. Hill. Raven Press, New York © 1983.

# Real-Time Ultrasound Technology

## Frank P. Leo

*Russell H. Morgan Department of Radiology and Radiological Science, Johns Hopkins Hospital, Baltimore, Maryland 21205*

The technology of real-time ultrasound has moved swiftly from a crude imaging tool to a refined, well-accepted imaging modality. Transducers have changed from a crude 64-element linear array to a high resolution 400-microelement system. Transducer design has also changed to accomodate the area of the body being examined. Since larger transducers are hard to use between ribs, small single-element mechanical sector transducers and small head phased array transducers have been developed. Several transducers have also been developed to produce high quality images of superficial structures ("small parts") such as the carotid arteries, thyroid gland, and testicles. The success of the engineering community in overcoming obstacles that hampered good image reproduction has advanced real-time ultrasound to the point where it has become the preferred imaging technique for many diagnostic studies.

In order to properly understand the workings of the newer real-time transducers, it is important to review a few selected features such as frequency and bandwidth, beam width, penetration, resolution, focal point, and beam steering. These functions, as they pertain to static transducers used for gray scale imaging, take on a new role when they are incorporated into real-time technology. The basic factors controlling transducer technology are (a) the width and thickness of the piezoelectric (PE) element, (b) its frequency and bandwidth, and (c) the lens assembly that controls the focusing of the beam. These factors, when manipulated and controlled under different conditions of "time," provide the responses necessary for "real-time" image generation.

### REAL-TIME TRANSDUCER PARAMETERS AND FUNCTIONS

When a crystal is initially "cut"[1] to a given frequency, the diameter of the crystal determines how many wavelengths of that frequency are incorporated. It stands to reason that a crystal of 6 wavelengths in diameter will not

---

[1] The term "cut" refers to the slice of PE material taken from the "grown" (fabricated) mother crystal. The angle of cut determines the mode of oscillation. The thickness and diameter of this slice determine the frequency and power of these oscillations.

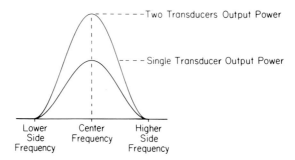

**FIG. 1.** Frequency spectrum drawing of two adjacent transducers of the same frequency and bandwidth, fired simultaneously. The output energy of the center frequency is higher than a single element.

have as long a "fresnel zone" (area where pulses of transmitted energy stay parallel to the face of the transducer) as a transducer of 10 wavelengths in diameter, which will penetrate more deeply than a transducer of 6 wavelengths in diameter even though they have the same frequency. This is due to the strength of the vibrations (intensity). The wider the transducer diameter, the more intensity there is in the beam and the farther it will travel. Manufacturers of static transducers usually have two separate transducers (13 mm and 19 mm diameter) of a given frequency to allow the user to obtain images of comparable resolution at different focal depths. The diameter of the transmitted transducer energy can also be varied by pulsing simultaneously more than one PE element, mounted next to each other. If these elements were of the same frequency and diameter, the resulting penetration would be deeper and the focal zone would also be deeper but the lateral resolution would be poorer because of the double width of the beam. If both of these transducers had identical frequency and bandwidth (referring to the center frequency and side frequency falloff) the frequency spectrum would be as shown in Fig. 1. If they had two different frequencies, i.e., 2.5 MHz (center frequency) and 3.5 MHz (center frequency), with a comparable

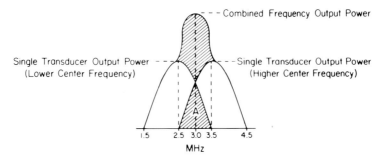

**FIG. 2.** Frequency spectrum drawing of two adjacent transducers of different frequencies, having the same bandwidth, fired simultaneously. The output energy is higher at the intermediate frequency.

bandwidth of about 2 MHz, the frequency spectrum created is as seen in Fig. 2. The larger amplitude output is the 3-MHz component caused by combining the frequency energy from the 2.5-MHz and 3.5-MHz PE elements in area A (Fig. 2). By proper filtering and by using frequency selection circuits, any of these 3 frequencies could be selected and utilized, but the highest amplitude frequency output would be the intermediate frequency (3-MHz component in this case).

## BEAM "SHAPING" AND BEAM "STEERING"

Terms such as phased array, electronic focus, electronic gating, delay transmissions, and beam shaping and steering are all names that in one way or another describe a transducer performing the same function. This function is to control the energy in the transmitted beam, by use of sophisticated electronics, to produce a desired controlled response. To further explain these controlled responses let us look at the lens assemblies on a single-element static transducer. The function of a concave lens is to bundle the energy in the transmitted field into a narrower diameter to provide a focal area within the beam. Fig. 3 (A and B) shows the energy in an unfocused transducer and a focused transducer. The concave "acoustic" lens is similar to a concave light lens that is used on a projector. If a convex lens was used (Fig. 4B) the light image would diverge and could not be focused.

Figure 4 (A and B) shows how the light rays enter the lens as a parallel beam but, because of the lens construction, these light rays bend as they go

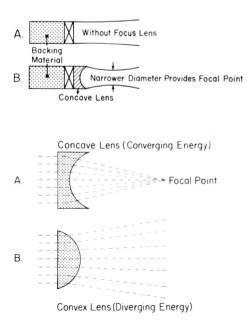

FIG. 3. A: Standard Gray Scale transducer beam profile without a concave focal lens. B: Standard Gray Scale transducer beam profile with a concave focal lens. The narrower diameter provides an area of higher intensity and better lateral resolution.

FIG. 4. A: When parallel sound energy is forced into a concave lens, the sound waves are bent (refracted) toward the thinner part of the lens, due to a change in velocity. This bending is always toward the thinner part of the lens. When these waves emerge they travel in a straight line and converge at a focal point. B: When parallel sound energy is forced into a convex lens, the sound waves are bent (refracted) toward the thinner part of the lens, due to a change in velocity. When they emerge they travel in a straight line and diverge.

through different thicknesses of the lens. This bending (refraction) is always toward the thinner part of the lens, because it has the least amount of resistance, and is a function of the change in velocity as the light travels through the lens medium. When these light rays leave the lens, they travel in a straight path. Sound waves react in the same manner as light waves. In the case of the concave lens, the small PE element on the back of a lens forces sound vibrations through the lens. These vibrations may appear parallel as they enter the lens, but due to the different thicknesses of the lens, their velocity changes as they travel through these different thicknesses causing them to bend toward the center. As these waves leave the lens, they travel in a straight line and converge to a focal area.

Real-time linear array transducers have many adjacent elements without a lens attached to the PE crystals. A focused beam is produced by varying the "firing" time of these parallel elements (Fig. 5) or by using a concave acoustic mirror. When a mirror is used, the focal area depends upon the concave bending of the mirror and how wide an area of transducer elements is being activated. When a "delay parallel firing" technique is used, the focal point

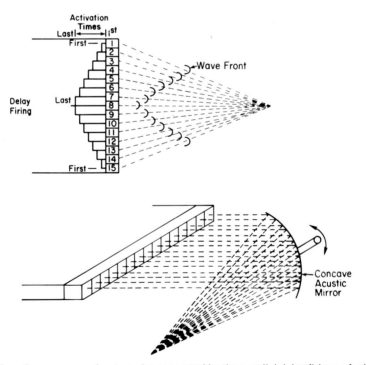

**FIG. 5. Top:** Concave wave front can be generated by the parallel delay firings of adjacent transducers to provide a focal area. The focal area is determined by the time between parallel firings. **Bottom:** Concave wave front can also be generated by reflecting a parallel wave front off a concave mirror. The focal point is determined by the width of the wave front and the curve of the mirror.

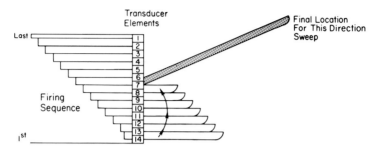

**FIG. 6.** "All electronic" controlled sector (phased array) provides a sweeping transmission in a form of a chevron display by single transducer firing followed by an adjacent transducer firing to move the beam towards the area of maximum deflection.

depends upon the time interval between the pulsing of the elements (which are parallel pulsed), time displaced from the center, and how many elements make up the concave wavefront. The more elements across the face of the activiated area, the wider the wavefront and the deeper the focal zone. The focal zone changes according to the lens and the width of the beam being controlled. In real-time transducer technology, electronic focus and electronic delay of transmission for focus controls the energy in the beam to provide "beam shaping" for good focus at a given area of interest.

"Beam steering" provides a different type of control and, unlike the parallel pulsed technique used for beam shaping, single transducer elements are fired sequentially to change slightly the direction of the transmitted concave beam of energy. The firing of single elements delayed in time provides a concave wave front that can vary the transmission spoke at predetermined locations across the face of the chevron. In Fig. 6, firing sequence from 14 to 1 provides a single displayed transmission at the shown location. Firing from 1 to 14 provides the displayed transmission at the maximum lower direction. Other firing sequences fill in other areas. This type of firing provides a sweeping response to the beam (noted by a "slice of pie" display on the screen of the monitor CRT). This display is not limited to the systems utilizing delay single firing elements, but is also found in many other real-time systems. A more pleasing name for the pie-shaped display that appears on the CRT, is a "chevron" image. This chevron display varies slightly in shape for each mode of real-time generation. Beam steering technology's prime function is to provide a sweeping action to the beam energy. This sweeping action (Fig. 6) is accomplished by the delayed firing of adjacent PE elements, but in a controlled sequence that combines the energy of an earlier fired element with the newly fired element in a time frame that is referred to as "being in phase" (Fig. 7). Combining maximum peaks of energy at only one side of a transmitted pulse causes the combined energy to move to the side of added energy. As more elements are fired "in phase," the moving energy sweeps an allowed distance, depending on how many elements are sequence fired for that direction of sweep. Each time elements

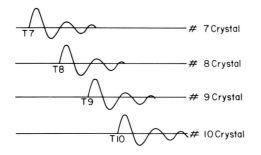

**FIG. 7.** A time frame to show the firing of each transducer to be at a maximum signal amplitude—a term that is generally referred to as "being in phase."

are fired they are slightly displaced in the direction of the sweep, and due to the speed of travel (1540 m/sec) completes the transmission and collects the echo responses before the next sequence is fired. One can see this firing and sweeping motion if the hard copy image is studied. The generation of energy starts at an apex (Fig. 8) and each firing is just slightly displaced and appears as a straight-line projection from the apex. It can also be noted that the further the signal penetrates from the transducer apex, the more it diverges. This is one of the drawbacks of most chevron generating systems. This divergence means that the axial and lateral resolution may not be the same at different depths within the chevron display.

To summarize, the diameter of the transducer determines the power output capabilities. Transducer diameters can be altered electronically by firing adjacent elements simultaneously so that the transmitted energy combines to form a broader field. This will provide deeper penetration and a deeper focal zone but poorer lateral resolution. Adjacent transducers of different frequencies can be fired simultaneously to make up the broader beam width, but proper filtering is required to select the maximum frequency output desired. The maximum frequency amplitude signal will provide a higher output and a narrower beam width. This type of mode is more flexible because the beam width is varied based on the frequency selected. A higher frequency will not penetrate as deeply, but will provide better lateral resolution owing to a narrower beam width. The attenuation of tissue for a given frequency is not changed, but having the flexibility to select a frequency to reach an area of interest with the best resolution is important clinically.

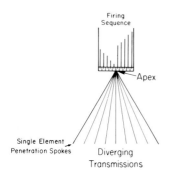

**FIG. 8.** The diverging transmissions that are associated with the chevron display systems. Both lateral and axial resolution is effected with depth penetration within the chevron.

Axial resolution [the ability to see two objects (interfaces) under each other in the direction of the penetrating beam as two separate objects] is also affected by frequency; the higher the frequency the better the axial resolution. The ability to delay fire pairs of elements on either side of a central PE element provides an additional focusing technology that can be extremely important in centering the focal area on a predetermined area of interest. This electronic lensing technique provides a concave beam front to produce an accurate and clearly defined area of focus. The technology to delay-fire single PE elements in phase and adjacent to each other in a controlled sequence provides an electronic means to sweep the transmitted energy in a manner that resembles the images produced by a mechanical sector device (to be discussed later). The final chevron display of each of these two systems is similar, but one is generated by mechanical motion controlled by a motor whereas the other contains no moving parts whatsoever. The technology of the single-element sector scanner also resembles the technology of a static transducer element performing a small arc scan. Keeping these transducer parameters and functions in mind, we will now apply them to the operations of modern "real-time" systems.

## LINEAR ARRAY SYSTEMS

Early linear array systems had 64 elements that were pulsed in sets of 4 to generate a single line of information on the monitor for each of the 4 pulsed elements. If the first 4 elements (1, 2, 3 and 4) were pulsed to generate the first line of a verticle displayed image, the next 4 (progress by one—2, 3, 4, and 5) were then pulsed to generate the second verticle line of the displayed image. This progression by one was continued until elements 61, 62, 63 and 64 were pulsed and they generated the 60th vertical line of the displayed image. A focusing capability was instituted by changing the pulsing sequence of the elements. For example, by turning up the far gain, the pulsing sequence activated 5 transducers instead of 4, thereby making the diameter of the transmitted beam wider and causing it to penetrate to a deeper focal area. The progression was still by one element and the 60 lines of information on the monitor were still maintained. If the area of interest was close to the skin line, the ultrasonographer would adjust the "near gain" to emphasize this area, thereby changing the pulsing sequence to 3. This narrower beam would not penetrate as deeply but would provide a near focal zone appropriate for this area of interest.

As technology further progressed, the linear array expanded to a transducer that consisted of 80 major elements made up of 400 microelements. Five microelements make up one major element and because of their miniature size could not be fitted in place as the earlier elements were constructed. These microelements are "grown" (a method of depositing a crystalline structure by a means of electrolysis) directly onto an electronic printed circuit board. In addition, modern linear array transducers have P.E. elements of two frequencies (Fig. 2) that produce higher and sharper fre-

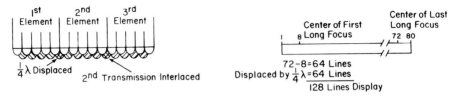

**FIG. 9. Left:** Dual frequency microelements provide maximum output of the intermediate frequency. The capabilities to shift the second series of transmissions by one microelement (¼ λ) provides an interlaced fill-in to the image. **Right:** Center element of a 16-wide element "long focus" transmission will provide 64 lines of data when "progression by one" is followed. The ¼λ shift will provide the second set of 64 lines when "progression by one" is also followed.

quency output. The microelements were pulsed (Fig. 9) in such a way as to produce 64 lines of information initially and then another 64 lines by shifting the frequency spectrum by one micro-element to give an image that had a total of 128 lines. This type of interlaced pulsing and shifting in itself does not produce good focal zones. Good focal zones are generated by tailoring the width of the transmitted beam by selecting 8, 12, or 16 full size elements (choice determined by depth of the area of interest) and by delaying the pulsing of these elements to provide a concave wavefront to match the focal zone (Fig. 10). Present linear array transducers produce good images with good focus and good depth penetration, i.e., to about 20.0 cm. Axial resolution is 0.5 mm whereas lateral resolution is 3.0 to 4.0 mm. These transducers are expensive; however, they are very reliable and durable unless they are dropped or mishandled.

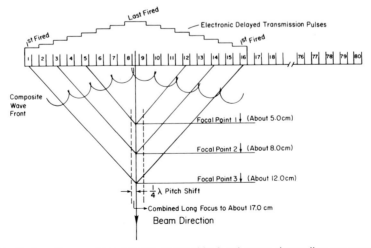

**FIG. 10.** Modern linear arrays provide selectable focal areas depending on number of adjacent transducers that are fired and the time delay between firings. The ¼λ pitch shift provides good quality filled-in images having 128 lines.

## SECTOR SCANNING DEVICES

These devices can be either mechanical or electronic and use single or multiple elements, employing either direct transmission of energy or a vibrating acoustic mirror which reflects the transmitted energy toward the patient. Each system has some good and bad points, but in general all produce fairly good images.

### Single Element Direct Transmission

The simplest type of sector scanner has only a single frequency PE element, aimed toward the patient, which sweeps mechanically in a given arc (60° to 120°) at a single or variable frame rate (Fig. 11). The gearing and drive coupling bearing from the DC motor to the transducer determines the arc of travel. The transducer head, in general, is filled with a liquid that approximates acoustically the impedance of tissue, but in most cases the interface between this fluid and the membrane and between the coupling gel and tissue causes some reverberation artifacts at the skin line. Almost all modern real-time scanners are computer-based devices, in which special programing can delete all near-field information including these artifacts so they are not seen. This area of deletion is between 0.5 and 1.0 cm, according to the field size selected, the type of sector device used, and the shape of the final "chevron" display. A sharp apex chevron has less of the near field deleted than a flat, squared-off apex display (Fig. 12). One should be aware of this when selecting real-time scanning devices for use in the near field, such as for the evaluation of "small parts." If a flat cutoff chevron system is used in the investigation of a superficial structure a water-path stand-off device should also be used to displace the skin-line data deeper into the chevron display. This avoids deletion of near-field data and places the skin-line data in the area of best focus (Fig. 13).

The function of the variable frame rate is to provide a variable scanning speed to assist in data gathering from the area of interest. In general, the

**TRANSDUCER (SERVO-SECTOR)**

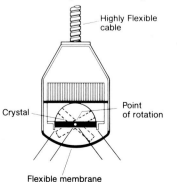

Highly Flexible cable

Crystal

Point of rotation

Flexible membrane

**FIG. 11.** Drawing of a modern direct transmission sector scanner. The transducer moves over a prescribed arc. The fluid-filled membrane provides good acoustic contact when acoustic gel is utilized. (Courtesy of Phillips Ultrasound Inc.)

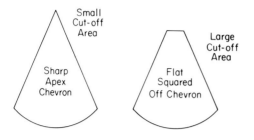

**FIG. 12.** Chevron sector scanner displays showing how the apex is corrected (via the computer) for skin-line artifacts. Sharp apex chevron has little skin-line correction; flat squared-off apex has more skin-line correction.

deeper the area of interest, the slower the frame rate utilized. When acquiring data from deep within the body, more time is needed for the echoes to reach the PE element and be interpreted. If a fast frame rate is used, an excessive amount of information is not interpreted fast enough to be utilized. The high frame rate, in most cases, creates spokes of "data dropout" for deep areas of interest and better images for near areas of interest. At high frame rates the internal computer lacks the capability to collect, process, and display the data at a sufficiently rapid rate. In some cases, by reducing the angle over which the data are gathered, i.e., from 100° to 50°, fill-in will occur but this technique is not always effective. If the transducer arc does not change, but the software (internal functions/commands of the computer) decides when the transducer starts and stops taking data based upon the arc selected, the dropout will still be there. We have found that some equipment that includes a sector scanner with a gray scale static system will have data dropout on a combined sector/gray scale device, but will not have dropout on an identical stand-alone sector system. On the full blown gray scale/real-time system, the speed of data gathering was initially designed for the static scanner and the real-time sector was an add-on device. The stand-alone sector was designed to acquire data at a faster rate and therefore the computer can handle higher frame rates. In addition, even though the data-gathering speed is correct for the system in question, the faster the frame rate, the poorer the depth resolution. This depth degradation is in addition to the poorer resolution caused by the diverging transmission spokes associated with a "chevron" display system.

### Single-Element Vibrating Mirror

The vibrating mirror type sector (Fig. 14) with a single stationary PE element is very similar to the direct transmission type sector device. The main difference is the extended path of travel of the sound vibrations from the PE element to the mirror where it is reflected through an output window. This device produces a chevron display that has a variable frame rate and a selectable sector angle, and the skin-line information is not cut off as much

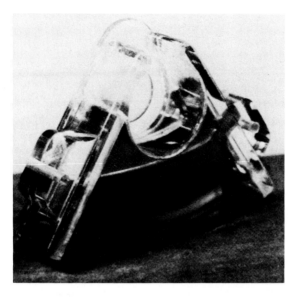

**FIG. 13.** Water path that is attached to a flat squared off apex sector scanner to provide skin-line data deeper in the chevron display. (Courtesy of A.T.L. Ultrasound, Inc.)

via computer software as with the direct sector scanner. The main problem with some of these systems is their lack of penetration and poorer resolution in comparison to the direct sector devices. Most direct transmission systems can penetrate a tissue equivalent material to about 15 cm using a 3.5-MHz PE element. This corresponds to an output of about 52.5 dB of usable power.[2] Most mirror type sectors penetrate to only about 13 cm (using the same frequency PE element) that equals a usable power output of about 45.5 dB. It is believed that the attenuation at the mirror plus the attenuation due to the extended path of travel within the transducer accounts for this lower power output. In some cases, if the gain of the system is raised to provide a higher output the system becomes noisy and will "fill in" the cystic area with echoes. To overcome this, some manufacturers have produced systems with high gain and low noise amplifying electronics built into the transducer head, which produce powers equivalent to the direct vibrating systems.

Phantom studies have shown that direct vibrating systems have an edge in resolution at this time. The axial resolution with a direct system is in the 0.5-mm range and the lateral resolution to the central areas of the chevron on a 16-cm field selection is about 5 to 6 mm. The mirrored systems in general have a 1-mm axial and a 6- to 7-mm lateral resolution in this same area of interest.

---

[2]Using a standard tissue phantom having an attenuation factor of 1 dB/cm/MHz.

### Rotary Head Multielement, Director Transmission Type of System

These systems have a constant frame rate based on the DC motor's revolutions per minute (rpm) (Fig. 16). The motor speed cannot be changed but if there are 3 PE elements that pass the transmission window each time the rotary wheel makes one revolution, by selecting 3, 2, or 1 element, the results are the same and the frame rate is changed. The fastest update of data occurs when all 3 elements are selected, but adequate images are obtained at the slower frame rate. The chevron display for this type of system is the flat squared-off type as seen in Fig. 12, where the skin-line area is deleted by software, but a water-path stand-off can be used to view skin-line areas (Fig. 13).

The rotary head construction yields a small-headed transducer that provides a satisfactory means to image between ribs. The gain and resolution of this type of system is also good. Gains in the order of 55 dB with an axial resolution of 0.5 mm and a lateral resolution of 4 to 5 mm in the central area of the chevron are common. One problem with some older models is mechanical burnout of the rotary head system. The system's rotary head must be turned off between patients or the rotating bearings will overheat and burn out. If a system is accidentally left on overnight with the head running, there is a good chance that the transducer assembly will not be in working order the next day.

Another manufacturer has provided a dual "port" rotary head sector scanner that incorporates two direct transmission transducers and two reflective transducers, all fixed on a rotating wheel. The two pairs of trans-

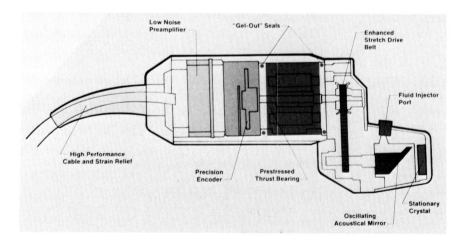

**FIG. 14.** Cutaway drawing of a mirror sector scanner showing transducer, vibrating mirror, motor, and high gain, low noise electronic package built into the transducer housing. (Courtesy of Technicare, Inc.)

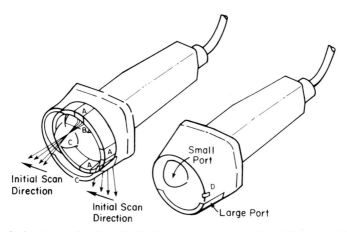

Initial Scan
Direction

Small
Port

Initial Scan
Direction

Large Port

**FIG. 15. Left:** A cutaway drawing of a dual port sector scanner that utilizes direct transmission and reflective transmission from a single rotating wheel that has 4 transducers mounted, two outboard and two inboard. **Right:** The outboard pair of transducers provide direct transmission through the large port, the inboard pair reflect off a mirror device and transmit through the small port. (Courtesy of G.E. Medical Systems, Inc.). A: Transducers; B: Acoustic mirror; C: Windows (small port and large port).

ducers face in opposite directions with one pair facing toward the outside of the rotary wheel and the other pair facing the inside of the rotary wheel. The outside pair provides a direct transmission of sound through a large "port," while the inside pair reflects the energy off a mirror before it leaves the probe through a small "port" facing out of the end of the probe assembly (Fig. 15). The internally constructed electronics provide high gain and low noise to ensure that both images are of equal quality and penetration.

### Multihead In-Line Sector, Direct Transmission

This multielement 3-transducer head provides a "wide field of view" based on a unique approach. Three transducer elements are arranged within the hand-held probe (Fig. 17) to perform a sector scan over a prescribed area and the results are computed and blended together to present an image that is the equivalent of 3 separate sectors side by side. This computer-based system has unique software to interpret the overlapped areas and correct any image misregistration due to interfaces seen at different angles from adjacent transducers. In addition, the single element at the curved forward corner of the transducer housing can be selected separately to perform individual sector scans in areas where the bulky size of the transducer restricts the acquiring of adequate images. An additional feature of this system is that there are many varieties of transducers that can be added to the basic system by incorporating interfacing electronics which have been constructed in "Draws" that can be easily installed into the system. This modular approach

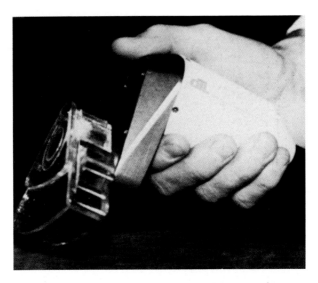

**FIG. 16.** A rotary sector scanner having 3 transducers of the same frequency. Each transducer rotates through a window of about 110°. The attached water path provides the displacement of skin line information deeper into the chevron display. (Courtesy of A.T.L. Ultrasound, Inc.)

ensures proper "matching" of the transducer designs for optimum performance and resolution with minimum adjustments to the rest of the system.

## MULTIFOCUSED ANNULAR ARRAY

The annular array system has several unique features and represents a system with exceptional gain, resolution, and focus. This system can have up to 6 round transducers of the same frequency, fitted one inside the other. A vibrating mirror is used along with a large water path contained within a large rubber membrane, which is in contact with the patient. Because of the large water path and large skin contact area, the chevron image is larger at the apex than with any other type of sector system. The operation of the system is a little cumbersome but adequate quality abdominal studies can be obtained. The 6 transducers provide 6 separate focal areas, which are individually selectable or can be combined to provide good focus from 2 to 20 cm. The large size and diameter of these transducers provides good power output, and losses due to mirror reflection and the long water path are not a problem as with other vibrating mirror systems. The vibrating mirror has two sweep modes (frame rates), one for normal real-time imaging and a slow rate to provide a final sweep prior to freeze framing, to give an image with

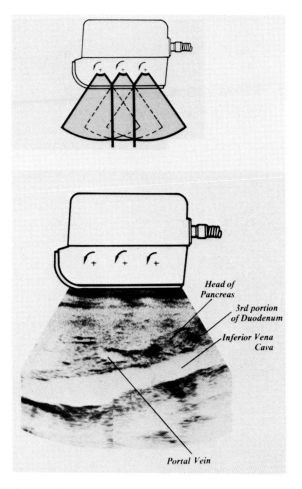

**FIG. 17.** A wide field of view transducer showing the 3 sectoring transducers and their overlapping fields. (Courtesy of Diasonics Ultrasound, Inc.)

good fill-in. Annular arrays, 19 mm in diameter, are presently being constructed with 4 inner-fitted PE elements of 3.5 MHz that provide good focus capabilities from about 3 cm to about 18 cm in depth. Figures 18A and 18B show how each PE element is fired in sequence to provide focus over a larger distance and improve lateral and axial resolution. The vibrating mirror is still utilized to perform the sweeping motion, but each transmitted pulse is focused by the delay in time of firing to provide the concave wavefront discussed earlier.

## ELECTRONIC SECTOR (PHASED ARRAY)

An electronic steering system that provides a means to deflect the transmitted beam energy in a sweeping direction, without any moving parts, is

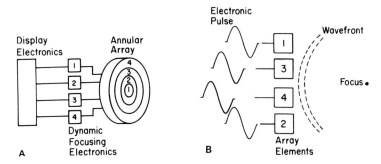

**FIG. 18. A:** Drawing of a modern 19 mm Annular Array having 4 inter-fitted 3.5 MHz transducers. The activation is from the center transducer out. **B:** Drawing showing how this delay firing results in beam shaping to provide a long focal zone from about 3 cm to 18 cm. (Courtesy Technicare Corporation.)

referred to as a "phased array" transducer (Fig. 6). This term refers to the firing of an adjacent transducer at a time when the previously fired element is at its peak of transmitted energy so that the two energies are added in phase and the transmitted energy is displaced a precise distance (Fig. 7). This adding of energy to only one side of the transmitted beam moves it in the direction of higher energy. An advantage of this system is that the transducer head is very small and can be used between the ribs, especially useful for cardiac studies. In addition, because the firing sequence is electronically controlled, the number of transducers that are fired at any one time can be controlled for variation of the concave wavefront allowing the focus to be varied. Until recently, these systems were not used for abdominal studies because of their expense and relatively poor penetrating power (10 to 12 cm). The resolution of these systems is only slightly inferior to a good mechanical direct sector device. This type of technology has great potential for technical expansion and in the future may replace the mechanical sector device altogether as it is more reliable. An electronic sector can be incorporated into a linear array system to provide both types of scanning by the simple turning of a switch on the control console of the system. Because of the large size of the linear array, there will probably be a special "cone down" water-path device attached to the transducer to provide a smaller access area while at the same time providing a soft, flexible contact point for better acoustic coupling (Fig. 19).

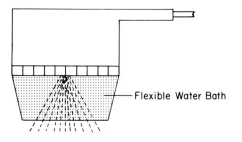

**FIG. 19.** Artist drawing of a combination linear/sector device that is possible due to the electronic capabilities for beam steering and beam delay firing for lensing control that are generated within the transducer.

## DOPPLER TECHNOLOGY

There are two basic reasons to utilize Doppler: the first is to define liquid flow direction and liquid flow rate, and the second is to define range (distance).

Direction and rate of flow through a vein or artery is assessed by using a continuous transmitted frequency from a PE element, directed toward the area of investigation. If the transmitted frequency energy is pointed toward the direction of flow (Fig. 20), the returned echo from this moving liquid causes the reflected frequency energy to be "drawn out" and have a longer wavelength and return at a lower frequency. If the transmitted beam is pointed against the direction of flow, the moving liquid flow causes the reflected frequency energy to be "shortened" to a shorter wavelength and it will return at a higher frequency. This basically is how police radar works. A police car is parked alongside the road. As a car moves away from the police car, the officer points his radar gun toward the back of the car. For simplicity sake, assume that the transmitted frequency is 1,000 cycles per second (cps). The returned frequency is lower than the transmitted frequency because the reflected energy is being returned from a moving interface that is "stretching" the contact point. How much lower than 1,000 cps is the returned frequency? This is a function of how fast the car is moving away from the radar gun. If the car is not moving, the returned frequency is the same as the transmitted frequency. If the car is moving at such a fast rate that the transmitted energy would not catch up to it in order to generate a reflection, the returned energy would be nonexistent. Therefore, the difference between the transmitted frequency and the returned energy frequency is a function of the car's rate of travel. The same analogy can be used to define how the returned frequency is higher than the transmitted frequency when the car is moving toward the police car's radar. The moving interface is now moving into the transmitted frequency, thereby moving the contact

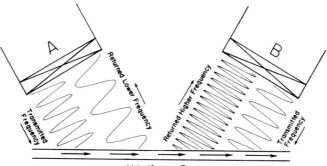

Vein/Artery Flow

**FIG. 20.** Doppler response when aimed with/against fluid flow in an artery or vein. Constant frequency transmission of the doppler results in a returned signal that is lower/ higher than the transmitted frequency.

point and shortening the duration between energy reflections making the return frequency higher. When flow and rate through an artery or vein is being analyzed, the transmitting PE element cannot be perpendicular to the vein because the returned echo is reflected from too small a cross-sectional area. The accepted angle for Doppler studies is about 20° from the vertical. This provides adequate reflective information to define flow rate.

The results of this transmitted Doppler frequency can be displayed as an audio signal that will be either below or above a standard 1000-cps rate (which is considered as "no flow") or on a strip chart record that will trace out a straight line in the center of the chart at 1,000 cps with a displacement to the left for a higher frequency or a displacement to the right for a lower frequency. The distance displaced from the center line is directly related to the rate of flow. The higher the flow, the greater the displacement. Doppler technology is becoming popular for peripheral vascular studies. Small parts transducers have been designed with high resolution that can simultaneously perform Doppler and measure flow velocities. Fast and dependable computers, that are a major portion of all real time ultrasound systems, have been programmed to perform parallel data reductions to present Doppler data and high resolution ultrasound images at the same time on the same video display.

## SMALL PARTS TRANSDUCERS

Small parts (SP) transducers, in general, are constructed using the single-sector PE element with direct transmission and a sufficiently large water path between the crystal element and the skin contact membrane to ensure no skin-line artifacts. The depth of the area of interest for SP systems is generally designed to be up to about 6 cm; therefore, the transducer element is constructed with an extremely short focus lens assembly. In addition, higher resolution is also necessary to provide adequate clarity for defining small interfaces, as well as "magnification" of the area of interest to ensure hard copy images that will display these smaller interfaces so they can be analyzed. SP sector transducers, therefore, have 5-MHz or 7-MHz PE elements with a diameter of 10 mm or 13 mm and a short focused lens assembly. The magnification is usually 1.5× or 2.0× normal. These parameters provide adequate depth penetration and resolution to properly visualize small areas of interest. Resolutions of less than 0.5 mm axially and 2 to 4 mm laterally are typical.

Linear array systems also have SP devices. These are also 5 MHz or 7 MHz and becaue of "microelement" construction can be fairly small in comparison to the larger standard size arrays. The standard 3.5-MHz linear array transducer has 10 to 12 cm of skin contact area whereas the SP linear array transducer has a 5 to 6 cm of skin contact area. The near focus requirements are provided by the electronic lensing functions that are incorporated into these newer designed systems. The magnification is generally 1.5×, and resolutions of 0.5 mm axially and 3 to 5 mm laterally are typical for these systems.

## MINERAL OIL VERSUS GEL

Mineral oil is widely used as a skin couplant because it does an adequate job and is low in cost. However, when mineral oil is used with real-time systems, the plastic membrane on the transducer becomes warped, and if it has a rubber membrane, this becomes soft, stretches, and finally leaks. Plastic and rubber membranes require the use of acoustic gels to provide adequate skin contact without causing chemical deterioration of these materials. If mineral oil is still being used for B-scans and a real-time study is also required, the skin area should be cleaned before the real-time study. On a daily basis the real-time machine, including the transducer and its cable, should be cleaned with an alcohol cloth.

## SAFETY

Many real-time systems are small and portable and are being used with increasing frequency in the operating room. It is necessary to isolate and insulate a patient during major surgery, but ultrasound safety standards do not currently mandate complete patient safety since they permit inadequate grounding. Transducer surfaces should be completely isolated from the ground, meaning that no metal part comes into contact with the patient or the sonographer holding the transducer. A simple way to check this is with an ohm meter. Place one of the leads of the meter to a chassis ground, or the third wire of the AC plug that is disconnected from the wall outlet, and probe all areas of the transducer including the cosmetic cover screws with the second meter lead. If any contact point of this second meter lead causes the meter to read even a very few ohms, then the transducer has an extended ground condition and should not be used in the operating room. Manufacturers are aware of this potential problem and new real-time transducers are being constructed with no ground extension to replace the older troublesome versions. At this point, it is still up to the user to determine whether a problem exists and to contact the manufacturer to correct this problem if it does.

## SERVICES AND CALIBRATION

It is not our intention to provide a "How to" section for keeping a real-time system in calibration and operation because there are areas where the user requirements dictate the accuracy of anatomic measurements. For example, the femur length provides a good indication of fetal age, but a slight error of a few millimeters can make a large difference in age. This length displayed horizontally on the hard copy unit ideally should measure the same distance if it were displayed in the vertical axis. It should also measure the same whether one uses a linear array system or a sector scanning device.

To verify real-time measurement accuracy requires the use of a real-time phantom. Like B-scan phantoms, real-time phantoms should have the same velocity as in tissue and should be made of a tissue-equivalent material with a given attenuation for a given frequency. In addition, they should allow the measurement of resolution at different depths of penetration and also provide accurately spaced pins over a distance of at least 16 cm in depth. With such a phantom, most real-time testing and calibration can be performed.

Figure 21 is an image taken with a linear array system of a real-time test phantom (R.M.I. Model 410), having nylon pins variably spaced at different depths (test modules) and they appear at 3 cm, 7 cm, and 12 cm in depth. The pins at each module are spaced 3,2,1, and 0.5 mm apart. There is also a line of pins spaced 2 cm apart from 2 cm in depth to 16 cm in depth. The attenuation of the acoustic material in the phantom is equivalent to tissue (a little less than 1 dB/cm/MHz) and the surface that the transducer comes in contact with is a flexible membrane.

The modules can be utilized for axial and lateral resolution with respect to depth. The 2-cm spaced pins can be used for accurate caliper measurements of large distances while the 3-mm and 2-mm spaced pins can be used to check accurate caliper measurements for small distances. The 2-cm pin spacing can be compared to the horizontal and vertical displayed centimeter markers to ensure that the camera CRT width and height adjust-

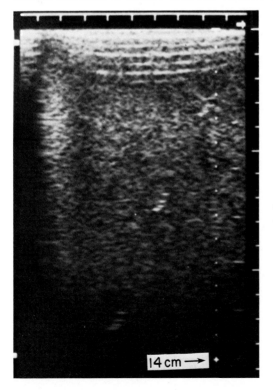

**FIG. 21.** A real-time phantom showing the 3 resolution modules and the 2-cm spaced pins. The deepest echo is noted 14 cm in depth.

14 cm →

ments are correct. If these CRT adjustments are not correct the calipers would give a wrong reading of the 2-cm pin spacing. If the calipers read the vertical centimeter markers correctly, but showed an error for the horizontal markers, the width (or horizontal linearity control) of the CRT is incorrectly adjusted. All measurements are taken on the final hard copy device, be it Polaroid or Multiformat camera. A system gain test can also be performed using the real-time phantom. Locate the distance from the image skin line to where the last echo appears in depth. Measure this distance with the calipers and then multiply this distance by the attenuation factor of the phantom (0.7 or 1.0 dB/cm) and multiply this result by the frequency of the transducer. In most cases the gain of a real-time system is between 40 and 50 dB. For example, the last echo in depth in Fig. 21 appeared at 14 cm using a 3.5 MHz transducer on a phantom that has an attenuation factor of 1.0 dB/cm/MHz. Therefore the gain of this system is $14 \times 1.0 \times 3.5 = 49$ dB.

In most cases the user decides if the equipment is calibrated correctly. Most service personnel are mainly concerned with the gross operational aspects of the equipment. Therefore, every real-time ultrasound user should acquire a real time test phantom to correct the problem. These fine tuning adjustments will give more accurate fetal measurements and therefore age determination. Measurements of fetal parameters can now be taken directly from the hard copy images by the use of a small computer system utilizing a "digitizing pad." This pad converts distances in a two-dimensional plane *(XY)* to counts by the use of a large multilined grid. A tracing device called a mouse is placed over the image that contains the area to be measured, e.g., a trunk circumference. The tracing device is hand controlled by the operator and moves around the area of measurement as counts are being collected by the computer each time the "mouse" crosses a grid crossing. Upon completion of the tracing, the operator prompts the computer to complete the computation and display the results. It is extremely important to have the image horizontal and vertical dimensions correct if accurate results are to be obtained. Small computers are being developed for ultrasound to perform measurements directly from the final hard copy image. These measurements are controlled by a "program" that works with the computer to perform all measurements automatically when prompted by the sonographer. These programs contain the appropriate curves that define fetal age, weight, and size, which prior to this time had to be hand-calculated by the sonographers.

In the very near future, complete measurement functions will be done directly by the computer within the real-time system, with faster and more accurate results. The data will be stored, in the form of an image, in a digital matrix (a grid) whose resolution is far better than the digitizing grid, and it will not be difficult to compute the number of pixels of the image that are in the area of interest. There will also be a means of inserting a programmed disk to prompt the internal computer to perform functions and other digital reductions that are presently being performed by outside computers. In general, the internal computer of most real-time systems is larger, faster, and more dependable than the small external type and can perform additional operations when programmed to do so. At present, some manufacturers are moving in this direction by providing a limited number of these measurements by keyboard prompting. Fetal head and trunk circumferences and femur lengths are readily available on newly designed systems.

## SUMMARY

Real-time systems have become a reliable sonographic imaging modality with good resolution and penetration that allow one to perform rapid ultrasound examination. The variety and flexibility of the many types of real-time transducers allows the diagnostician to tailor the choice of transducer to the area of investigation. Body structures and access windows to see within the body have dictated the design of real-time transducers. Equipment manufacturers who have followed the "modular" design approach, in which many varieties of transducers can be interfaced into the main data reduction computer, see the importance of this approach and have warded off obsolescence.

New real-time transducers will be designed to improve reliability and image resolution. It is likely that mechanical sector scanners will be replaced by a pure electronic controlled sector (phase array) which is more costly, but more reliable. B-scan transducers have been designed incorporating a real-time sector within a static image to study smaller areas of interest. All manufacturers of B-scan systems are aware that real-time attachments are necessary and desirable and at present most of them are producing dual systems. It is likely that new, small diameter annular arrays will also become popular because of their good focusing and penetrating power. In the future these may be used with the B-scan systems as the primary B-scan transducer. These advances, and many more, will push real-time ultrasound to new heights. Are you ready?

## ACKNOWLEDGMENTS

I wish to express my sincere thanks to Mrs. Lois E. Akehurst for the monumental amount of typing and revisions that were necessary in writing the text, and to Mr. Leroy Warthen, artist and magic man, who made my ideas of drawings take shape and become a reality.

Ultrasound Annual 1983, edited by R. C. Sanders and M. Hill. Raven Press, New York © 1983.

# Ultrasound in Tropical Diseases

Yacov Itzchak, Zalman Rubinstein, and Ruth Shilo

*Tel-Aviv University School of Medicine, Sheba Medical Center, Tel-Hashomer, Israel 52621*

Increased worldwide air travel, brought about by tourism and immigration, has resulted in the dissemination of many diseases formerly regarded as "tropical" and that previously were confined to large but localized endemic areas. The physician working in nonendemic areas must now be aware of these diseases and their protean manifestations. Many of these conditions become manifest long after the initial infestation and often after the patient has left the endemic area. Delay in arriving at the correct diagnosis is thus common. Spread of the disease from the infected carrier to persons who have never been in endemic areas further complicates the diagnostic process.

The establishment of ultrasound (US) and computed tomography (CT) as integral parts of the physician's diagnostic armamentarium has, for the first time, allowed detailed visualization of the major abdominal areas affected by many of these so-called tropical diseases. The most common conditions for which sonography can identify infestation of the affected organ are: echinococcosis, amebiasis, ascariasis, and schistomiasis. Other rare infestations will also be briefly mentioned.

## HYDATID DISEASE (ECHINOCOCCOSIS)

There are two forms of this disease, one caused by *Echinococcus granulosis* and the other by *Echinococcus multilocularis*. The former is the most common type and gives rise to the so-called cystic hydatid disease, whereas the latter causes the relatively uncommon alveolar form of the disease, which involves predominantly the skeletal system (19, 24).

The primary host of *E. granulosis* is the dog, with sheep or cattle acting as the intermediary host (14, 16, 26). Infection is transmitted to man by ingestion of the egg. The larvae then form in the gastrointestinal tract before penetrating the intestinal mucosa and entering the portal venous system. Filtering of these larvae occurs first in the liver and then in the lung, which accounts for the frequent involvement of these organs. The larvae that remain viable can develop into the hydatid cyst which is typical of this disease.

One or more separate cysts may develop and each of the so-called parent cysts may have numerous smaller daughter cysts within the capsule. The daughter cysts arise from the germinal epithelium, which is the endocyst or true cyst wall. The expanding parent cyst compresses the surrounding tissue of the host organ, which gives rise to the ectocyst or false capsule. The liver is the organ most frequently involved.

The number and size of the cysts vary considerably and calcifications may occur in the wall of the cyst many years after the initial infection. Although complete cyst wall calcification usually indicates inactive disease, other viable noncalcified cysts may be present in the same organ. Partial and rarely complete calcification of the parent cyst wall may occur while the daughter cyst within remains viable. Prior to the introduction of ultrasound and computed tomography, the diagnosis of hepatic hydatid disease depended on the demonstration of cyst wall calcification on plain radiographs (3, 7). Isotope scanning and angiography showed an avascular space-occupying lesion without being able to indicate its cystic nature or to demonstrate the pathognomic daughter cyst within (2, 5).

Hydatid disease of the abdomen almost invariably affects the liver (7). Involvement of the kidneys, retroperitoneum, or peritoneal cavity are well-recognized but rare manifestations (3, 26). The sonographic characteristic of a hydatid cyst in the abdomen depends on many factors such as the size of the cyst, whether it is single or multiple, unilocular or multilocular, and its location (Figs. 1–10). The presence of calcification or secondary infection also influences the picture (8, 11, 25). The uncomplicated cyst usually appears as a fluid-filled, sonolucent mass with well-defined smooth borders and good through transmission (Fig. 4). The most common finding is that of a single parent cyst containing multiple daughter cysts. Sonographically, the single parent cyst with its well-defined capsule can be identified with the daughter cysts incorporated within it (Fig. 1). These daughter cysts give the parent cyst a multilocular appearance. The cyst has a similar appearance on computed tomography (Fig. 3) (20). In the early stage of the disease, the daughter cysts appear as small 2- to 3-mm highly echogenic solid masses (11). At this stage, they consist only of growing walls, and occasionally the parent cyst may be completely filled with these multiple small growing cysts (11, 16). The mass, instead of being cystic, may be full of high level echoes due to the multiple reflecting surfaces of the daughter cyst (Fig. 5). As they enlarge, the typical fluid-filled cystic pattern appears (Fig. 6). These daughter cysts are round, but as they increase in size within the confines of the parent cyst, which already has a relatively fixed size or even a partially calcified capsule, the pressure on the growing daughter cysts increases. They thus compress each other and their shapes become oval or elongated (8, 11). This, in part, may account for the internal radiating septa seen within the parent cyst (Fig. 1). The daughter cysts may retain their rounded appearance if the parent cysts can expand freely, such as occurs when the

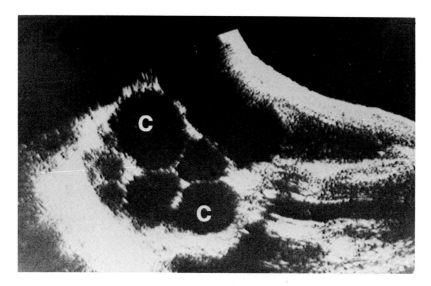

**FIG. 1.** Hydatid cyst (parent cyst with multiple daughter cysts). Sonogram through left lobe of liver shows a well-rounded cyst with multiple large daughter cysts (C) within it compressing each other to give a multilocular appearance.

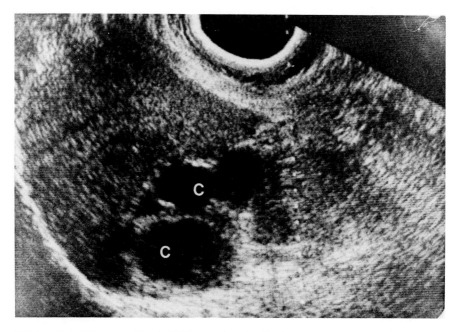

**FIG. 2.** Hydatid cyst in the right kidney. Longitudinal sonogram through the liver and right kidney. Multiple fluid-filled lesions (C) involving the upper pole of the right kidney are seen. These could not be differentiated from simple cysts of the kidney.

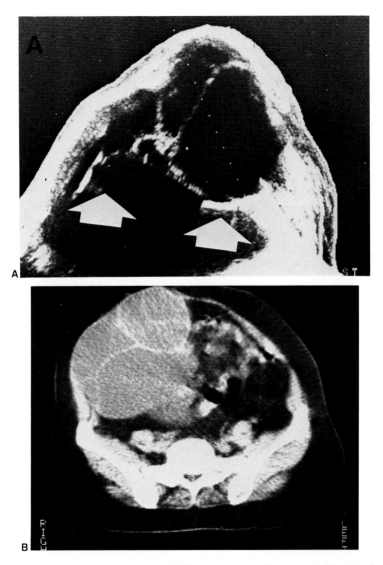

**FIG. 3.**  Intraperitoneal hydatid cysts. **A:** Transverse scan through a mid-abdominal ventral hernia. A 12-cm fluid-filled mass with multiple septae is present *(arrows).* **B:** CT scan shows the same appearance of multiple daughter cysts within a parent hydatid cyst.

disease spreads into the peritoneum or retroperitoneum (Fig. 7) (11). The detection of such daughter cysts indicates that the disease is still active even when the parent cyst is calcified.

In other instances, liver involvement consists of multiple parent cysts situated in both lobes, causing hepatomegaly. Sonographically, multiple

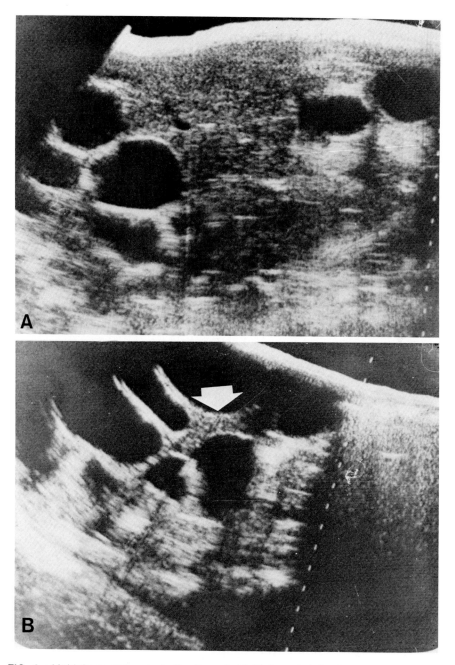

**FIG. 4.** Multiple parent cysts in the liver. **A:** Multiple well-defined separate fluid-filled cysts of various sizes are present in the liver. **B:** Some of the cysts are compressed by others and thus lose their rounded appearance. There is liver tissue between the cysts *(arrow),* indicating that they are multiple parent cysts and not daughter cysts.

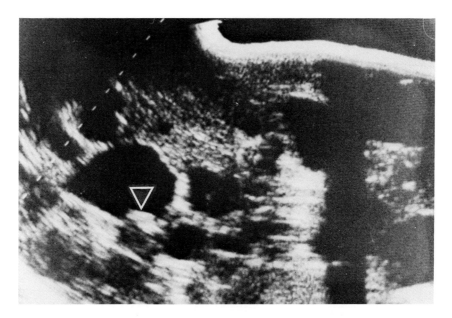

**FIG. 5.** Small daughter cyst developing within a parent cyst. Multiple fluid-filled hydatid cysts in the right lobe of the liver. In one of them, a small reflecting pole *(arrowhead)* is seen attached to the wall of the parent cyst. This probably represents a developing daughter cyst.

cysts with thick walls are seen occupying different parts of the liver (Fig. 4). The detection of liver tissue between the cysts clearly indicates that each cyst is a separate parent cyst and not multiple daughter cysts within a single parent cyst (Fig. 1) (11). In rare cases, a hydatid cyst may be single, without thick walls, and unaccompanied by demonstrable daughter cysts within (8, 11). Detection of such a lesion creates a diagnostic dilemma since differentiation between a simple cyst and a hydatid cyst then becomes virtually impossible. Detection of shell-like calcification in a thick wall around the cyst, if demonstrated, can indicate the true hydatid nature of the cyst (Fig. 10). Two hypotheses have been proposed to explain the apparent lack of daughter cysts in these cases. First, if calcification is present, this may indicate that the disease is inactive, and death and disintegration of the daughter cysts may have already occurred. Alternatively, previous unrecognized secondary infection of the cyst may have caused a disintegration of the daughter cysts without wall calcification of the parent cyst (8, 11).

A hydatid cyst with secondary infection may give rise to a number of different patterns on the ultrasound scan. Examination of the cysts during the acute onset of secondary infection may show a cyst that has a variable number of internal echoes which may give it the appearance of a solid mass.

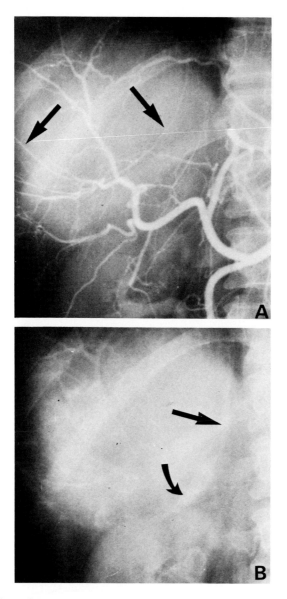

**FIG. 6.** Hydatid cyst (parent cyst with multiple small daughter cysts). **A:** Selective hepatic angiography, arterial phase, showing displacement of vessels *(arrows)* by a large avascular mass *(arrows)*. **B:** Parenchymal phase, a thick wall is demonstrated surrounding the mass *(arrows)*.

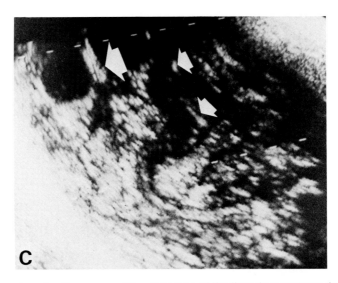

**FIG. 6C. continued:** Sonogram of the right lobe of the liver demonstrates the avascular mass to be cystic in nature with multiple internal echoes. It contains some small cystic areas *(arrows)* indicating the hydatid nature of this mass. (Proven at operation.)

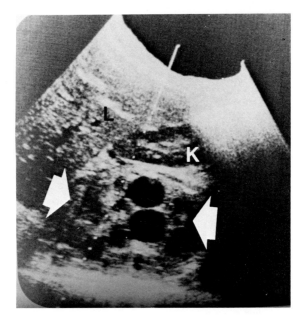

**FIG. 7.** Retroperitoneal hydatid parent cyst with daughter cysts. An oblique sonogram through the right abdomen in a patient with a palpable mass, showing it to be a multilocular fluid-filled lesion *(arrows)*. The mass is dorsal to the right kidney (K) and below the liver (L) and is separated from both organs. The well-rounded regularly-shaped fluid-filled lesions represent multiple daughter cysts in a retroperitoneal hydatid cyst.

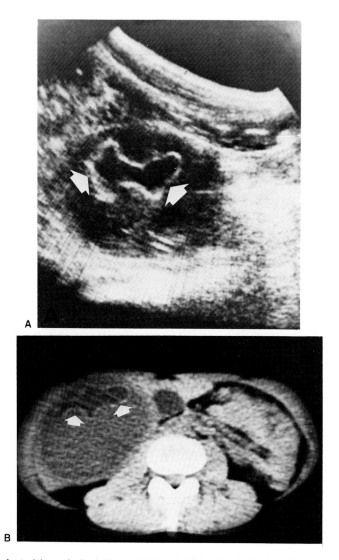

**FIG. 8.** Infected hepatic hydatid cyst (intermediate stage). **A:** Longitudinal sonogram through the liver. A 10-cm well-defined mass with some internal echoes and with good through transmission is identified. An irregular membrane *(arrows)* is seen within the fluid-filled mass. **B:** Transverse CT scan of the mass showing the same appearance as in (A). Note fluid density inside the membrane *(arrows)* compared to the rest of the mass.

There may also be membranes of various shapes within the cyst which can have a bizarre appearance (Fig. 8). These membranes usually indicate disintegration of the daughter cysts while the echoes within the cyst are caused by the presence of infected particles. At a later stage, following complete

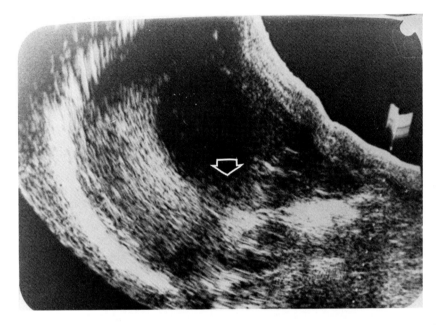

**FIG. 9.** Infected hepatic hydatid cyst. Longitudinal sonogram through the right lobe of the liver in a febrile patient. A large oval mass is demonstrated with sharp borders. The mass is mostly fluid-filled with some reflecting particles *(arrow)* in it. An infected hydatid cyst was found at operation.

disintegration of these particles, the hydatid cysts may then come to resemble simple cysts (Fig. 9).

In rare instances, a parent cyst may rupture and result in dissemination of the daughter cysts into surrounding areas. A cyst lying in close proximity to the bile ducts can compress or displace them and can produce obstructive jaundice if rupture into the ducts occurs. Occasionally, a hydatid cyst situated at the periphery of the liver can mimic a lesion in an adjacent organ (Fig. 10).

## AMEBIASIS

Infestation with *Entamoeba histolytica* is one of the most widespread diseases in the world (14, 16, 26). Ingestion of the protozoa *E. Histolytica* in contaminated water or food results in the organism becoming lodged in the caecum and colon. In most instances, the patient is asymptomatic and the organism confines itself to the gastrointestinal tract. The patient at this stage is a carrier and can infect other people. Pathologically, there is mucosal and submucosal inflammation of the caecum and colon giving rise to the clinical picture of colitis (10). The spectrum of colonic involvement may vary from a

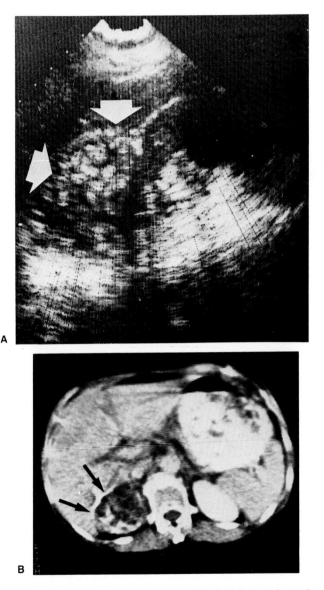

**FIG. 10.** Hydatid cyst mimicking a right adrenal mass. **A:** A 5-cm echogenic mass is seen located superior to the kidney and inferior to the liver *(arrows)*. **B:** On the CT scan a calcified rim is seen *(arrows)*. An adrenal mass was suspected, but at operation a subcapsular hepatic hydatid cyst with calcified walls and multiple daughter cysts was found.

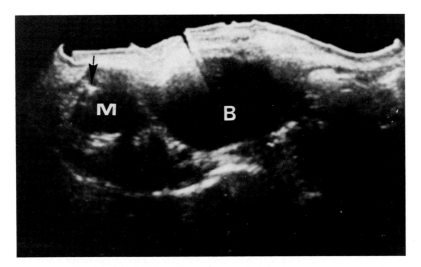

**FIG. 11.** Ameboma. Transverse sonogram of the lower abdomen. A 4-cm mass (M) is present in the right lower abdomen. It is homogeneous in nature and contains minimal low level echoes. High level echoes are seen at the top of the mass due to the contents of the colon. Bladder (B). Amoeba was present in the stool. The mass disappeared following antiamoebic therapy.

mild, almost subclinical colitis to severe fulminating toxic megacolon (19). A more chronic and localized form of the disease causes an inflammatory mass or ameboma to form in the wall of the colon.

Sonographically, an ameboma appears as a well-organized, partially solid mass with some internal echoes and good through transmission (Fig. 11). Follow-up studies during and after specific antiamebic therapy may show the degree of response, and with complete recovery the previously demonstrated mass should disappear. Spread of the organism from the colon to the portal venous system results in infection of the liver. Such involvement can occur at any stage of the disease, and it is important to note that the liver may be affected without overt colonic involvement. Stool cultures, usually positive in patients with acute colitis, may be negative in patients in whom liver involvement is the primary manifestation of the disease. An abscess can develop in any part of the liver and may have a rapid or insidious onset. The abscess may be single or multiple, and the right lobe of the liver is involved in approximately 75% of cases (Fig. 12). Deposition of the organisms occurs in the capillaries of the portal veins and so most amebic abscesses are situated in the periphery of the liver (18). The abscess is formed by the liquefying necrosis of hepatocytes with only a minor surrounding inflammatory and fibrotic response. This lack of host reaction may explain the formation of extremely large abscesses containing liters of so-called "anchovy" pus and also the ease with which these abscesses may rupture (Fig. 13).

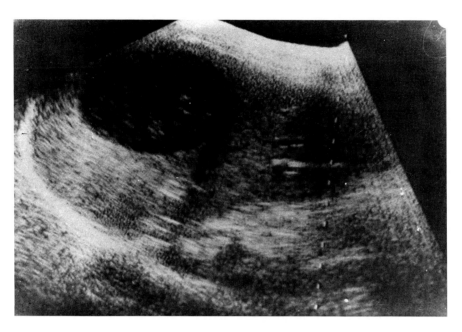

**FIG. 12.** Hepatic amoebic abscess. Large homogeneous mass in the right lobe of the liver. Note good delineation between the lesion and the liver parenchyma. The mass contains internal echoes and has good through transmission. Anchovy pus was aspirated from the mass.

Several sonographic features have been reported, which suggest that an abscess is amebic in nature (18, 23). Most of the lesions detected by ultrasound are spherical or ovoid with an average diameter of more than 7 cm (Figs. 12, 14). In the majority of cases, the abscess does not have a significant wall echo, but exhibits an abrupt transition between the normal surrounding hepatic parenchyma and the fluid-filled mass (Figs. 12, 14). In rare instances, the mass may demonstrate a highly reflective wall of varying thickness that may be either completely circumferential or segmental (Fig. 15). Many of these lesions when scanned at a normal gain setting appear anechoic or hypoechoic, but have fine low-level echoes at a high gain setting with some enhancement behind the lesions (Fig. 14) (18, 23). This pattern can be explained, in part, by the nature of the thick "anchovy sauce" pus within the abscess.

The presence of these features in a single case can suggest the diagnosis of an amebic abscess. In one series, such typical findings were noted in over one-third of cases while over half had at least three of the above five features (18). Some cases have unusual sonographic findings including an irregular shape and border and a heterogeneous echo pattern within the lesion (Fig. 16). Ultrasound in such instances is of limited value in determining the etiology of such lesions. However, it can determine the presence of an

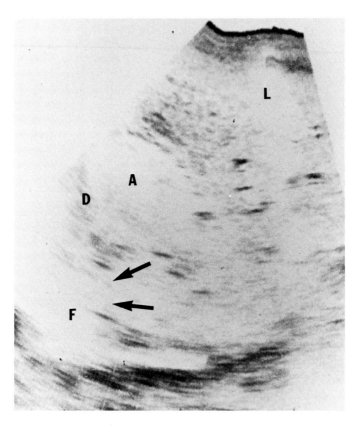

**FIG. 13.** Rupture of a hepatic amebic abscess through the diaphragm. A longitudinal sonogram through the right lobe of the liver shows an abscess beneath the diaphragm (D). The abscess has broken through *(arrows)* the diaphragm and fluid (F) can be identified in the right pleural space. (Courtesy M. C. Hill.)

abscess in the appropriate clinical setting, i.e., fever, hepatic tenderness, and a high hemagglutination titer. After the initiation of treatment, the sonographic findings of amebic abscess can vary widely. The abscess may enlarge, become smaller, or remain unchanged (4, 18). Alteration of the internal echo pattern may also occur with treatment (Fig. 16). Most treated abscesses eventually resolve completely and the sonogram will then be normal; however, "hepatic cysts" have been reported to persist.

Rupture of an untreated abscess is not infrequent and most commonly occurs into either the peritoneal cavity, subphrenic space, or through the diaphragm into the pleural cavity, and may even involve the lung parenchyma and bronchial tree (Fig. 13) (13). Extension into the biliary tree pericardium or through the skin are rare complications. Untreated amebic liver abscesses have a mortality rate approaching 100% and even treated cases

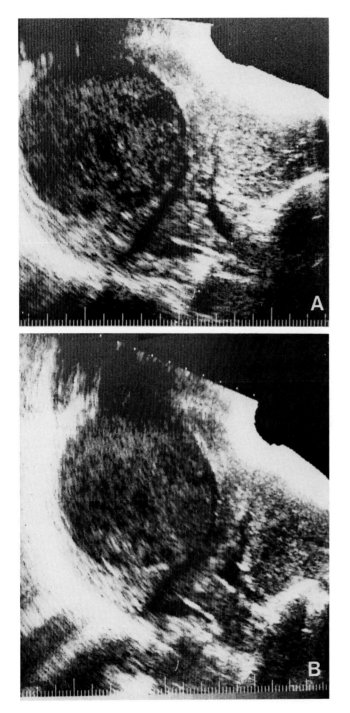

**FIG. 14.** Hepatic amoebic abscess with normal and high gain settings. A well-demarcated 7-cm mass is present in the right lobe of the liver. With a normal gain setting, the mass has less internal echoes (A) than when a high gain setting is used (B). This finding is frequently present in amoebic abscesses.

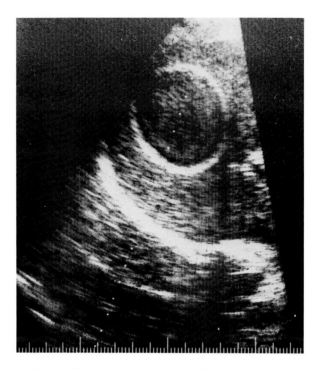

**FIG. 15.** Hepatic amoebic abscess with a thick wall. A 6-cm mass is seen in the right lobe of the liver. It has a thick capsule that separates it from the rest of the liver. This is a relatively infrequent appearance of a hepatic amoebic abscess.

have a mortality of approximately 10%. It is thus obvious that early and accurate diagnosis followed by treatment is essential for this potentially lethal disease. Percutaneous aspiration using US or CT guidance should be reserved for cases where the diagnosis is uncertain, or if a superimposed pyogenic infection is suspected. It should also be performed when response to drug therapy is inadequate or when impending rupture is considered likely.

## SCHISTOSOMIASIS

Schistosomiasis (bilharzia) is a disease that is widespread throughout the world. Three species of flukes are known to infect man. *Schistosoma haematobium* involves primarily the lower urinary tract while *Schistosoma mansoni* and *Schistosoma japonica* involve mainly the colonic mucosa (14). The immature worms or cercariae exist in fresh water streams. Infection occurs when the cercariae penetrate the skin of humans and migrate via the lymphatic or venous system to the general circulation. In the liver, it matures into the adult form and lives in pairs. The female worm, once

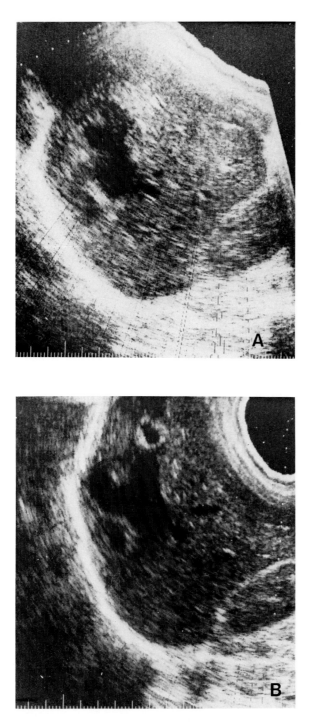

**FIG. 16.** Changes in size, configuration, and sonographic pattern during therapy of hepatic amoebic abscess. **A:** An irregular cystic mass with some internal echoes is demonstrated in the right lobe of the liver. **B:** 1 week after the start of specific therapy. The mass increased in size and the number of internal echoes had decreased.

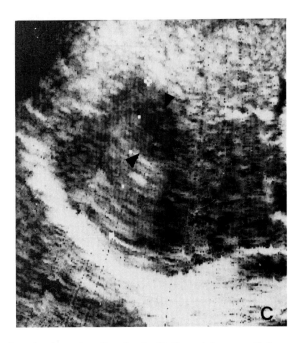

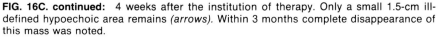

**FIG. 16C. continued:**  4 weeks after the institution of therapy. Only a small 1.5-cm ill-defined hypoechoic area remains *(arrows)*. Within 3 months complete disappearance of this mass was noted.

fertilized, migrates in a retrograde fashion into the terminal venous radicles of the bladder, ureters, and colon. The ova deposited by the female worm penetrate the mucosa and thus infect the urine and feces. Discharge of infected excreta into water allows the cycle to continue.

In *S. hematobium* infection, the trapped ova cause thickening and eventual calcification of the ureters and bladder wall. Strictures of the distal ureter lead to hydroureter and hydronephrosis in many patients. Some ova travel back to the liver via the portal venous system where they penetrate the walls of the smaller portal veins and lodge in the periportal connective tissue. Here they cause an intense fibrotic response resulting in obstruction of the portal venous system with portal hypertension (17). The entire process occurs over a period of many years, and the true bilharzial nature of the disease may not be readily apparent as the original infection may have been forgotten or may not have even been noticed by the patient. The presinusoidal portal hypertension that occurs with hepatic schistosomiasis results in the development of splenomegaly and portasystemic venous collaterals. Gastrointestinal hemorrhage from esophageal varices or splenomegaly causing a mass in the left upper abdomen usually prompts the patient to seek medical attention (15).

Ultrasound examination of these patients is often performed in the later stages of the disease, and a large spleen with increased echogenicity is the commonest finding (Fig. 17A). Dilated splenic and portal veins with multiple collaterals can be seen (Fig. 17A). The liver may be normal in size or smaller than expected with foci of increased echoes secondary to diffuse fibrosis (Fig. 17B). Good correlation has been reported between the portal venous pressure and the diameter of the portal and splenic veins as measured on the ultrasound scan (1).

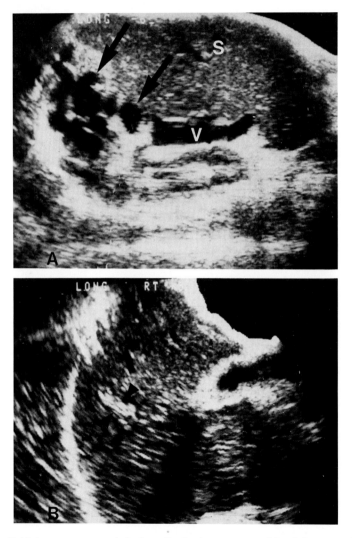

**FIG. 17.** Schistozoma mansoni. **A:** Longitudinal sonogram of the left upper abdomen shows a huge spleen (S) with increased echogenicity and a dilated splenic vein (V) with dilated short gastric collaterals *(arrows)*. **B:** Longitudinal sonogram of the right lobe of the liver shows it to be small with a coarse echo pattern compatible with fibrosis *(arrows)*.

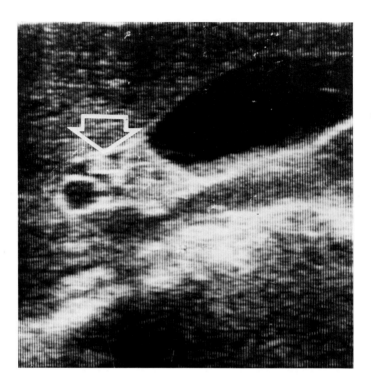

**FIG. 18.** Ascaris in the common hepatic duct. An echogenic ascaris worm *(arrow)* is present in a dilated hepatic duct anterior to the portal vein. (Courtesy R. C. Sanders.)

## ASCARIASIS

The roundworm, *Ascaris lumbricoides,* infests the gastrointestinal tract and has a worldwide distribution. The ova are ingested from contaminated food or water. They discharge larvae into the small bowel, which penetrate the mucosa and enter the lymphatic or venous system. From there, they migrate to the lungs where they exit through the alveoli to reach the bronchi. Traveling up the bronchi and trachea, they are swallowed, and the worms mature in the proximal small bowel where they can live for many months (10). The worms may present clinically in the feces or in vomitus. A bolus of the worms may produce a small bowel obstruction which has a well-known radiographic appearance. On occasion, a single adult worm may migrate up the common bile duct and even enter the gallbladder to produce biliary colic and on occasion acute cholecystitis (Fig. 18). Ascariasis has also been reported to involve the pancreatic duct. Thus, it can present with signs and symptoms of pulmonary, gastrointestinal, biliary, or pancreatic disease.

Biliary ascariasis is encountered mainly in children, and clinical jaundice is rare, but the liver enzymes are often elevated. A child in an endemic area who has acute abdominal pain and tenderness compatible with biliary tract disease should be suspected of having biliary ascariasis (21). Sonography is the procedure of choice for evaluating the biliary tract of such patients while intravenous cholangiography should be reserved for those cases where the ultrasound examination is inadequate or equivocal. A false negative diag-

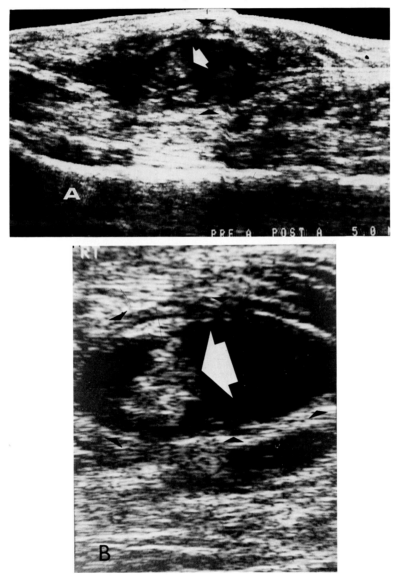

**FIG. 19.** Trichinella spiralis in striated muscle. **A:** Longitudinal scan (5-MHz transducer) and **B:** high resolution (10 MHz) of the muscles of the right leg. An encapsulated oval lesion *(black arrows)* containing fluid is demonstrated in the soleus muscle. Within the cyst a small mass is attached to the capsule *(white arrows).*

nosis has been reported to occur where there is some anatomic variation of the biliary tract (22). Real-time scanning helps to resolve these problems and probably increases the accuracy of the study. The sonographic characteristics of biliary ascariasis consists essentially of the demonstration of worms within the common bile duct or gallbladder (Fig. 18) (6, 21, 22). In the common bile duct, the worm appears as a thick, long echogenic interface containing a central sonolucency ("strip sign") that most likely represents its digestive tract (22). In the gallbladder, a coiled-up echogenic worm with the "strip sign" can be demonstrated. In follow-up studies, sonography can be used to confirm the efficacy of medical treatment and to assess whether the worm has been completely evacuated from the biliary tree.

## TRICHINIASIS

Trichiniasis, although rare in the tropics, is a parasitic disease of worldwide distribution, characterized by gastrointestinal symptoms, edema of the face, muscular pains, and fever (14, 16). The cause of the disease is the roundworm *Trichinella spiralis* and infection occurs when raw or inadequately cooked pork containing encysted larvae is ingested. The larvae penetrate the mucosa of the duodenum and jejunum and mature and mate within a few days. The females burrow deeply into the intestinal wall where they discharge their larvae, and this process continues for about 4 to 6 weeks (26). These minute larvae (0.1 mm) are carried by the lymphatics and portal circulation to the systemic blood stream and then to the various tissues and organs of the body. Only those larvae that reach striated muscle survive. Here they cause a myositis by penetrating the individual muscle fibers where they grow in length. Eventually, they coil up and within three months their encystment is complete. In this state, they remain viable for several years. These cysts can be identified on plain radiographs owing to the presence of calcification in their walls. In animals, these encysted larvae are the source for continued infection when the meat is eaten by the next host.

High resolution ultrasound scanning has been able to demonstrate the parasites within striated muscle (12). An oval cystic mass with a thick capsule may be identified within the muscle (Fig. 19). Direct biopsy of the lesion using US guidance demonstrates the parasite.

## LIVER FLUKES

*Clonorchis sineunsis* (chinese liver fluke) and *Opisthoreehis viverrini* are two flukes, found in Southeast Asia, which can lodge in the biliary tract. The infestation occurs by eating raw or partially cooked fish. The cercariae in

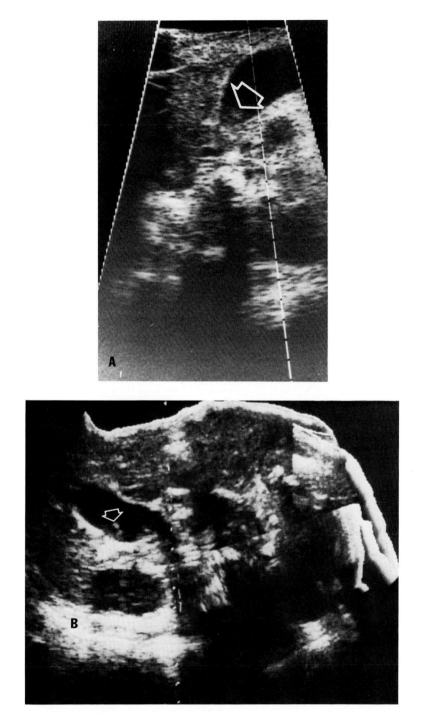

**FIG. 20.** Chinese liver flukes in the gallbladder. Longitudinal **(A)** and transverse **(B)** scans show an echogenic ball *(arrow)* within the gallbladder. Percutaneous gallbladder puncture yielded infected material. A subsequent contrast study of the bile ducts showed multiple liver flukes. (Courtesy R. C. Sanders.)

both flukes migrate from the intestinal tract to the liver via the portal system, and penetrate the liver tissue to enter the bile ducts (9, 16). In heavy infestations, hepatomegaly with an abnormal liver parenchyma and dilated bile ducts with thick walls has been described. The parasites may settle in the gallbladder causing a mobile echogenic mass (Fig. 20).

## REFERENCES

1. Abdel-Latif, Z., Abdal-Wahab, F., and El-Kady, N. M. Evaluation of portal hypertension in cases of hepatosplenic schistosomiasis using ultrasound. *J. Clin. Ultrasound,* 9:409–412, 1981.
2. Baltaxe, H. A., and Fleming, R. J. The angiographic appearance of hydatid disease. *Radiology,* 97:599–604, 1970.
3. Bloomfield, S. A. Protean radiological manifestations of hydatid infestation. *Australias Radiol.,* 10:330–343, 1966.
4. Breathnach, S. M., Metreweli, C., Joplin, G. F., and Hall, A. P. Ultrasound and the monitoring of treatment of amoebic liver abscess. *Trans. R. Soc. Trop. Med. Hyg.,* 72:647–649, 1978.
5. Deutsch, V., and Garti, I. The angiographic diagnosis of Echinococcosis of the liver and spleen. *Clin. Radiol.,* 22:466–471, 1971.
6. Eisenscher, A., and Sauget, Y. Aspect ultrasonore des ascardidiosis et distomatoses des vioes biliares. *J. Radiol.,* 61:319–322, 1980.
7. Gonzalez, L. R., Marcos, J., and Illanas, M. Radiologic aspects of hepatic echinococcosis. *Radiology,* 130:21–27, 1979.
8. Hadidi, A. Ultrasound findings in liver hydatid cysts. *J. Clin. Ultrasound,* 7:365–368, 1979.
9. Ho He. Clonorchiasis. In: *Tropical Radiology,* edited by H. Middlemiss, pp. 140–141. Intercontinental Medical Book Corp., New York, 1961.
10. Hunter, G. W., III, Frye, W. W., and Swartzwelder, J. C. *A Manual of Tropical Medicine.* W.B. Saunders, Philadelphia, 1966.
11. Itzchak, Y., Rubinstein, Z., Heyman, Z., and Gerzof, S. Role of ultrasound in the diagnosis of abdominal hydatid disease. *J. Clin. Ultrasound,* 8:341–345, 1980.
12. Itzchak, Y, Graif, M., and Heyman, Z. Ultrasound in trichinella spirallis. (Report of a case.) To be published.
13. Landay, M. S., Seitawan, H., Hirsch, G., Christensen, E. E., and Conrad, M. R. Hepatic and thoracic amebiasis. *AJR,* 135:449–454, 1980.
14. Manson-Bahr, P. *Manson's Tropical Diseases,* 17th ed. Balliere, Tindal, and Cassell, London, 1976.
15. Mousa, A. H., Atta, A. A., El-Rooby, A., et al. Bilharziasis. In: *Hepatosplenic Schistosomiasis,* edited by F. K. Mostofi pp. 15–47. Springer Verlag, New York, 1967.
16. Noble, E. R., and Noble, G. A. *Parasitology, the Biology of Animal Parasites,* 4th ed. Lea and Febiger, Philadelphia, 1976.
17. Philips, J. F., Cockrills, H., Jorge, E., et al. Radiographic evaluation of patients with schistomiasis. *Radiology,* 114:31–37, 1966.
18. Rallo, P. W., Colleti, P., Riun, M. F., and Halls, J. Sonographic findings in hepatic amebic abscess. *Radiology,* 145:123–126, 1982.
19. Reeder, M. M., and Hamilton, L. C. Radiological diagnosis of tropical diseases of the gastrointestinal tract. *Radiol. Clin. North Am.,* 7:57–81, 1969.
20. Scherer, U., Weinzieri, M., and Strum, R. Computed tomography in hydatid disease of the liver—a report on 13 cases. *J. Comput. Assist. Tomogr.,* 2:612–617, 1978.
21. Schulman, A., Roman, T., Dalrymple, R., Fataars, A., and Morton, P., Sonography of biliary worms (ascariasis). *J. Clin. Ultrasound,* 10:77–78, 1980.
22. Schulman, A., Loxton, A. J., Heydenreyh, J. J., and Abdurhaman, K. E. Sonographic diagnosis of biliary aseriasis. *AJR,* 139:485–489, 1980.

23. Sukov, R. S., Cohen, L. S., and Sample, W. F. Sonography of hepatic amebic abscesses. *AJR,* 134:911–915, 1980.
24. Thompson, W. M., Chisholm, D. P., and Tank, R. Plain film roentgenographic findings in alveolar hydatid disease—*Echinococcus multilocularis. AJR,* 116:345–358, 1972.
25. Vicary, F. R., Cusick, G., and Shirley, I. M. Ultrasound and abdominal hydatid disease. *Trans. R. Soc. Trop. Med. Hyg.,* 72:29–37, 1977.
26. Woodruff, A. W. (Ed.) *Medicine in the Tropics.* Churchill Livingstone, London, 1974.

*Ultrasound Annual 1983*, edited by R. C. Sanders and M. Hill. Raven Press, New York © 1983.

# Ultrasound of the Prostate

## Matthew D. Rifkin and Alfred B. Kurtz

*Thomas Jefferson University, 1015 Walnut Street, Philadelphia, Pennsylvania 19107*

The prostate gland is the most common reproductive structure to develop neoplastic growth in the older age male population. Benign prostatic enlargement affects over 80% of men past their fifth decade (9, 45), and prostatic carcinoma is the second most common male cancer (42). Previously, the identification of these diseases had been limited to the clinical symptomatology of urinary frequency, dysuria and difficulty in attaining a normal urine stream, and to the physical findings of diffuse enlargement or focal mass. Evidence of prostatic malignancy with spread included elevated serum acid phosphatase, retroperitoneal and pelvic lymphadenopathy, and sclerotic bone lesions (5, 29, 43).

In addition to ultrasound, direct prostatic visualization has been performed radiographically with plain films of the pelvis, excretory urography, and computed tomography. The plain film has usually been nondiagnostic, revealing only punctate calcifications of the gland suggestive of chronic prostatitis or healed necrosis. The urogram frequently demonstrates extrinsic bladder compression or irregularity of the bladder wall from an enlarged gland, but differentiation between benign and malignant lesions is usually not possible. The computed tomogram has been able to define overall prostatic size and, if malignancy is present, to evaluate local extension and distant metastasis, particularly to the retroperitoneum and the liver (7, 43). Direct diagnosis of intrinsic prostatic abnormalities and differentiation between benign and noninvasive malignant disease, however, has not been consistently possible.

Prostatic ultrasound has allowed direct visualization of both the internal glandular structures and the surrounding tissues (11, 12). At first, the suprapubic abdominal approach through a distended urinary bladder was used exclusively. The development of specialized endosonographic probes has permitted transurethral (10, 20, 30) and transrectal placement of the ultrasound transducer, providing higher resolution images of the prostate. The prototype endoscanning equipment was initially evaluated in the early 1970s (22, 25, 44, 46, 47) and has become commercially available in the past few years.

These various ultrasound imaging modalities have allowed extensive in-depth evaluation of the prostate and its various disease processes. It is the purpose of this chapter to perform an in-depth analysis of prostatic ultrasound. After the normal anatomy of the prostate and surrounding structures are discussed, the techniques and analysis of the prostate will be evaluated.

## ANATOMY

The normal prostate (Fig. 1) is situated in the pelvic cavity and measures 4 cm in maximum transverse diameter, 2 cm in anteroposterior dimension, and 3 cm in cephalocaudad projection. It is enveloped by a thin fibrous capsule and weighs about 20 g (Figs. 2, 3) (13, 24).

The prostate is situated immediately superior to the urogenital diaphragm, between the symphysis pubis anteriorly and the rectum posteriorly. A collection of veins, fat, and the anterior prostatic fascia are located between the prostate and the symphysis pubis (Figs. 2, 3). The urinary bladder is cephalad and slightly anterior to the gland, its position varying slightly with distension. The inferior and posterolateral margins of the gland are bordered by the urogenital diaphragm and the levator ani and the obturator internus muscles, respectively (Fig. 3).

The mature prostate is divided into five major and a few variable insignificant minor lobes. The major lobes include: (a) the anterior, situated from the anterior margins to the prostatic urethra, (b) the middle, separated by the prostatic urethra anteriorly and the ejaculatory ducts posteriorly, (c) the posterior, extending from the ejaculatory ducts to the posterior margin of the

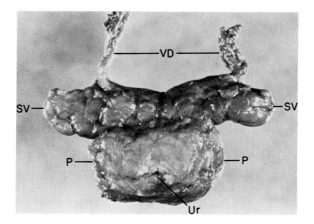

**FIG. 1.** Gross anatomic specimen of the prostate, seminal vesicles, and vas deferens. An anterior view of a normal-sized prostate (P) from a cadaver demonstrating the prostatic urethra (Ur) at the anterior, proximal portion of the gland. The seminal vesicles (SV) and the vas deferens (VD) are symmetrically paired structures placed on the superior portion (the base) of the prostate gland.

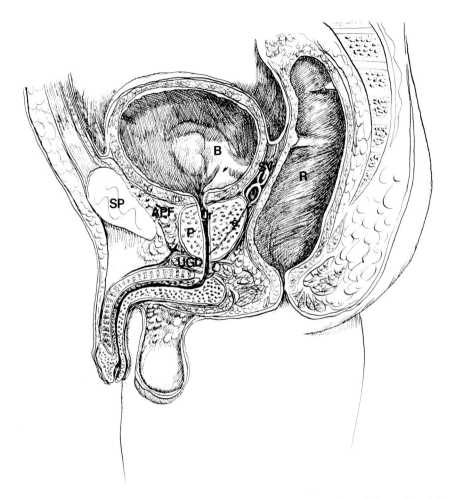

**FIG. 2.** Anatomic drawing of the male pelvis. Midline sagittal drawing of the male pelvis showing the prostate gland (P) situated anterior to the rectum (R) and posterior to the symphysis pubis (SP) and anterior prostatic fascia (APF). The seminal vesicles (SV) are between the fluid-filled urinary bladder (B) and the rectum. The prostatic urethra (Ur) and the ejaculatory ducts (e) join at the caudad portion of the prostate. UGD, urogenital diaphragm.

prostate, and (d) the two symmetrical lateral lobes contiguous with the other divisions dorsal to the prostatic urethra and comprising the majority of the gland. Superiorly the lateral lobes are connected by a fibrous band, the isthmus. The posterior surface of the gland (composed of the posterior and two lateral lobes) is wedge-shaped with a thin midline septum, the posterior sulcus. There are additional minor accessory lobes, the subcervical and subtrigonal, which are poorly defined in the adult. The apex of the gland is the most caudad portion abutting the urogenital diaphragm.

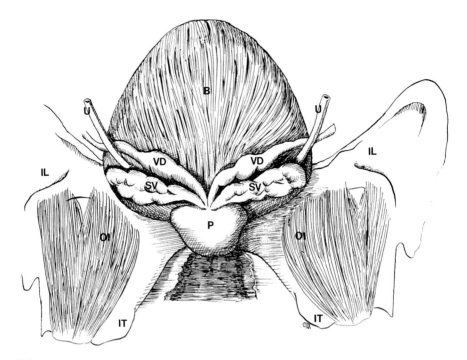

**FIG. 3.** Anatomic Diagram of the Prostate. Posterior anatomic view of the prostate showing the prostate (P), the seminal vesicles (SV), and the vas deferens (VD) situated posterior
to the fluid-filled urinary bladder (B). The obturator internus (OI) and levator ani muscles
are lateral to the prostate. IL, iliac bone; IT, ischial tuberosity; U, ureter.

The prostatic urethra courses in the midline of the gland, separating the
anterior and posterior portions. As it drains into the penile urethra, it as-
sumes a more anterior position. The ejaculatory ducts are bilaterally symmetrical structures, originating at the confluence of the vas deferens and
seminal vesicles. They are situated just lateral to the midline in the posterior
aspect of the prostate and drain into the caudad portion of the prostatic
urethra (Fig. 2).

The microstructure of the gland has 16 to 32 ducts composed of tubular
alveolar structures which converge upon and open into the prostatic urethra
(49). The cells are simple or pseudostratified columnar epithelium, although
cuboidal and squamous cells are seen occasionally in the normal patient.
The glandular epithelium is diffusely separated by connective tissue and
often encased by involuntary smooth muscle.

The seminal vesicles are lobulated structures located superiorly on the
cephalic portion of the prostate gland (Figs. 1–3). They extend laterally and
superiorly, immediately anterior to the rectum. The vas deferens are situated medial to the seminal vesicles. Both the vas and seminal vesicles insert
in the medial portion of the base of the prostate (the cephalad portion).

## ULTRASOUND OF THE PROSTATE

Numerous sonographic approaches have been used to evaluate the prostate. The suprapubic is the most easily available and is performed by scanning from the anterior abdominal wall and angling down through a filled urinary bladder. This approach has the advantage of using standard gray-scale ultrasound equipment, both contact and real-time (sector and linear array), with optimum results obtained with the use of either 3.5- or 5.0-MHz transducer. In addition, images can be obtained in transverse, longitudinal, and oblique orientation (Figs. 4, 5).

The transperineal approach also allows the use of standard ultrasound equipment. It is performed with direct contact of the transducer on the perineum and is angled cranially. A distended urinary bladder is essential. The visualization of the gland is limited, however, since the prostate cannot be differentiated from surrounding structures unless it is markedly enlarged or distinct echogenic foci are noted (Fig. 6).

Endosonoscopic approaches using ultrasound transducers attached to transurethral and transrectal probes are now felt to be the most promising methods for accurate evaluation of the prostate and may allow the differentiation of benign from malignant pathology (38). The transurethral examination is used infrequently, however, since there are: (a) risks associated

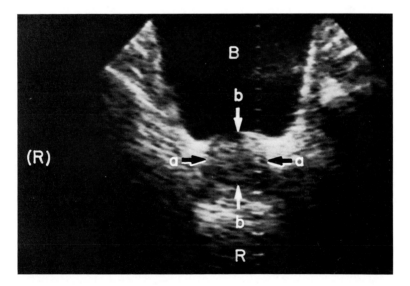

**FIG. 4.** Transversely oriented abdominal ultrasound of the prostate gland. Transverse image through a fluid-filled urinary bladder (B) demonstrates a normal-sized prostate gland *(arrows)* situated in the midline, anterior to the rectum (R). The transverse dimensions are denoted by the arrows (a) and the anterior–posterior dimensions are demarcated by the arrows (b). (R), patient's right side; R, rectum.

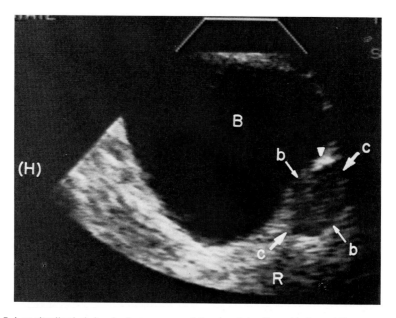

**FIG. 5.** Longitudinal abdominal sonogram of the prostate. Examination of the prostate by an anterior suprapubic abdominal approach angled inferiorly through a fluid-filled urinary bladder (B) demonstrates the normal-sized gland *(arrows)*. The anterior–posterior dimensions are denoted by the arrows (b) and the cephalocaudad size by arrows (c). A benign echogenic focus without shadowing is noted involving the anterior portion of the gland *(arrowhead)*. R, rectum; (H), toward patient's head.

with the need for heavy sedation or general anaesthesia, (b) possible postexamination infections or nonspecific urethritis, and (c) more accurate and technically simpler evaluations by the transrectal approach. The endosonoscopic rectal studies require specially designed probes utilizing either radial static imaging (3, 10, 14, 15, 23, 32–35) or longitudinal linear array real-time equipment (37, 38, 40, 41). Both systems are commercially available, with the latter having been introduced more recently. While there are limitations in scanning, the transrectal approach does not require sedation and does not have an increased risk of infection.

The earliest radial scan units were produced by Aloka (Japan), one unit utilizing a specially designed chair. The probe (covered by a rubber condom) was placed through a central hole in the seat of the chair. With the patient sitting in the chair, the transducer was inserted into the rectum and advanced until the prostate was imaged. More recently, Aloka and Bruel & Kjaer (Denmark) have manufactured commercially available radial scanners that do not require the use of a chair. Instead, the examination can be performed with the patient in the lithotomy, knee–chest or lateral decubitus position. With either type of instrumentation, however, the urinary bladder

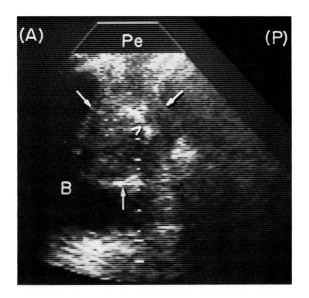

**FIG. 6.** Ultrasound of the prostate using the perineal approach. Real-time perineal (Pe) examination of the prostate *(arrows)* demonstrates a slighty enlarged gland *(arrows)* protruding into a fluid-filled urinary bladder (B). A benign echogenic focus within the prostate *(arrowhead)* is noted. A, anterior aspect of patient; P, posterior aspect of patient.

should be distended prior to the examination. After a digital rectal examination is performed to exclude any obstructing lesion, the anus and probe are adequately lubricated with gel. Following insertion of the endoscope, non-aerated water is placed into the condom to maximize acoustic coupling between the probe and the rectal wall. The apex of the prostate is visualized inferiorly in transverse projection (Figs. 7, 8). The probe is then moved superiorly at 0.5-cm sequential intervals (Fig. 9) until the seminal vesicles are imaged (Fig. 10).

The real-time examination utilizes a commercially available transrectal endoscope with the transducer crystals arranged in a longitudinal fashion (Fig. 11). Manufactured by the Toshiba Corporation (Japan) for use with their linear array real-time units, the probe has an insertable portion and a handle separated by a thick ridge. A condom is placed over the insertable portion of the probe and is secured at the ridge. Similar to the radial scanning technique, the patient is placed in the lithotomy, lateral decubitus or knee–chest position and, following a digital rectal examination, the tip of the probe is lubricated and placed into the rectum until the prostate is visualized. The urinary bladder should be distended during examination. The prostate is imaged in long axis. The transducer images the midline and is then rotated clockwise and counterclockwise to evaluate the right and left

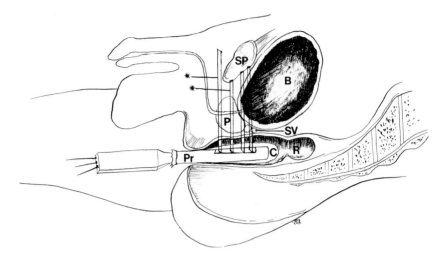

**FIG. 7.** Anatomic drawing—radial scan. The probe (Pr) with a condom (C) over the tip is placed into the rectum (R). The prostate (P), the seminal vesicles (SV), and the fluid-filled urinary bladder (B) are visualized. Multiple transverse images of the prostate from the apex to the seminal vesicles are obtained (*). SP, symphysis pubis.

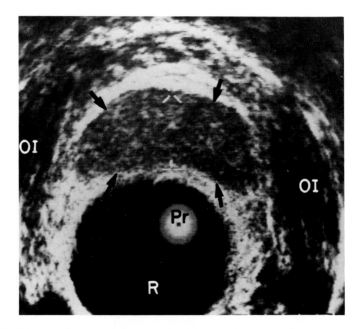

**FIG. 8.** Radial scan of a normal prostate gland. A normal prostate gland *(arrows)*, demonstrating normal homogeneous low level echogenicity is seen with a transrectal probe (Pr). The obturator internus muscles (OI) are noted as bilaterally symmetrical structures of low level echogenicity bordering the prostate. R, rectum. (From Dr. Bruno Fornage.)

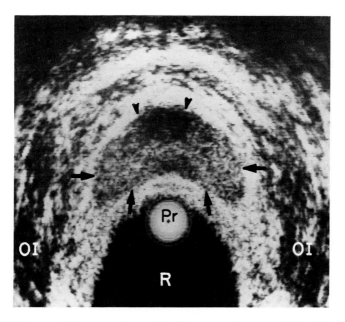

**FIG. 9.** Radial scan of the normal prostate. Transverse images obtained by transrectal probe (Pr) demonstrates the prostate *(arrows)* to be symmetrically shaped, bordered by the obturator internus muscles (OI). On radial scans, a slightly less echogenic area is occasionally imaged anteriorly in the midline *(arrowheads)*, a normal finding. R, rectum. (From Dr. Bruno Fornage.)

lateral lobes (Fig. 12). If the entire cephalo-caudad length of the gland is not encompassed in one image, the probe is then inserted further to evaluate the superior aspect of the gland. The anterior prostatic fascia, the prostatic capsule, the symphysis pubis, the urinary bladder, and seminal vesicles are routinely visualized with this method.

While the focal zones of the various transducers are different, all the transducers have lengths of focus so that the entire prostate is clearly defined. To place prostatic lesions within the sharpest zone of focus, up to 100 cc of nonaerated water can be placed in the potential space between the condom and the transducer crystals to allow the correct separation of the gland from the transducer.

## EVALUATION OF PROSTATE SIZE

Accurate estimation of the prostate is invaluable so that the clinician and surgeon can plan proper medical and surgical intervention in patients with bladder outlet obstruction (19). The surgical approach varies, depending

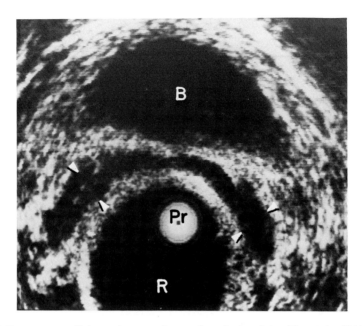

**FIG. 10.** Transverse radial scan images of normal seminal vesicles. The probe (Pr) inserted deeper into the rectum (R) reveals the seminal vesicles to be symmetrically paired hypo-echoic structures *(arrowheads)*. The urinary bladder (B) is distended. (From Dr. Bruno Fornage.)

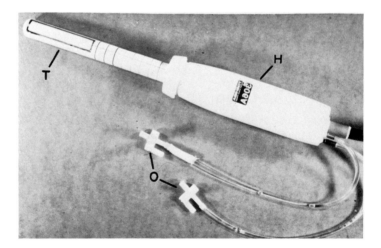

**FIG. 11.** Linear array probe. Commercially available probe manufactured by the Toshiba Corporation demonstrates the larger handle (H) and the thinner insertable portion of the instrument with the transducer crystals (T) in a longitudinal fashion at the tip. Two tubes with stopcocks (O) in the distal portion of the probe allow introduction of fluid through a condom placed over the tip and secured at the mid-portion of the instrument.

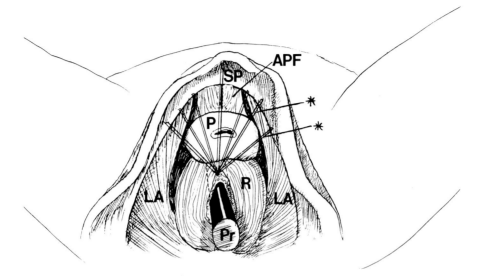

**FIG. 12.** Anatomic drawing of perineum. Exposed perineal view of the male pelvis projecting cephalad demonstrates the endoscopic probe (Pr) located in the rectum (R). The prostate (P) and the centrally placed prostatic urethra are noted. After a midline section of the prostate is obtained, the probe is rotated clockwise and counterclockwise to visualize the lateral segments and lateral lobes of the prostate (image projected noted by (*). SP, symphysis pubis; LA, levator ani muscles; APF, anterior prostatic fascia.

upon prostatic size. The smaller gland, less than 50 to 60 g, can be adequately and effectively resected using a transurethral approach (1). The larger gland, however, is often incompletely or inadequately removed by this method (28). Instead, open prostatectomy, using either the suprapubic or retropubic approach, is often required for large glands. These open procedures are technically more difficult with a small gland since inadequate resection may result.

Clinically, digital rectal palpation of the prostate is accurate in estimating symmetrical enlargement. Not uncommonly, however, the gland may focally enlarge anteriorly, posteriorly, or cephalically (either intravesically or posterior to the bladder). In these cases, the clinical digital examination and radiographic studies of the prostate have been shown to be inaccurate (1).

Prostatic ultrasound examination has proven to be very accurate in estimating both the dimensions and weight of the gland (27). The suprapubic sonogram is the simplest method. The gland is seen in all three dimensions—anteroposterior, lateral, and cephalocaudal (Figs. 4, 5). The prostatic size in cubic centimeters (cm$^3$) is estimated by assuming that the prostate is a sphere, using the formula $\frac{4}{3}\pi R^3$. Since the specific gravity of prostatic tissue is between 1 and 1.05 g/cm³, the prostatic size multiplied by the specific gravity gives the weight in grams (18).

A second, more simplified but equally accurate method for evaluating prostatic size has been developed in France. The suprapubic abdominal approach is again used but only the transverse image is needed. A single diameter of the largest section of the prostate is obtained when the gland is spherical (Fig. 4) and an average of the two largest dimensions is used if the gland is more triangular or ovoid in shape (Fig. 13). The prostate size obtained on these examinations correlates with the weight of the entire gland (Table 1) (1).

The transrectal examination has also been used for preoperative evaluation of gland size. This technique requires more complicated arithmetic computation. During routine transrectal radial scanning, the prostate is examined from apex to base in 0.5-cm intervals. Electronic planimetric calculation of the area of each section is obtained and all sections summated (16).

It is evident, therefore, that whereas both transrectal and transabdominal sonography will accurately assess prostatic size, the transabdominal approach is simpler to use and requires no special equipment. The transrectal

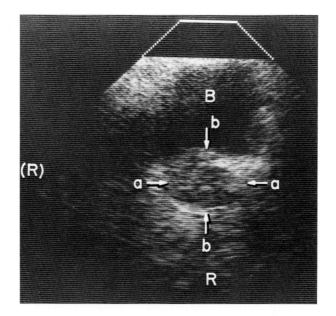

**FIG. 13.** Ovoid-shaped prostate seen on abdominal approach. A normal homogeneous prostate gland *(arrows)* is noted between the fluid-filled urinary bladder (B) and the rectum (R). Anterior–posterior dimensions are noted by arrows (a) and the transverse size by arrows (b). (R), toward patient's right; R, rectum.

TABLE 1. *Suprapubic abdominal examination: correlation of prostate weight to transverse average diameter of the prostate*[a]

| Degree of size | Diameter (cm) | Weight (g) |
|---|---|---|
| I | 3.0–3.8 | 30 |
| II | 3.8–4.5 | 30–50 |
| III | 4.5–5.5 | 50–80 |
| IV | 5.5 | 85 |

[a]Reproduced from ref. 1., with permission.

scan, however, may better detect intrinsic prostatic adenomas causing bladder outlet obstruction, even in the normal-size gland (3, 15, 38).

## NEOPLASIA

There are many different neoplastic processes that affect the prostate. Benign enlargement can be either a focal or a diffuse process. The five histologic variations of hyperplasia are: stromal, fibromuscular, muscular, fibroadenomatous, and fibromyoadenomatous (9). Acoustically, these processes are indistinguishable with currently available equipment.

Prostatitis is usually a diffuse process. Following appropriate medical therapy, prostate calcifications (stones) may form.

Malignant degeneration of the prostate is histologically most commonly adenocarcinoma. Transitional and squamous cell carcinoma and leiomyosarcoma, although rare, may also be seen as primary lesions of the gland.

Despite the numerous sonographic studies of the prostate, there has been little direct correlation of acoustically detected focal lesions, both benign and malignant, with pathology. Instead, assumptions have been made that a focal abnormality noted on ultrasound must be the malignant pathologic area (3, 10–12, 14, 15, 23, 30, 33–35). Recent evidence refutes these presumptions (38). A technique (to be discussed under biopsies) has been developed that accurately allows needle placement within the central portion of any abnormal prostatic foci. These biopsies have yielded more accurate histologic evaluation of the prostate (8, 17, 21, 36, 37).

## SUPRAPUBIC ABDOMINAL ULTRASONOGRAPHY

The suprapubic transabdominal approach for ultrasonic evaluation of the prostate can accurately delineate the size and shape of the prostate and is particularly accurate when the gland is enlarged. However, its major limitation is its inability to fully image the small and the minimally enlarged gland. The normal gland when visualized is homogeneous with low-level acoustic reflections (Figs. 4, 5). Both benign and malignant lesions demonstrate focal areas of increased (Fig. 14) or decreased (Fig. 15) echogenicity. Malignant degeneration with extension outside the prostatic capsule may be defined when the gland is adequately visualized (5). Retroperitoneal adenopathy or other evidence of metastases can also be detected.

Benign disease may present with diffuse glandular enlargement (Fig. 16) or with focal lesions (Fig. 17), areas being either hypo- or hyperechoic. The bright and thick echoes seen in the hyperechoic lesions do not always represent calcium. Recent evidence, using the longitudinal linear array units with guided biopsies (discussed below), has shown that these foci are usually not calcifications.

## TRANSRECTAL ULTRASONOGRAPHY

The use of transrectally placed sonoendoscopic probe allows greater in-depth evaluation of the prostate and surrounding structures. This is true for both radial, transversely oriented static images and longitudinal oriented linear array real-time devices.

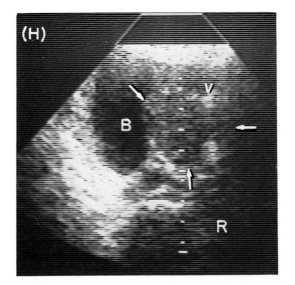

**FIG. 14.** Longitudinal abdominal sonogram of an enlarged prostate with a benign echo-genic focus. An enlarged prostate gland *(arrows)* is noted impinging upon a partially fluid-filled urinary bladder (B). Benign echogenic focus without shadowing *(arrowhead)* is imaged at the apex of the gland. R, rectum; (H), toward patient's head.

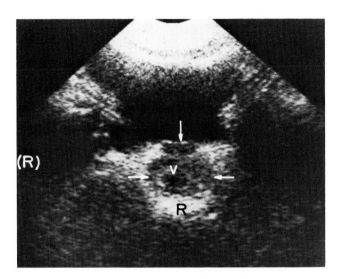

**FIG. 15.** Transverse abdominal sonogram of a hypertrophied prostate gland. The slightly enlarged prostate *(arrows)* is imaged with a well-defined hypoechoic focus *(arrowhead)* representing benign adenomatous change. R, rectum; (R), toward patient's right.

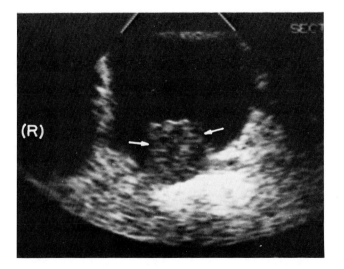

**FIG. 16.** Enlarged prostate gland with intravesical extension. A transverse image of the prostate obtained by suprapubic sonogram demonstrates an enlarged gland *(arrow)* impinging upon the urinary bladder. (R), toward patient's right.

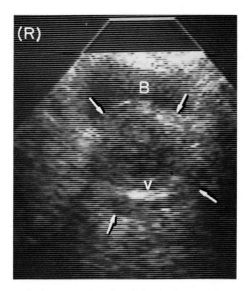

**FIG. 17.** Benign prostatic hypertrophy. An abdominal scan demonstrates an enlarged prostate gland *(arrows)* impinging upon the urinary bladder (B). A benign, highly echogenic focus without shadowing *(arrowhead)* is noted in the posterior portion of the gland. (R), toward patient's right.

The apparent benefits of the radial scan are:

1. The entire gland can be imaged regardless of its size and position (Figs. 8, 9).
2. The prostatic capsule is clearly identified and disruptions caused by invasion defined (Fig. 18).
3. The seminal vesicles can be adequately demonstrated superiorly (Fig. 10).
4. The lateral musculature, the levator ani, and obturator internus muscles are clearly defined. In cases of carcinoma, extension into these structures can be clearly evaluated (Figs. 8, 9, 10, 18).

The apparent benefits of the longitudinally oriented scan are:

1. The entire gland can be imaged regardless of its size and position.
2. The prostatic capsule is clearly identified and disruptions caused by invasion defined (Fig. 19).
3. The seminal vesicles can be identified but are often not as clearly seen as on radial scans (Figs. 20, 21).
4. The accurate guidance of percutaneous biopsies.
5. Prostatic calculi are accurately defined (Fig. 33).

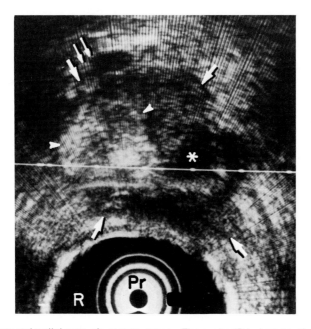

**FIG. 18.** Transrectal radial scan of prostate cancer. The probe (Pr) placed in the rectum (R) demonstrates a transverse image of an acoustically inhomogeneous enlarged prostate gland *(arrows)*. There is an asymmetric echogenic focus involving the right lateral aspect of the prostate *(arrowheads)* which represents carcinoma invading the anterior margin *(double arrows)*. The mass is also deviating the prostatic urethra (*) enlarged from previous resection. (From Dr. Bruno Fornage.)

## ACOUSTIC CHARACTERIZATION BY ENDOSONOSCOPIC STUDIES

The normal gland measures approximately 3 × 3 cm and has acoustically homogeneous, low level echogenicity (Fig. 20). When empty the prostatic urethra may be seen as a hyperechoic linear longitudinal reflection from its apposed fibrous walls (Fig. 22). The visualization of these reflections appears to be beam-angle dependent. When the urethra is identified partially distended with urine (Figs. 23, 24), the urethral walls may not be perpendicular to the beam and the reflections not as pronounced (Figs. 23, 24). Linear acoustic reflections may also be seen from the walls of the ejaculatory ducts (Figs. 22, 23). In patients who have undergone previous transurethral prostatic resection, irregularity and enlargement of the proximal portion of the urethra can be identified (Fig. 25).

The seminal vesicles are homogeneously hypoechoic structures of lower acoustic reflectivity than the prostate gland. On the radial scans they are clearly acoustically differentiated and are usually distinctly separate from the prostate (Fig. 10). On the longitudinal linear array examination, they

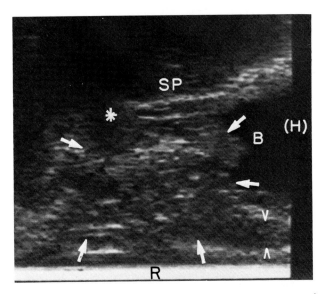

**FIG. 19.** Longitudinal linear array of prostatic carcinoma. The linear array is oriented so that the probe, placed in the rectum (R), transmits sound anteriorly toward the symphysis pubis (SP). The study is performed with the distended urinary bladder (B). The prostate gland is irregular *(arrows)* with scattered echogenic foci. The anterior margin is poorly seen (*) suggesting invasion. The seminal vesicles *(arrowheads)* are defined at the superior margin of the prostate abutting the rectum. (H), toward patient's head.

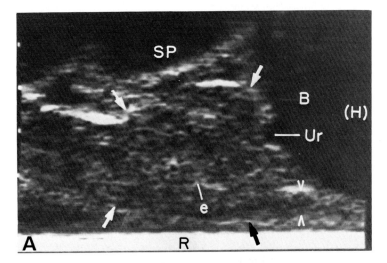

**FIG. 20A.** Longitudinal linear array transrectal images of the normal prostate. A midline examination demonstrates the prostate to be normal-sized *(arrows)*. The prostatic urethra (Ur) is noted extending from the fluid-filled urinary bladder (B). A small portion of the ejaculatory duct (e) is seen as a linear echogenic line. The symphysis pubis (SP) is noted with distal shadowing caused by loss of sound transmission through bone. The seminal vesicles *(arrowheads)* are noted superiorly.

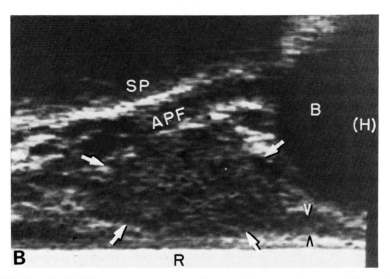

**FIG. 20B.** Longitudinal linear array transrectal image of the normal prostate. The probe is rotated slightly clockwise. The normal prostate becomes slightly rounded *(arrows)*. The homogeneous echogenic texture is unchanged. The anterior prostatic fascia (APF) is seen between the prostate's anterior margin and the symphysis pubis (SP).

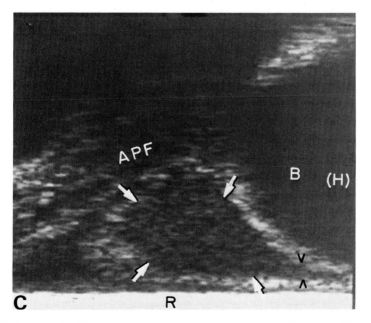

**FIG. 20C.** Longitudinal linear array transrectal image of the normal prostate. The probe is rotated slightly more clockwise and demonstrates more of the lateral lobe. The gland retains its homogeneous low level echogenic texture and is more triangular in shape *(arrows)*.

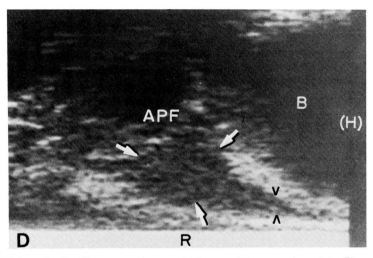

**FIG. 20D.** Longitudinal linear array transrectal image of the normal prostate. The probe is rotated maximally clockwise to visualize the most lateral portion of the gland. The prostate becomes smaller and rounded *(arrows)*. The seminal vesicles are still defined *(arrowheads)*. (H), toward patient's head; R, rectum.

may not be as clearly demarcated from the prostate, but can often still be defined by their subtle acoustic differences (Figs. 20, 21).

## BENIGN DISEASE

The prostate in benign disease will usually have clearly demarcated capsular margins. Focal adenomatous nodules, if located at the prostatic margins, may cause a localized bulge in the capsule (Fig. 26). Invasion of the capsule and involvement of the surrounding muscle and fascia should, however, never be seen.

Benign enlargement of the prostate may be diffuse or focal. Diffuse abnormalities will demonstrate glandular enlargement with echogenicity that is either normally homogeneous or diffusely inhomogeneous (Fig. 27). Differentiation of the latter process from prostatitis (Fig. 28) is usually impossible. Focal prostatic lesions may be hypoechoic (Fig. 26), acoustically mixed (Fig. 29), or hyperechoic (Figs. 30–33). The margins of these focal abnormalities may be well demarcated (Figs. 26, 29) or poorly defined (Figs. 31–33). It is of interest that only 50% of all these focal lesions demonstrated on transrectal sonography will be seen on the abdominal approach (38).

Purely hypoechoic lesions are uncommon. These are usually solid lesions, although cysts may be noted (Fig. 34). If cystic, they may be either congenital from Mullerian duct remnants or may be due to dilatation of the prostatic duct from obstruction in adenomatous hyperplasia (47). Acoustically, these benign lesions will have sharp back walls, no internal echoes, and enhanced

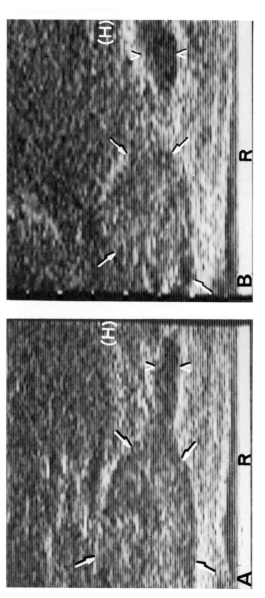

**FIG. 21.** Linear array transrectal sonogram of a normal prostate and seminal vesicles. **A:** The probe is rotated clockwise. A well-defined acoustically homogeneous normal prostate (*arrows*) and the seminal vesicles (*arrowheads*) are noted. **B:** While the most lateral portion of the lateral lobes are sonographically unremarkable, the seminal vesicles are distinctly separate from the prostate in this patient. (H), toward patient's head; R, rectum.

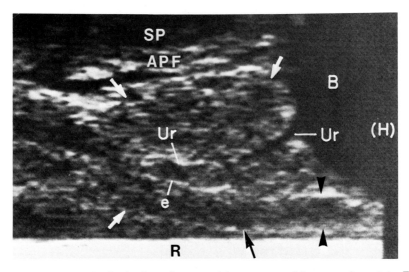

**FIG. 22.** Midline longitudinal oriented transrectal sonogram of the normal prostate. The prostatic urethra is defined in its superior cephalad portion (Ur) filled with fluid. In its nondistended portion it is represented by linear echoes from its acoustically reflective walls. An ejaculatory duct (e) is also noted as linear acoustic reflections posterior to the prostatic urethra. (H), toward patient's head; B, urinary bladder; R, rectum; APF, anterior prostatic fascia; SP, symphysis pubis; *arrows*, prostate; *arrowheads*, seminal vesicles.

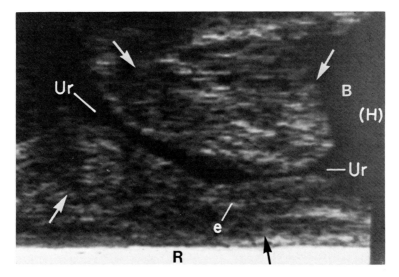

**FIG. 23.** Normal fluid-filled prostatic urethra during voiding. A longitudinal real-time image demonstrates the prostatic urethra (Ur) is completely distended with fluid during this voiding study. The ejaculatory duct (e) is seen transiently as a linear parallel structure posterior to the urethra. R, rectum; (H), toward patient's head; *arrows*, prostate.

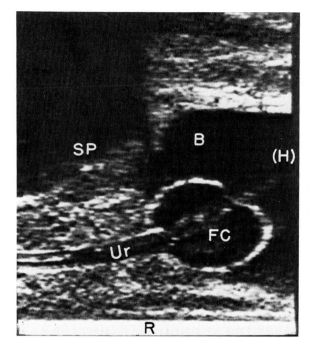

**FIG. 24.** Foley catheter in place in the urinary bladder. A Foley catheter (FC) with its fluid-filled balloon is imaged in the urinary bladder (B). The fluid-filled catheter is also imaged extending through the prostatic urethra (Ur) on this longitudinally oriented image. (H), toward patient's head; SP, symphysis pubis; R, rectum.

posterior through transmission. Solid hypoechoic lesions may have irregular margins.

Acoustically mixed lesions with anechoic areas are often seen in benign disease (Figs. 26, 29). The mixed lesions may demonstrate smooth or irregular margins.

The majority of focal lesions in benign prostatic hypertrophy will be hyperechoic. These acoustically reflective changes can be further divided into echo brightness and echo thickness. Focal echogenic areas are at times indistinct and can be scattered anywhere throughout the gland (38).

Echo thickness can be classified as foci that are either solitary and focal, or multiple and scattered:

    I. 1 to 2 mm in thickness (Figs. 28, 38).
   II. 2 to 3 mm in thickness (Fig. 37).
  III. 3 to 4 mm in thickness (Fig. 31).
  IV. Greater than 4 mm in thickness (Figs. 30, 32).

Echo brightness has been classified as:

    I. Slightly more echogenic than the normal prostatic tissue (Figs. 36 and 38).

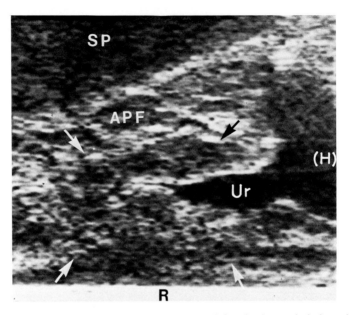

**FIG. 25.** Transurethral resection defect. There is a defect in the cephalad portion of the prostatic urethra (Ur), denoting previous transurethral resection of the prostate. SP, symphysis pubis; APF, anterior prostatic fascia; (H), toward patient's head; R, rectum; *arrows, prostate.*

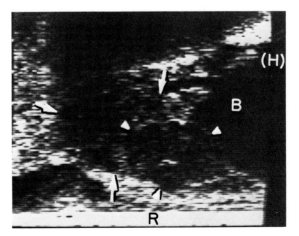

**FIG. 26.** Benign prostatic nodule. Transrectal longitudinal linear array examination demonstrates the prostate *(arrows)* to be slightly enlarged. An acoustically mixed, mostly hypoechoic nodule *(arrowheads)* is noted distorting both the posterior margins of the prostate and the margins of the urinary bladder (B). The seminal vesicle is not affected. (H), toward patient's head; R, rectum.

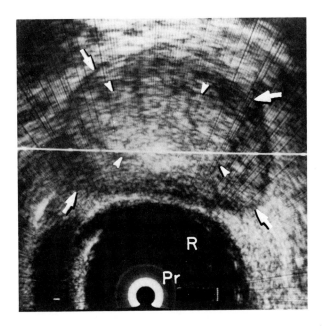

**FIG. 27.** Diffuse prostatic enlargement. Transrectal radial scan demonstrates the prostate gland to be enlarged *(arrows)* with diffuse echogenic changes scattered throughout most of the gland *(arrowheads)*. R, rectum; Pr, probe.

II. More echogenic than Class I, less echogenic than Class III (Figs. 31 and 37).

III. As acoustically reflective as the surrounding prostatic capsule (Figs. 32 and 33).

IV. More echogenic than the prostatic capsule (Fig. 30) (38).

The vast majority of benign lesions will have both Class III and IV echo thickness and Class III and IV brightness (Figs. 30, 32, and 33). Twenty-five percent of foci, however, will have Grade I and II echo thickness and echo brightness (Fig. 28) (38). The etiology of these bright, thick echogenic foci can be found in histologic correlation. Thirty percent have acoustic shadowing and correlate with calcification (Fig. 33). The remaining 70% do not (Fig. 30, 31, and 32) and have been shown to have no calcification on histologic evaluation (38). Preliminary evidence suggests that these echogenic foci may instead be related to corpora amylacea, a proteinaceous material.

The seminal vesicles, when inflamed, will demonstrate enlargement and decreased echogenicity (Fig. 35). This may be bilateral but is usually a unilateral process.

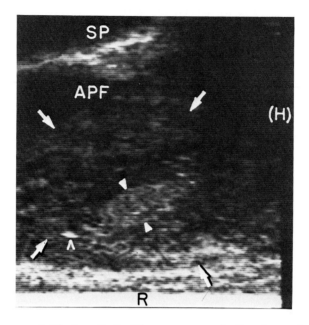

**FIG. 28.** Diffuse prostatitis. Longitudinal linear array examination demonstrates the prostate to be enlarged *(arrows)* with diffuse areas of highly echogenic *(open arrowhead),* moderately echogenic *(closed arrowhead),* and hypoechoic structures scattered throughout the gland. These findings are consistent with prostatitis, but may be seen similarly in diffuse benign prostatic enlargement. R, rectum; (H), toward patient's head; APF, anterior prostatic fascia; SP, symphysis pubis.

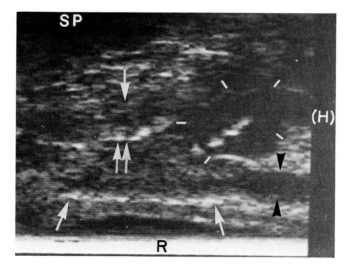

**FIG. 29.** Benign adenomatous nodule. Longitudinal linear array prostatic sonogram demonstrates a minimally enlarged prostate *(arrows).* The prostatic urethra *(double arrows)* is distorted by a nodule of mixed echogenicity *(lines).* SP, symphysis pubis; (H), toward patient's head; *arrowheads,* seminal vesicles.

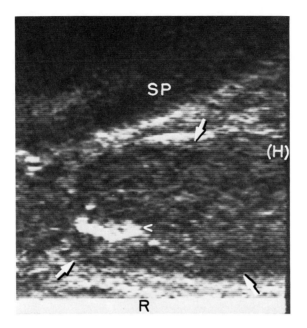

**FIG. 30.** Benign echogenic focus in an enlarged prostate. Transrectal longitudinal linear array sonogram demonstrates a slightly enlarged prostate *(arrows)* with a bright echogenic focus *(arrowhead)* representing Grade III thickness, Grade IV brightness. There is no shadowing noted. Benign disease without calcification was demonstrated on histologic evaluation. R, rectum; SP, symphysis pubis; (H), toward patient's head.

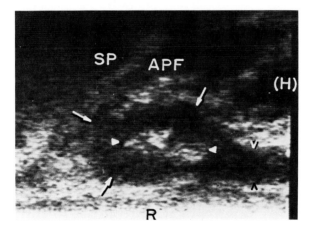

**FIG. 31.** Benign prostatic disease in a normal-sized prostate. Transrectal linear array real-time examination of the prostate demonstrates a normal-sized gland *(arrows)* with normal seminal vesicles *(open arrowheads)*. An echogenic focus in the central portion of the gland *(closed arrowhead)* with Grade IV echogenic thickness and Grade III echogenic brightness is demonstrated. No acoustic shadowing is noted. No calcification was noted on histology. R, rectum; SP, symphysis pubis; APF, anterior prostatic fascia; (H), toward patient's head.

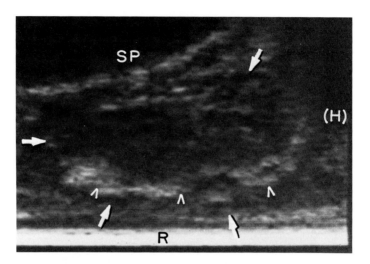

**FIG. 32.** Benign prostatic disease. Diffuse echogenic foci *(arrowheads)* involving the entire posterior portion of the prostate *(arrows)* demonstrate Grade IV echogenic thickness and Grade III echogenic brightness. No acoustic shadowing is demonstrated. SP, symphysis pubis; (H), toward patient's head; R, rectum.

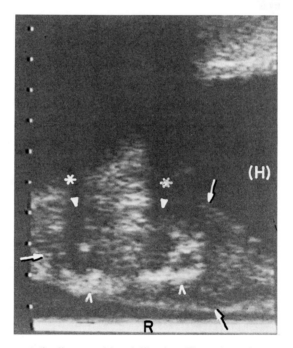

**FIG. 33.** Benign prostatic disease with calcification. The enlarged prostate *(arrows)* has multiple echogenic foci with shadowing *(arrowheads and asterisks)*. The echogenic foci have Grade III echogenic brightness and Grade IV echogenic thickness. R, rectum; (H), toward patient's head.

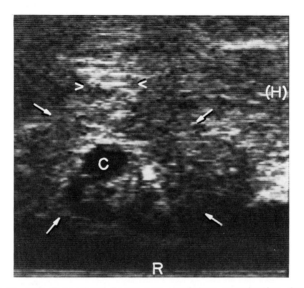

**FIG. 34.** Prostatic cyst. Transrectal linear array real-time examination demonstrates a minimally enlarged prostate *(arrows)* with a centrally placed cyst (C). The cyst has the classic acoustic appearances of a fluid-filled mass, no internal echoes, sharp walls, and enhanced through transmission *(arrowheads)*. R, rectum; (H), toward patient's head.

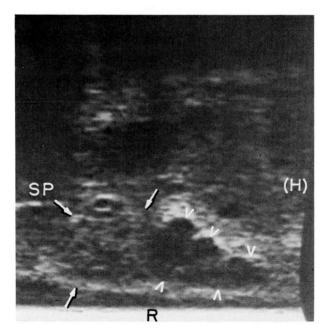

**FIG. 35.** Unilateral seminal vesiculitis. The right seminal vesicle *(arrowheads)* is enlarged, lobulated, and more hypoechoic than normal. The adjacent prostate *(arrows)* is normal. SP, symphysis pubis; (H), toward patient's head; R, rectum.

## CARCINOMA OF THE PROSTATE

Carcinoma of the prostate has been thought to be almost exclusively confined to the posterior lobes. Recent pathologic evidence, however, has demonstrated that all the peripheral prostatic tissues are more likely to develop cancer than the central portions, which are more prone to develop adenomas (26). Thus, the anterior, lateral, and posterior lobes appear to have an equal propensity to develop carcinoma.

Before the advent of imaging, particularly ultrasound, the posterior lobes and posterior portion of the lateral lobes were the only areas that were clinically detectable. Subclinical carcinoma was usually found only on autopsied specimens or as secondary findings during histologic evaluation of transurethral or suprapubic prostatectomy specimens. It had been felt that these unsuspected lesions, classified as noninvasive Grade I carcinomas, were clinically insignificant. Recent evidence has suggested, however, that these lesions may metastasize early and thus may be more ominous than previously thought (6).

Using the transrectal approach, reports have shown the ability to detect the focal area representing cancer in up to 95% of cases (14, 15, 38, 47). However, the ultrasound diagnosis of malignancy has extensive overlap with benign disease and so the differentiation of benign from malignant lesions is not always possible. There will be a number of histologically benign lesions that mimic carcinoma on the sonogram.

Malignancy will demonstrate acoustic alteration of the normal homogeneous echogenicity of the gland. The majority of lesions are hyperechoic with the echogenic changes localized to either small areas (Figs. 36–38) or scattered throughout the gland (Fig. 39). The majority of cancers are of low level echo thickness and echo brightness, predominantly in Grade I and II category and are usually poorly defined (3, 15, 23, 38). Mixed echogenic lesions may be seen in up to 25% of cancers (Fig. 37), whereas purely hypoechoic carcinomas are rare. It is quite unusual for shadowing to be caused by carcinoma, and when both are imaged, it is more likely a cancer developing in an area adjacent to the calcification.

Patients with proven carcinoma have been followed with transrectal ultrasound to evaluate the success of treatment (4, 41). A decrease in the size of both the entire gland and the focally abnormal area is indicative of response to therapy (4, 41).

Differentiation between benign and malignant lesions in many cases may be suggested if a constellation of findings is present (Table 2) (38): (a) A benign lesion will not invade the capsule. (b) A malignant lesion should not have Grade IV thickness or brightness. (c) A malignant lesion will usually have some echogenic foci and will not be purely hypoechoic. (d) A malignant lesion should not cause acoustic shadowing.

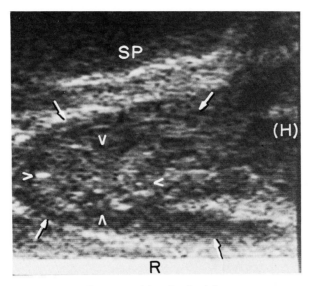

**FIG. 36.** Prostatic carcinoma. Transrectal longitudinal linear array sonogram demonstrates a minimally enlarged prostate *(arrows)* with poorly defined nonpalpable echogenic areas scattered throughout the apex of the gland *(arrowheads)*. Echogenic thickness and brightness are Grade I in this patient, with locally invasive carcinoma. SP, symphysis pubis; (H), toward patient's head; R, rectum.

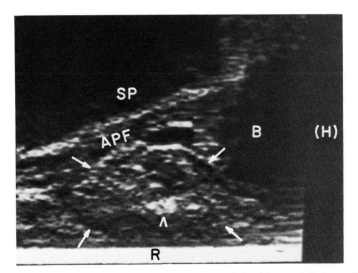

**FIG. 37.** Invasive adenocarcinoma. The prostate is normal sized *(arrows)*. Echogenic areas are noted throughout the mid and anterior portions of the gland with one bright echogenic focus *(arrowhead)*. This locally invasive adenocarcinoma has echogenic brightness and thickness ranging from Grade I to Grade III. APF, anterior prostatic fascia; SP, symphysis pubis; B, bladder; (H), toward patient's head; R, rectum.

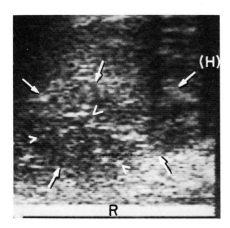

**FIG. 38.** Adenocarcinoma of mixed echogenicity. This poorly defined prostate *(arrows)* is slightly enlarged. There is a mixed echogenic area involving the posterior portion of the gland *(arrowheads)* with Grade I echogenic thickness and brightness scattered between areas of decreased echogenicity. (H), toward patient's head; R, rectum.

Malignant invasion from the prostate into the seminal vesicles may be noted on both radial and longitudinal transrectal examination and occasionally by the suprapubic approach. It is felt that capsular and pelvic sidewall invasion may be more accurately noted on radial scans (Fig. 11) than on the longitudinal linear array examination.

In summary, preliminary evaluation with both transrectal radial and trans-

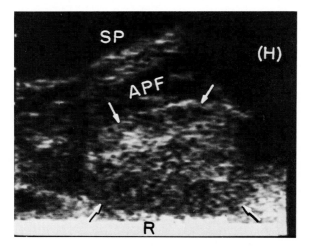

**FIG. 39.** Diffuse invasive adenocarcinoma. This clinically unsuspected normal-sized prostate *(arrows)* has marked areas of increased echogenicity scattered throughout the entire gland. This was a cribiform-type invasive adenocarcinoma. R, rectum; APF, anterior prostatic fascia; SP, symphysis pubis; (H), toward patient's head.

TABLE 2. *Suggestive acoustic criteria for focal lesions of the prostate—criteria developed by transrectal ultrasound examinations[a]*

|                      | Benign | Malignant |
|----------------------|--------|-----------|
| Thick echogenic foci | Yes    | No        |
| Thin echogenic foci  | Maybe  | Yes       |
| High reflective foci | Yes    | No        |
| Low reflective foci  | Maybe  | Yes       |
| Shadowing            | Yes    | No        |
| Purely hypoechoic    | Maybe  | No        |

[a]Reproduced from ref. 38, with permission.

rectal longitudinal scanning of the prostate gland demonstrates the following differences:

1. Radial scans define the margins more adequately than does the longitudinal linear array scan.
2. Radial scans define the seminal vesicles more accurately than does the longitudinal linear array image.
3. Longitudinal scans will define the size of the prostate as well as radial scans and is technically simpler to use.

## BIOPSY OF THE PROSTATE

Because the definitive diagnosis of prostatic carcinoma can only be ascertained with tissue diagnosis, biopsy of the prostate gland is still imperative in all suspicious cases. When focal prostatic alterations are noted on ultrasound, tissue extraction is required. Because digitally guided transperineal or transrectal prostate biopsies have a high degree of inaccuracy and since clinically nonpalpable lesions cannot be biopsied with satisfactory guidance, techniques have been developed to evaluate and procure tissue from specific areas of the prostate.

Patients who have undergone previous anterior perineal resection resulting in closure of the rectum can undergo transperineal biopsy guided by a transducer placed on the abdomen (39). However, clinically unsuspected lesions may not be noted on the abdominal prostatic ultrasound and the small gland may not be adequately identified (38).

Transperineally guided biopsy is of limited value. It can be performed with a sector scan with a biopsy guide that allows oblique insertion of the needle (ATL, Technicare, Diasonics) and is used only in patients who cannot be examined transrectally. In addition, as previously discussed, an enlarged gland or brightly echogenic foci is required to detect the prostate.

Biopsy guidance utilizing the radial scan has been developed (17, 21). Because this imaging modality utilizes static scans in transverse projection and the biopsy needle is placed in a longitudinal orientation, the needle cannot be visualized in its entirety as it is placed into the lesion. The need to change the path of the needle cannot be ascertained prior to final placement. This limitation is most obvious in biopsies of clinically unsuspected lesions.

Techniques have been developed utilizing the longitudinal linear array equipment with transperineal biopsy (8, 36–38). After the patient is examined with the transrectal ultrasound and a focal disruption identified, the patient is placed in the lithotomy position and a biopsy needle is placed in the midline of the perineum. Under ultrasonic guidance, the needle is placed in the prostate gland and with direct visualization of the needle throughout the procedure it is inserted into the area to be biopsied (Figs. 40–42). Thus, the biopsy is performed under direct and continuous ultrasonic guidance with either a small gauge needle for cytologic evaluation or a large bore needle, i.e., a tru-cut (Travenol) needle, for tissue extraction and histologic diagnosis. Accuracy with both types of needles appears to be similar (8, 37). The benefits of this procedure are that it enables adequate needle placement in areas of focal disruptions; and clinically unsuspected lesions, especially in small glands, can be accurately biopsied.

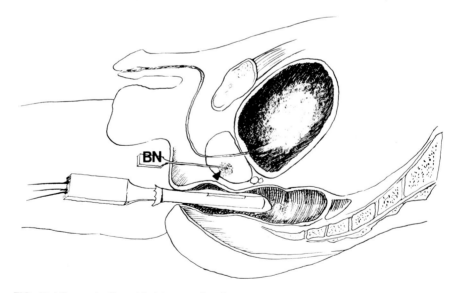

**FIG. 40.** Ultrasonically guided transperineal prostatic biopsy. With the probe placed into the rectum, the prostate and the abnormal area of the prostate *(arrowhead* to *shadowed area)* is visualized. The biopsy needle (BN) is placed into the perineum in the midline and ultrasonic guidance, advanced to the area of abnormality in the prostate. The biopsy is also performed under direct, continual ultrasonic guidance.

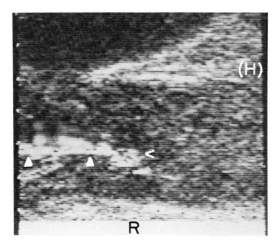

**FIG. 41.** Ultrasonically guided transperineal prostatic biopsy—adenocarcinoma. The biopsy needle *(closed arrowhead)* is placed through the perineum and guided by the transrectal probe placed in the rectum (R) to an echogenic focus *(open arrowhead)* which proved to be Grade II adenocarcinoma. (H), toward patient's head.

## SUMMARY

In conclusion, ultrasonic evaluation of the prostate has permitted evaluation of the size and acoustic texture of the gland. It appears that the transrectal approach is more accurate in defining focal abnormalities, and although a specific tissue diagnosis cannot be ascertained by ultrasound alone, this

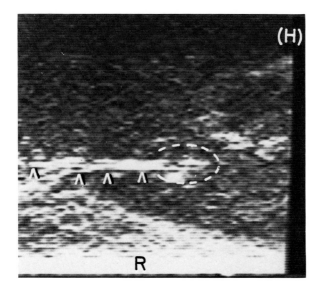

**FIG. 42.** Ultrasonically guided transperineal prostatic biopsy—adenocarcinoma. The biopsy needle *(arrowheads)* is placed into an area of increased echogenicity *(circled)* which proved to be Grade I adenocarcinoma. R, rectum; (H), toward patient's head.

technique has allowed accurate placement of biopsy needles within specific areas for diagnosis of both clinically suspected as well as unsuspected lesions.

## ACKNOWLEDGMENTS

The authors would like to thank Dr. Bruno Fornage of the Institut Jean Godinot, Rheims, France for his contribution of Figs. 8, 9, 10, 18, and 27, and JoAnn Anderson for her editorial assistance.

## REFERENCES

1. Aguirre, C. R., Tallada, M. B., Mayayo, T. D., Perales, L. C., and Romero, J. M. Evaluation comparative du volume prostatique par l'echographie transabdominale, le profil uretral et la radiologie. *J. Urol. (Paris)*, 86(8):675–679, 1980.
2. Bissada, N. K., Finkbeiner, A. E., and Redman, J. F. Accuracy of preoperative estimation of resection weight in transurethral prostatectomy. *J. Urology*, 116:201–202, 1976.
3. Brooman, P. J. C., Griffiths, G. J., Roberts, E., Peeling, W. B., and Evans, K. Per rectal ultrasound in the investigation of prostatic disease. *Clin. Radiol.*, 32:669–676, 1981.
4. Carpentier, P. J., Schroeder, F. H., and Blom, J. H. Transrectal ultrasonography in the followup of prostatic carcinoma patients. *J. Urology*, 128:742–746, 1982.
5. Denkhaus, H., Dierkopf, W., Grabbe, E., and Donn, F. Comparative study of suprapubic sonography and computed tomography for staging of prostatic carcinoma. *Urol. Radiol.*, 5:1–9, 1983.
6. Dhom, G., and Hohbach, Ch. Pathology and classification of prostate malignancies: Experience of the German prostate cancer registry. In: *Prostate Cancer*, edited by G. H. Jacobi and R. Hohenfellner. Williams & Wilkins, Baltimore, 1982.
7. Lee, D. J., Leibel, S., Shiels, R., Blitt, B., Sanders, R., Siegelman, S., and Order, S. The value of ultrasonic imaging and CT scanning in planning the radiotherapy for prostatic carcinoma. *Cancer*, 45:724–727, 1980.
8. Fornage, B. D., Touche, D. H., Delglaire, M., Farous, M. J. C., and Simatos, A. Real-time ultrasound-guided prostatic biopsy using a new transrectal linear-array probe. *Radiology*, 146:547–548, 1983.
9. Franks, L. M. Benign prostatic hyperplasia: gross and microscopic anatomy. In: *Benign Prostatic Hyperplasia*, edited by J. T. Grayhack, J. D. Wilson, and M. J. Scherbenske, pp. 63–89. NIH Workshop. PHEW Publication (NIH) 76–1113, 1975.
10. Gammelgaard, J., and Holm, H. H. Transurethral and transrectal ultrasonic scanning in urology. *J. Urology*, 124:863–868, 1980.
11. Greenberg, M., Neimen, H. L., Brandt, T. D., Falkowski, W., and Carter, M. Ultrasound of the prostate. *Radiology*, 141:757–762, 1981.
12. Greenberg, M., Neimen, H. L., Vogelzang, R., and Falkowski, W. Ultrasonic features of prostatic carcinoma. *J. Clin. Ultrasound*, 10:307–312, 1982.
13. Gray, H. *Gray's Anatomy*, 28th ed., edited by C. M. Goss. Lea & Febiger, Philadelphia, 1966.
14. Harada, K., Igari, D., and Tanahashi, Y. Gray scale transrectal ultrasonography of the prostate. *J. Clin. Ultrasound*, 7:45–49, 1979.
15. Harada, K., Tanahashi, Y., Igari, D., Numata, I., and Orikasa, S. Clinical evaluation of inside echo patterns in gray scale prostatic echography. *J. Urology*, 124:216–220, 1980.
16. Hastak, S. M., Gammelgaard, J., and Holm, H. H. Transrectal ultrasonic volume determination of the prostate—A preoperative and postoperative study. *J. Urology*, 127:1115–1118, 1982.
17. Hastak, S. M., Gammelgaard, J., and Holm, H. H. Ultrasonically guided transperineal biopsy of the diagnosis of prostatic carcinoma. *J. Urology*, 128:69–71, 1982.

18. Henneberry, M., Carter, M. F., and Neiman, H. L. Estimation of prostatic size by suprapubic ultrasonography. *J. Urology*, 121:615–616, 1979.

19. Hohenfellner, R. Suprapubic prostatectomy In: *Prostatic Disease*, edited by H. Marberger, H. Haschenk, H. K. A. Schirmer, J. A. C. Colston, and E. Witkin. Alan R. Liss, New York, 1976.

20. Holm, H. H., and Northeved, A. A transurethral ultrasonic scanner. *J. Urology*, 111:238–241, 1974.

21. Holm, H. H., and Gammelgaard, J. Ultrasonically guided precise needle placement in the prostate and the seminal vesicles. *J. Urology*, 125:385–387, 1981.

22. King, W. W., Wilkiemeyer, R. M., Boyce, W. H., and McKinney, W. M. Current status of prostatic echography. *J. Am. Med. Assoc.*, 226(4):444–447, 1973.

23. Kohri, K., Kaneko, S., Akiyama, T., Yachiku, S., and Kurita, T. Ultrasonic evaluation of prostatic carcinoma. *Urology*, 17(2):214–217, 1981.

24. Leissner, K. H., and Tisell, L. E. The weight of the human prostate. *Scand. J. Urol. Nephrol.*, 13:137–142, 1979.

25. Lerski, R. A., Barnett, E., and Morley, P. Ultrasound equipment for intra-rectal imaging of the prostate. *Br. J. Radiol.*, 52:225–226, 1979.

26. McNeal, J. E. Origin and development of carcinoma in the prostate. *Cancer*, 23:24–34, 1969.

27. Miller, S. S. and Garvie, W. H. H. The evaluation of prostate size by ultrasonic scanning: A preliminary report. *Br. J. Urol.*, 45:187–191, 1973.

28. Melchoir, J., Valk, W. L., Foret, J. D., and Mebust, W. K. Transurethral prostatectomy: Computerized analysis of 2,223 consecutive cases. *J. Urology*, 112:634–642, 1974.

29. Murphy, G. P. The diagnosis of prostatic cancer. *Cancer*, 37:589–596, 1976.

30. Nakamura, S., and Niijima, T. Transurethral real-time scanner. *J. Urol.*, 125:781–783, 1981.

31. Peeling, W. B., Griffiths, G. J., Evans, K. T., and Roberts, E. E. Diagnosis and staging of prostatic cancer by transrectal ultrasonography. A preliminary study. *J. Urol.*, 51:565–569, 1979.

32. Resnick, M. I., Willard, J. W., and Boyce, W. H. Recent progress in ultrasonography of the bladder and prostate. *J. Urol.*, 117:444–446, 1977.

33. Resnick, M. I., Willard, J. W., and Boyce, W. H. Ultrasonic evaluation of the prostatic nodule. *J. Urol.*, 120:86–89, 1978.

34. Resnick, M. I., Willard, J. W., and Boyce, W. H. Transrectal ultrasonography in the evaluation of patients with prostatic carcinoma. *J. Urol.*, 124:482–484, 1980.

35. Resnick, M. I. Noninvasive techniques in evaluating patients with carcinoma of prostate. *Suppl. J. Urol.*, 17(3):25–30, 1981.

36. Rifkin, M. D., Kurtz, A. B., and Goldberg, B. B. Technique for ultrasonically guided transperineal prostatic biopsy. *Am. J. Roentgenology*, 139(4):745–747, 1983.

37. Rifkin, M. D., Kurtz, A. B., and Goldberg, B. B. Prostate biopsy utilizing transrectal ultrasound guidance: diagnosis of clinically nonpalpable cancers. *J. Ultrasound Med.*, 2(4):165–167, 1983.

38. Rifkin, M. D., Kurtz, A. B., and Goldberg, B. B. Endoscopic ultrasonic evaluation of the prostate utilizing a transrectal probe: prospective evaluation and acoustic characterization. *Radiology (in press)*.

39. Schapira, H. E. Prostatic needle biopsy in patients after abdominoperineal resection. *Urology*, 20(1):76–77, 1982.

40. Sekine, H., Oka, K., and Takehara, Y. Transrectal longitudinal ultrasonotomography of the prostate by electronic linear scanning. *J. Urol.*, 127:62–65, 1982.

41. Shapeero, L. G., Friedland, G. W., Shortliffe, L. D., and Torti, F. M. Real-time transrectal ultrasonography of cancer of the prostate: diagnosis and response to therapy. Presented at The Radiological Society of North America, Scientific session, November 28–December 2, 1982.

42. Silverberg, E. Cancer statistics 1983. *Cancer—A Cancer Journal for Clinicals*, 33:9–25, 1983.

43. Sukov, R. J., Scardino, P. T., Sample, W. F., Winter, J., Confer, D. J. Computed tomography and transabdominal ultrasound in the evaluation of the prostate. *J. Comput. Assist. Tomogr.*, 1(3):281–289, 1977.

44. Taylor, W. B., Hunt, J. W., Foster, F. S., Blend, R., and Worthington, A. A high-resolution transrectal ultrasonographic system. *Ultrasound Med. & Biol.*, 5:129–138, 1979.
45. Walsh, P. C. Benign prostatic hyperplasia. In: *Campbell's Urology*, 4th ed., edited by T. H. Harrison, R. F. Gittes, A. D. Perlmutter, T. A. Stamey, and P. C. Walsh, pp. 949–964, W. B. Saunders, Philadelphia, 1979.
46. Watanabe, H. Kaiho, H., Tanaka, M., and Terasawa, Y. Diagnostic application of ultrasonotomography to the prostate. *Invest. Radiol.*, 8(5):548–559, 1971.
47. Watanabe, H., Igari, D., Tanahashi, Y., Harada, K., and Saitoh, M. Transrectal ultrasonotomography of the prostate. *J. Urol.*, 114:734–739, 1975.
48. Watanabe, H., Saitoh, M., Mishina, T., Igari, D., Tanahashi, Y., Harada, K., and Hisamichi, S. Mass screening program for prostatic diseases with transrectal ultrasonotomography. *J. Urol.*, 117:746–748, 1977.
49. Weyrauch, H. M. *Surgery of the Prostate*. W. B. Saunders, Philadelphia, 1959.

*Ultrasound Annual 1983*, edited by R. C.
Sanders and M. Hill. Raven Press, New York
© 1983.

# Prenatal Diagnosis of Craniospinal Anomalies

*,†D. Graham, †J. L. Chezmar, and †R. C. Sanders

*Department of Obstetrics and Gynecology and †The Russell H. Morgan
Department of Diagnostic Radiology, The Johns Hopkins Medical Institutions,
Baltimore, Maryland 21205*

Abnormalities of the neural tube (neural tube defect—NTD) are among the most common structural anomalies of the fetus and among the most severe in their clinical significance. The incidence of such defects varies in different geographic areas; in the United States the incidence is 1 per 1,000 live births but anomalies occur as often as 4 to 7 per 1,000 live births in certain areas of the United Kingdom. Until recently, the majority of such anomalies were first diagnosed at the time of delivery but with the development of high resolution real-time ultrasound technology most of these problems can be diagnosed as early as 12 to 14 weeks of gestation. Prenatal diagnosis allows the option of pregnancy termination, prenatal intervention for alleviation of certain conditions, or early delivery with definitive surgery of the neonate. The timing, route, and place of delivery can be chosen to maximize fetal outcome and minimize potential trauma to the fetus and mother. This chapter reviews the sonographic anatomy of the normal fetal neural tube and the diagnosis of the more commonly encountered anomalies.

## NORMAL SONOGRAPHIC ANATOMY

When bistable ultrasound techniques were first used clinically in the assessment of gestational age, the fetal cranium was routinely visualized in each instance; however, little intracranial anatomy could be recognized, with the exception of the falx. Increased gray scale resolution and the availability of real-time equipment allows a rapid examination of the fetal cranium while displaying a considerable amount of intracranial anatomy (51).

In the first trimester, the small size of the fetus prevents visualization of normal intracranial anatomy. The cranium can be recognized from approximately 8 to 9 weeks but it is not until 10 to 12 weeks that intracranial structures can be identified. At this time, the choroid plexuses which are highly echogenic and which fill the lateral ventricles are readily visualized

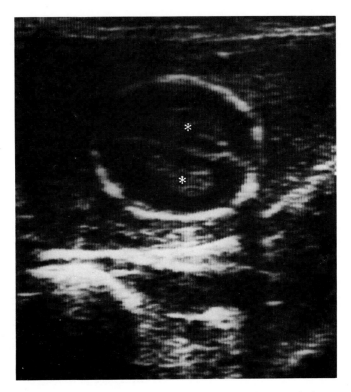

**FIG. 1.** Choroid plexus. Transverse section of the head in early second trimester showing the large echogenic choroid plexus (*).

(Fig. 1). Since the fetal head is usually scanned in a series of transverse planes in an effort to identify the correct plane for measurement of the biparietal diameter (BPD), the intracranial anatomy is usually studied in this "axial" plane, differing from the sagittal and coronal planes of visualization used in neonatal echoencephalography. If the fetal head is examined from the base of the skull in a rostral direction the intracranial structures may be visualized in a systematic fashion.

### BASE OF SKULL

A transverse scan at the base of the skull will demonstrate the sphenoid wings anteriorly and the petrous pyramids posteriorly as four echogenic lines coming together at a central point.

### Choroid Plexus

The choroid plexuses are readily visualized from early in the second trimester as echogenic structures on either side of the midline. The lateral ventricles in the early second trimester are proportionately much larger than they are in later pregnancy and the choroid plexus fills most of the lateral ventricle. Crade et al. (7), after examining feti from 8 to 22 weeks, showed that the width of the choroid plexus occupied 80 to 90% of the cerebral axial dimension at 12 weeks, falling to 60 to 70% at 17 weeks and 50 to 60% at 20 weeks. In addition, the choroid plexus becomes less readily visualized as pregnancy advances.

### Lateral Ventricles

The lateral ventricles may be visualized from early in the second trimester. At this stage, the ventricles are relatively large, becoming proportionately smaller as pregnancy advances. The bodies of the lateral ventricles may be seen as paired linear echogenicities parallel to the midline (Fig. 2) at a level slightly higher than that used for measurement of the BPD. The frontal horns are visualized as small paired echogenicities parallel to the midline anteriorly (Fig. 3), while the occipital horns are more difficult to visualize (10, 30), are variable in width, and are seen as paired linear echogenicities posteriorly.

Lateral ventricular size may be measured prenatally to detect hydrocephalus prior to any abnormal increase in head size. Normal standards have been published by Denkhaus (10), Dunne (13), Fiske (16), Johnson (32), Jeanty (30), and Hadlock (20). Denkhaus measured the ratio of the lateral ventricles (measured at the frontal or temporal horns) and compared this to

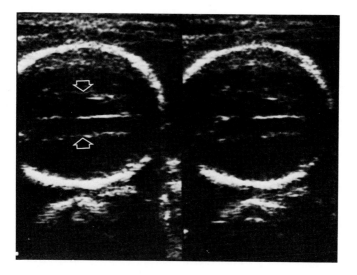

**FIG. 2.** Lateral ventricles. Transverse section of the head at a level higher than the thalami showing the lateral ventricles *(open arrows)*.

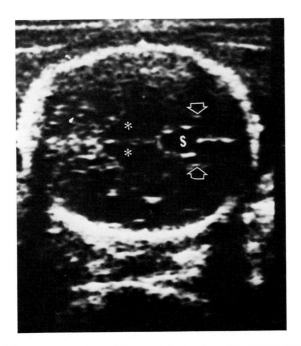

**FIG. 3.** Thalami. Transverse section of the head at a level used for measuring the biparietal diameter showing the Thalami (*), the cavum septum pellucidum (S) and the frontal horns of the lateral ventricles *(open arrows)*. The third ventricle is seen as a thin slit in the middle of the thalami.

the BPD. Jeanty, Dunne and Johnson, and Fiske produced curves of the measurement of the frontal horns, ventricular bodies, atria, or occipital horns against the transverse diameter of the head in the same plane. This is called the lateral ventricle/hemispheric width (LV/HW) ratio. Similar curves were found by all, vis, the LV/HW is greater earlier in gestation, falling as pregnancy advances and reflecting greater growth of the cerebral hemispheres at this time (41, 50). At 15 weeks the LV/HW width has a mean of 56% and a range of 40 to 71%. At 21 weeks it should be below 50% and at term should be no greater than 35% with a mean of 28% and a range of 23 to 35% (32).

## Posterior Fossa

The cerebellum is readily visible as a bilobed structure with an echogenic border (Fig. 4), becoming more prominent as pregnancy advances. McLeary (45) measured the diameter of the cerebellum and correlated this with the BPD and found a fairly linear relationship.

Immediately superior to the cerebellum, the tentorium may be seen as a V-shaped area of echogenicity.

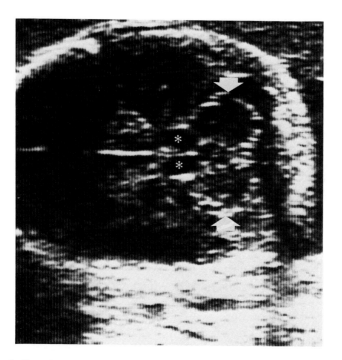

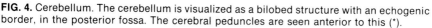

**FIG. 4.** Cerebellum. The cerebellum is visualized as a bilobed structure with an echogenic border, in the posterior fossa. The cerebral peduncles are seen anterior to this (*).

### Cerebral Peduncles

The cerebral peduncles are seen as a heart-shaped structure with its apex directed posteriorly, anterior and superior to the cerebellum (Fig. 4). Anterior to the cerebral peduncles, one may see the pulsations of the basilar artery with a real-time examination.

### Thalami

At a slightly higher level and more anterior to the cerebral peduncles are seen the diamond-shaped hypoechoic thalami (Fig. 3). Between the thalami is seen a linear echogenicity or a thin slit-like structure representing the third ventricle (Fig. 3).

### Sylvian Fissure

At the same level as the thalami and approximately two-thirds of the distance between midline and calvarium, the Sylvian fissure is seen as a linear echogenicity paralleling the echoes from the calvarium. Real-time examination usually shows the pulsations of the middle cerebral artery within the fissure. It is important not to mistake the Sylvian fissure for the wall of the body of the lateral ventricle, which is at a slightly higher level.

### Cavum Septum Pellucidum

Anterior to the thalami in the midline is a small box-like structure which previously was thought to represent the third ventricle and is now considered to be the cavum septum pellucidum (Fig. 3). This structure should be visualized on the plane used for measurement of the BPD.

## CRANIAL ANOMALIES

### Anencephaly

Anencephaly is the commonest of the neural tube defects, with an incidence of approximately 1 in 1,000 (52, 63) and a significant female to male preponderance of 4:1. As with other neural tube defects, it is significantly more common in certain areas of the United Kingdom.

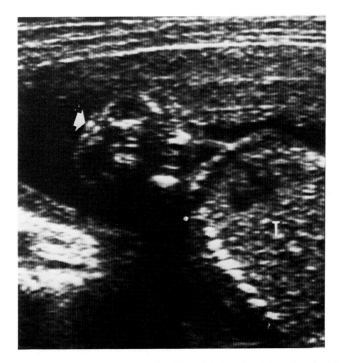

**FIG. 5.** Anencephaly. Longitudunal study of a midtrimester fetus showing the cranial remnant *(arrow).* The fetal trunk (T) is well visualized.

Anencephaly results from failure of closure of the cephalic portion of the neural tube, occurring between the 2nd and 3rd weeks of development. The anatomic result is an absence of cerebral tissue although portions of the midbrain and brainstem are usually present. The cranial vault is also absent but basal portions of the frontal, parietal, and occipital bones usually develop (2, 38).

Sonographically, it may be recognized as early as 12 to 14 weeks of pregnancy owing to replacement of normal cranial structures by a small nubbin of tissue, representing the facial structures, base of the brain, and remaining brain tissue (Fig. 5). It may be detected during a routine scan performed for gestational age assessment or there may be some other factor leading one to suspect NTD, e.g., polyhydramnios, previous history of an affected infant, or elevated maternal serum alpha-feto-protein (AFP) in a screening program. Later in pregnancy the absence of the normal cranial vault is quite obvious and X-ray confirmation is usually not necessary. However, care should be taken not to misinterpret the deeply engaged head as anencephaly.

Since approximately 50% of anencephalics have associated anomalies of the central nervous system (CNS) (8, 38, 52) the spine should be carefully examined. Other anomalies may be seen including hypoplastic or absent adrenals, (14), talipes equinovarus, umbilical hernia, harelip, and cleft palate (55).

## Hydrocephalus

Since normal lateral ventricles can now be recognized from early in the second trimester, the diagnosis of dilated ventricles may be made at a very early stage of pregnancy, prior to an abnormal increase in head size. Previously this diagnosis could not be made until late in the course of the disorder, with the finding of a significant head-to-trunk discrepancy or a head size greater than 11 cm.

There are a number of potential causes of hydrocephalus *in utero*. Communicating (nonobstructive) hydrocephalus is the most common type and has a recurrence rate of 1 to 4% (53). Obstructive hydrocephalus may be secondary to aqueductal stenosis [which may occur as an X-linked (29) or autosomal recessive (47) abnormality] or by obstruction to cerebrospinal fluid (CSF) flow through the foramina of the fourth ventricle, e.g., secondary to prenatal infections. The result is an increase in CSF pressure, which leads to an increase in ventricular size and secondarily to an increase in head size (Fig. 6). It is very important, however, to correlate the lateral ventricular ratio to the correct gestational age. Where there is already an abnormal increase in the head size, the BPD cannot be used for gestational age assessment, and some other parameter, e.g., the femur length, should be used.

One of the earliest signs of ventricular enlargement may be dilatation of the occipital horns (13, 32, 33) but measurement of this portion of the ventri-

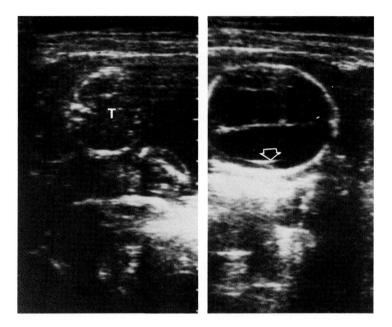

**FIG. 6.** Hydrocephalus. The head of this second trimester fetus shows marked ventricular dilatation with only a small amount of cortex remaining *(open arrow)*. There is already a significant discrepancy between the size of the head and the trunk (T).

cles is more cumbersome to obtain and subject to more variation than the LV/HW ratio (10, 30). The next change appears to be the visualization of the medial border of the ventricle which is not normally seen because it is not in the optimal plane of the ultrasound beam. With ventricular dilatation, the medial walls become more parallel to the plane of the falx and then five echogenic lines rather than three may be seen. Where the ventricles are dilated, reverberations in the half of the cranium nearest to the skin may obscure the ventricle and may give the false appearance of an asymmetric hydrocephalus.

Where hydrocephalus is diagnosed prenatally, it is important to measure the width of the remaining cortex since this is of prognostic importance. Early prenatal diagnosis not only allows the option of pregnancy termination but also allows the possibility of prenatal intervention by placing a shunt into the dilated ventricle and allowing the CSF to drain into the amniotic fluid. Birnholz and Frigoletto (3) treated hydrocephalus *in utero* by repeated aspirations of CSF. This technique, however, increases the risk of injury to vital intracranial structures and also becomes more difficult in the third trimester as the calvarium becomes thicker. Clewell et al. (6) successfully implanted a ventricular-amniotic shunt in a fetus with hydrocephalus and a family history consistent with X-linked hydrocephalus. This shunt remained patent until approximately 34 weeks of pregnancy when the infant was delivered by cesarean section. The aim of this procedure is to maximize the potential for brain growth (6). Although there is experimental evidence that antenatal CSF diversion in rhesus monkeys improves outcome (48), similar results have not been proven in humans because of the lack of sufficient information. Indeed, mild to moderate ventricular dilatation may be seen early in pregnancy, which may not progress or which may in fact regress. Because of this, caution is advised in the use of such drastic *in utero* procedures.

Hydrocephalus may be associated with other anomalies such as spina bifida, encephaocele, and Dandy-Walker cyst. The remainder of the neural axis should be scanned carefully to detect such lesions.

## Hydranencephaly

Hydranencephaly is a rare condition of uncertain etiology in which some prenatal insult leads to infarction of the cerebral tissues supplied by the anterior and middle cerebral arteries. Suggested etiologies have included occlusion of the internal carotid arteries (11, 42, 43), *in utero* infections (1, 12, 65), venous thrombosis (57), or a defect in vascular ontogenesis (57). Associated anomalies are uncommon.

The result of the prenatal insult is the replacement of normal cerebral tissue by membraneous fluid-filled sacs. The midbrain, basal ganglia, and infratentorial structures are usually present since they are supplied primarily by the posterior circulation. In some patients, remnants of the basal aspects of the frontal, temporal, and occipital lobes are recognizable. The falx may be absent to varying extents (57).

Sonographically, hydranencephaly is recognized as a replacement of the normal supratentorial structures by fluid (Fig. 7). The width of the head itself is not usually significantly enlarged as it is with hydrocephalus. Where the falx is absent, a midline echo may not be seen (15). If it is seen, it may be deviated if the hemispheres are asymmetrically involved (11). At the base of the brain, one characteristically sees the brainstem and basal ganglia. Remnants of the basal portions of the cerebral tissues may also be seen. It is important to differentiate hydranencephaly from severe hydrocephalus and from holoprosencephaly. With severe hydrocephalus, one will see more marked enlargement of the head and one can usually still visualize remaining cortical tissue, whereas with holoprosencephaly (qv) there is an irregular ventricular cavity surrounded by cortical tissue. The prognosis of hydranencephaly is poor with most affected infants dying in the neonatal period, although a few live for several years (40).

Polyhydramnios was an associated feature in a case reported by Fleischer (17), and it was postulated as being due to a depressed swallowing reflex.

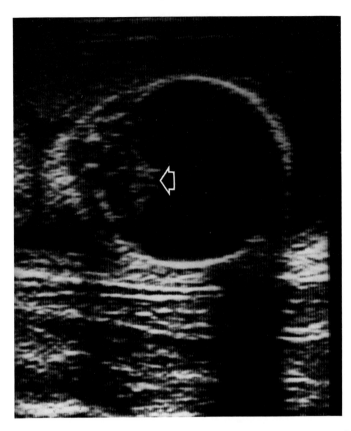

**FIG. 7.** Hydranencephaly. A coronal section through the head of this second trimester fetus shows replacement of normal cranial tissue by fluid. The basal ganglia and midbrain structures are visualized *(arrow)*.

## Holoprosencephaly

Holoprosencephaly is a rare condition in which the prosencephalon fails to cleave and evaginate, resulting in a spectrum of defects from rudimentary olfactory bulbs to severe anomalies involving fusion of the cerebral hemispheres and a single, large, irregular cerebral ventricle (4). The corpus callosum and septum pellucidum may be rudimentary or absent (27). Midline defects are commonly seen and include cleft lip and/or palate or cyclopia (34). The lesion may be seen in association with trisomy 13 or 15 (9) and with a partial chromosome deletion (27). Infants with trisomy of the D group are more likely to have cardiac as well as a number of other congenital anomalies (27).

Sonographically, in the more severe varieties, one sees a single irregular ventricular cavity with a remaining cortex of varying width (Fig. 8). The head size is usually not significantly increased.

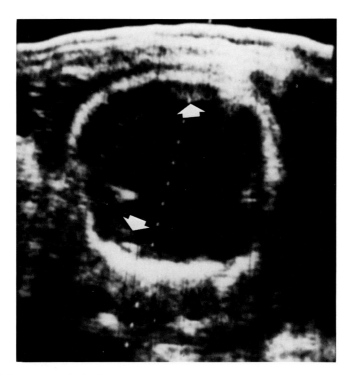

**FIG. 8.** Holoprosencephaly. A transverse section shows a dilated single ventricle with a varying amount of remaining cortex *(arrows).*

## Microcephaly

Microcephaly is an abnormally small head that may occur secondarily to an abnormality of the calvarium (craniosynostosis) or failure of development of the brain (micrencephaly) due to genetic mutations, chromosomal abnormalities, or environmental factors such as prenatal infections (64). The main clinical importance of microcephaly is in its frequent association with micrencephaly and mental retardation. Where the head is smaller than 3 standard deviations below the mean with no defect secondary to premature cranial synostosis (5, 39), mental retardation has been shown to be a frequent association. When the head is between 2 and 3 standard deviations below the mean, however, the correlation with mental retardation is less frequent (64).

Sonographically, microcephaly may not be diagnosed until late in pregnancy by failure to visualize a satisfactory BPD and an abnormal head-to-trunk ratio, with the trunk larger than the head prior to 36 weeks. Alternatively a head circumference or BPD more than 3 standard deviations below the mean for gestational age is found (gestational age can be assessed by some parameter such as the femoral length) (Fig. 9).

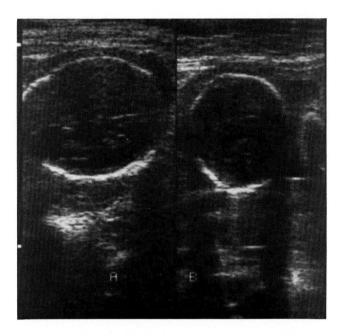

**FIG. 9.** Microcephaly. In this twin pregnancy there is a significant difference in the head size of the normal twin *(left)* and the affected twin with microcephaly *(right)*.

### Encephalocele

Encephalocele is a complex malformation involving herniation of cerebral tissue and/or meninges through a defect in the cranial bones (Fig. 10). The bony defect is usually in the midline with approximately 75% being in the occipital area, 15% in the frontal area, and the remainder in the parietal area. Sonography provides an accurate method of diagnosing this malformation. It allows assessment of the size and composition of the lesion and the underlying bony defect along with evaluation of the intracranial anatomy and any associated anomalies such as spina bifida. Several appearances may be seen sonographically (19, 49):

(a) A cystic mass adjacent to the skull, representing a meningocele rather than an encephalocele.

(b) A solid mass, often showing convolutions and representing herniated cerebral tissue.

(c) A combination of the above, representing meningoencepholocele.

(d) An underlying cranial bone defect (cranium bifidum).

(e) The BPD may be small for the gestational age (26).

The differential diagnosis of a juxtracranial mass such as an encephalocele will include a teratoma, cystic hygroma, and iniencephaly (54). Teratoma is more likely to have a solid or complex appearance whereas the cystic hygroma is characteristically a multiseptated cystic lesion.

When encephalocele is diagnosed the fetal spine should be carefully scanned to detect any associated spinal defects that might be present. The fetal kidneys should also be scanned since encephalocele and infantile polycystic kidneys may coexist in the Meckel-Gruber syndrome (encephalocele, polycystic kidneys, and polydactyly) (46, 62). Since this condition is inherited as an autosomal recessive trait, it is important that it be identified to allow counseling in subsequent pregnancies.

An encephalocele has been decompressed prenatally using real-time sonographic guidance in order to facilitate vaginal delivery (19).

### Acrania

Acrania differs from anencephaly in that while there is partial or complete absence of the cranial bones, there is complete (but abnormal) development

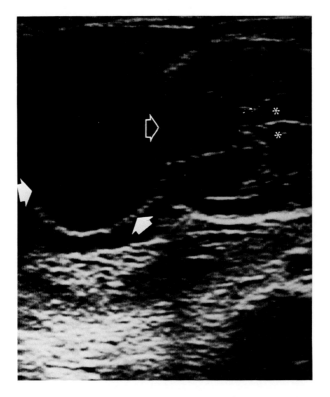

**FIG. 10.** Encephalocele. A transverse section of the head shows a large cystic mass *(closed arrows)* adjacent to a bony defect in the cranium *(open arrow)*. This communicates with the dilated lateral ventricles. The thalami are also seen (*).

of cerebral tissue resulting from abnormal mesodermal and ectodermal differentiation rather than faulty closure of the neural tube (44). Sonographically, acrania is seen as an absence of normal calvarial echoes with a mass of cerebral tissue adjacent to the base of the skull.

### Dandy-Walker Malformation

Dandy-Walker malformation is a condition of unknown etiology with cystic dilatation of the 4th ventricle and is associated with abnormal development of the cerebellum and hydrocephalus (21, 23). Associated abnormalities such as aqueductal stenosis, agenesis of the corpus callosum, and systemic anomalies may be found in up to 68% of affected infants (21). Whereas the mortality rate was previously reported as 50%, recent results after operative therapy are more promising (36, 58).

Sonographically, the Dandy-Walker malformation is seen as a cystic mass in the posterior fossa (Fig. 11). Remnants of the cerebellum may be visible and associated hydrocephalus is often present. Hatjis (24), in reporting a case first diagnosed at 25 to 26 weeks, noted a progressive increase in the size of the cystic structure and gradual development of hydrocephalus. In the case reported by Kirkinen (36), however, the relative dimensions of the cerebral ventricles, cortical tissue, and the cystic 4th ventricle remained relatively constant in the 3rd trimester.

### Iniencephaly

In iniencephaly there is a complex malformation involving faulty closure of the occipital bones and a spinal defect of variable extent involving the

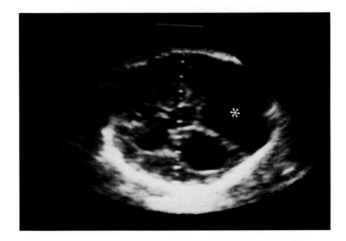

**FIG. 11.** Dandy-Walker malformation. A transverse section shows cystic dilatation of the fourth ventricle (*), together with hydrocephalus.

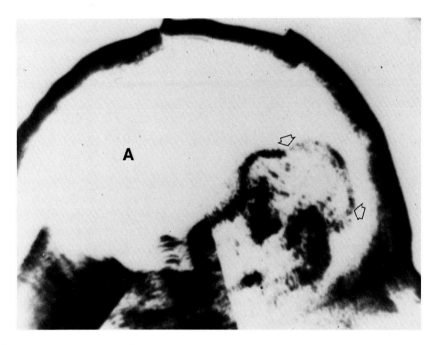

**FIG. 12.** Iniencephaly. In this transverse section of the neck there is a large mass of neural tissue *(arrows)* adjacent to a v-shaped spinal canal. There is also polyhydraminios (A).

cervical and upper thoracic spine. A mass of skin-covered neural tissue lies adjacent to these defects and there is characteristically hyperextension of the head (Fig. 12).

## Periventricular Calcification

The cytomegalovirus (CMV) is the most common cause of a congenital infection in the United States. It may pass transplacentally and lead to hematogenous spread throughout the fetus. When the virus spreads to the brain, there may be direct tissue destruction and subsequent formation of calcified areas which are typically, (but not invariably) periventricular in distribution (56). This may be seen prenatally as periventricular areas of echogenicity that may have acoustical shadowing and the ventricles may be dilated (18).

## Intracranial Tumors

Although intracranial tumors are a very frequent cause of childhood malignancy, they are rarely present at birth (28). The most common congenital tumors are gliomas and teratomas (31). The latter may reach a large size *in utero* and have been reported to cause dystocia because of cephalopelvic disproportion (60, 61). Prenatal sonographic diagnosis of intracranial teratoma has been reported by Hoff (28) as replacement of normal recognizable intracranial structures by a disordered array of echoes compatible with a large solid mass. Early diagnosis permitted prompt termination of pregnancy by a cesarean section.

### Intracranial Hemorrhage

Although intracranial hemorrhage is a rather common postnatal finding in premature infants it has not been diagnosed prenatally until recently. Kim (35) reported an *in utero* diagnosis of intraventricular hemorrhage visualized as a large dilated ventricular system filled with echogenic material and a large intracerebral hematoma lateral to the body of a lateral ventricle. The examination was performed at 29 weeks of gestation because of fetal death *in utero.*

### ANATOMY OF THE SPINE

The fetal spine may be visualized on longitudinal section as two relatively parallel lines of echoes from as early as the late first trimester and is more readily visualized as pregnancy advances. The two rows of echoes are the posterior ossification centers of the vertebrae. There is a normal flaring of

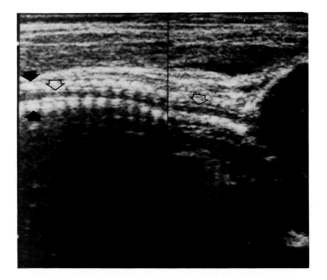

**FIG. 13.** Longitudinal spine. A longitudinal section of the spine shows the parallel groups of echoes from the ossification centers *(closed arrows).* Within these two rows of echoes are seen faint linear echogenicities which represent the nonossified borders of the spinal canal *(open arrows).*

the parallel rows of echoes in the cervical spine, a less marked flaring in the lumbar spine, and then a tapering in the sacrum. On transverse section in early pregnancy three separate ossification centers are seen, one for the vertebral body and the two posterior centers. In later pregnancy, a complete ring of echoes is visualized. Occasionally, on longitudinal section, two faint linear echogenicities are seen paralleling the ossification centers of the spine. While these have been described as representing the spinal cord, they are more commonly due to visualization of the nonossified borders of the spinal canal (Fig. 13).

With spina bifida, there is a failure of closure of the posterior elements of the vertebral body and there may be an associated exposed mass of neural tissue, the meningocele. Such defects may occur along the length of the spine but are much more common in the lumbar area. They result from failure of closure of the neural tube at approximately 3 to 4 weeks and may be variable in size and extent. They range from a small spina bifida cystica with no exposed neural tissue to myelomeningocele in which several segments are usually involved with exposed spinal cord and nerve roots. The resulting neurological defect depends on the extent of the lesion, the amount of involved neural tissue, and the postnatal treatment.

Sonographic diagnosis of spina bifida requires meticulous scanning of the spine in both the longitudinal and transverse planes. Each segment of the spine down to the sacrum should be examined transversely to determine the integrity of the posterior neural arch and whether there is a soft tissue mass adjacent to the back. While movement of the fetal lower extremities may be seen *in utero,* this does not appear to correlate with subsequent postnatal

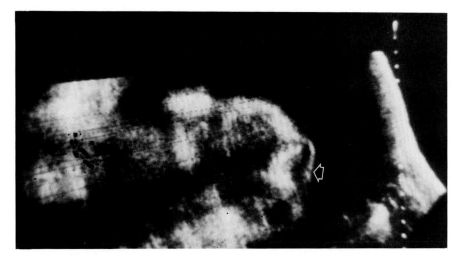

**FIG. 14.** Spina bifida. A transverse section of the lower lumbar spine shows a thin membrane covering *(arrow)* adjacent to a V-shaped spina bifida. Polyhydramnios is present.

neurological development. Spina bifida is seen in longitudinal section as a localized widening of the parallel echoes (care must be taken not to misinterpret the normal cervical widening) and as a V- or U-shaped spine in transverse section, with or without an associated soft tissue mass (Fig. 14).

## REFERENCES

1. Altshuler, G. Toxoplasmosis as a cause of hydranencephaly. *Am. J. Dis. Child,* 125: 251–252, 1973.
2. Bergsma, D. *Birth Defects: Atlas and Compendium.* Williams and Wilkins, Baltimore, 1973.
3. Birnholz, J. C., Frigoletto, F. D. Antenatal treatment of hydrocephalus. *N. Engl. J. Med.,* 313: 1021–1023, 1981.
4. Bishop, K., Connolly, J., Carter, C. H. et al. Holoprosencephaly. A case report with no extracranial abnormalities and normal chromosome count and karyotype. *J. Pediatr.,* 65: 406, 1964.
5. Book, J. A., Schut, J. W., and Reed, S. C. A clinical and genetical study of microcephaly. *Am. J. Ment. Ret.,* 56: 637, 1953.
6. Clewell, W. H., Johnson, M. L., Meier, P. R., et al. A surgical approach to the treatment of fetal hydrocephalus. *N. Engl. J. Med.,* 306: 1320–1325, 1982.
7. Crade, M., Patel, J., and McQuown, D. Sonographic imaging of the glycogen stage of the fetal choroid plexus. *AJR,* 137: 489–491, 1981.
8. Cunningham, M. E., and Walls, W. J. Ultrasound in the evaluation of anencephaly. *Radiology,* 118: 165–167, 1976.
9. Demyer, W. Holoprosencephaly (cyclopia-arhinencephaly). In: *Handbook of Clinical Neurology,* Vol. 30, edited by P. J. Vinken and G. W. Bruyn, pp. 431–478, North Holland, Amsterdam, 1977.
10. Denkhaus, H., and Winsburg, F. Ultrasonic measurement of the fetal ventricular system. *Radiology,* 131: 781–787, 1979.
11. Dublin, A. B., and French, B. N. Diagnostic image evaluation of hydranencephaly and pictorially similar entities, with emphasis on computed tomography. *Radiology,* 137: 81–91, 1980.
12. Dublin, A. B., and Marten, D. F. Computed tomography in the evaluation of herpes simplex encephalitis. *Radiology,* 125: 133–134, 1977.
13. Dunne, M. G., and Johnson, M. L. The ultrasonic demonstration of fetal abnormalities in utero. *J. Reprod. Med.,* 23: 195–206, 1979.
14. Erez, S., and King, T. M. Anencephaly: A survey of 44 cases, *Obstet. Gynecol.,* 27: 601–604, 1966.
15. Fiske, C. E., and Filly, R. A. Ultrasound evaluation of the normal and abnormal fetal neural axis. *Radiol. Clin. North Am.,* 20: 285–296, 1982.
16. Fiske, C. E., Filly, R. A., and Callen, P. W. Sonographic measurement of lateral ventricular width in early ventricular dilatation, *J. Clin. Ultrasound,* 9: 403–405, 1981.
17. Fleischer, A., and Brown, M. Hydramnios associated with fetal hydrancephaly. *J. Clin. Ultrasound,* 5: 41–43, 1977.
18. Graham, D., Guidi, S. M., and Sanders, R. C. Sonographic features of *in utero* periventricular calcification due to cytomegalovirus infection. *J. Ultrasound Med.,* 1: 171–172, 1982.
19. Graham, D., Johnson, T. R. B. Jr., and Sanders, R. C. The role of sonography in the prenatal diagnosis and management of encephalocele. *J. Ultrasound Med.,* 1: 111–115, 1982.
20. Hadlock, F. P., Deter, R. L., and Park, S. K. Real-time sonography: Ventricular and vascular anatomy of the fetal brain *in utero. AJR,* 136: 133–137, 1981.
21. Hart, N. M., Malamud, N., and Ellis, W. G. The Dandy-Walker syndrome. *Neurology,* 22: 771, 1972.
22. Harwood-Nash, D. C. Congenital craniocerebral abnormalities and computed tomography. *Semin. Roentgenol.* 12: 39–51, 1977.
23. Harwood-Nash, D. C., and Fitz, C. R. Abnormal skull. In: *Neuroradiology in Infants and Children.* Mosby, St. Louis, 1976.

24. Hatjis, C. G., Horbar, J. D., and Anderson, G. C. The *in utero* diagnosis of a posterior fossa intracranial cyst (Dandy-Walker cyst). *Am. J. Obstet. Gynecol.,* 140: 473–475, 1981.
25. Heimburger, R. F., Patrick, J. T., Fry, F. O., et al. Pathological confirmation of ultrasound brain tomograms. In: *Ultrasound in Medicine,* Vol. 3A, edited by D. White and R. E. Brown, pp. 829–832, Plenum, New York, 1977.
26. Hidalgo, H., Bowie, J., Rosenberb, E. R., et al. *In utero* sonographic diagnosis of fetal cerebral anomalies. *AJR,* 139: 143–148, 1982.
27. Hill, L. M., Breckle, R., and Bonebrake, C. R. Ultrasonic findings with holoprosencephaly. *J. Reprod. Med.,* 27: 172–175, 1982.
28. Hoff, N. R., and Mackay, I. M. Prenatal ultrasound diagnosis of intracranial teratoma. *J. Clin. Ultrasound,* 8: 247–249, 1980.
29. Holmes, L. B., Nash, A., Zurhein, G. M., et al. X-linked aqueductal stenosis. Clinical and neuropathological findings in two families. *Pediatrics,* 51: 697, 1973.
30. Jeanty, P., Dramaix-Wilmet, M., Delbeke, D., et al. Ultrasonic evaluation of fetal ventricular growth. *Neuroradiology,* 21: 127–131, 1981.
31. Jellinger, K., and Plassmann, M. S. Conatal intracranial tumors. *Neuropaediatrie,* 4: 46, 1973.
32. Johnson, M. L., Dunne, M. G., Mack, L. A., et al. Evaluation of fetal intracranial anatomy by static and real-time ultrasound. *J. Clin. Ultrasound,* 8: 311–318, 1980.
33. Johnson, M. L., Mack, L., Rumack, C. M., et al. B-mode echoencephalography in the normal and high risk infant. *AJR,* 133: 375, 1979.
34. Khan, M., Rozdilsky, B., and Gerrard, J. W. Familial holoprosencephaly. *Dev. Med. Child Neurol.,* 12: 71, 1970.
35. Kim, M. S., and Elyaderani, M. K. Sonographic diagnosis of cerebroventricular hemorrhage *in utero. Radiology,* 142: 479–480, 1982.
36. Kirkinen, P., Jouppila, P., Valkeakar, T., et al. Ultrasonic evaluation of the Dandy Walker Syndrome. *Obstet. Gynecol.,* 59: 18–21, 1982.
37. Korobkin, R. The relationship between head circumference and the development of communicating hydrocephalus in infants following intraventricular hemorrhage. *Pediatrics,* 56: 74, 1975.
38. Kossoff, G., Garrett, W., and Radovanovich, G. Grey scale echography in obstetrics and gynecology. *Aust. Radiol.,* 18: 63–111, March 1974.
39. Kurtz, A. B., Wapner, R. D., Rubin, C. S., et al. Ultrasound criteria for the *in utero* diagnosis of microcephaly. *J. Clin. Ultrasound,* 8: 11, 1980.
40. Lee, T. G., Warren, B. H. Antenatal diagnosis of hydranencephaly by ultrasound: correlation with ventriculography and computed tomography. *J. Clin. Ultrasound,* 5: 271–273, 1977.
41. Lemire, R. J., Loeser, J. D., Leech, R. W., et al. *Normal and Abnormal Development of the Human Nervous System,* p. 95, Harper & Row, New York, 1975.
42. Lindenberg, R., and Swanson, P. D. Infantile hydranencephaly. A report of five cases of infarction of both cerebral hemispheres in infancy. *Brain,* 90: 839–850, 1967.
43. Mack, L. A., Rumack, C. M., and Johnson, M. L. Ultrasound evaluation of cystic intracranial lesions in the neonate. *Radiology,* 137: 451–455, 1980.
44. Mannes, E. J., Crelin, E. S., Hobbins, J. S., et al. Sonographic demonstration of fetal acrania. *AJR,* 139: 181–182, July 1982.
45. McLeary, R. D., and Kuhns, L. R. Ultrasonography of the fetal cerebellum. *Proceedings of AIUM/SDMS Annual Convention, Denver, 1982.*
46. Mecke, S., and Passarge, E. Encephalocele, polycystic kidneys and polydactyly as an autosomal recessive trait simulating certain other disorders, the Meckel Syndrome. *Ann. Genet.,* 14: 97, 1971.
47. Mehne, R. G. Three hydrocephalic newborns. *Arch. Pediatr.,* 78: 67, 1961.
48. Michejda, M., Hodgen, G. D. *In utero* diagnosis and treatment of nonhuman primate fetal skeletal anomalies I. Hydrocephalus. *JAMA,* 246: 1093–7, 1981.
49. Miskin, M., Rudd, N. L., Disthe, M. R., et al. Prenatal ultrasonic diagnosis of occipital encephalocele. *Am. J. Obstet. Gynecol.,* 130: 585–587, 1978.
50. Moore, K. L. *The Developing Human. Clinically Oriented Embryology.* W. B. Saunders, Philadelphia, 1977.
51. Morgan, C. L., Trough, W. S., Haney, A., et al. Applications of real-time ultrasound in

obstetrics: The linear and dynamically focussed phased arrays. *J. Clin. Ultrasound, 7:* 108–114, 1979.
52. Penrose, L. S. Genetics of anencephaly. *J. Ment. Defic. Res.,* 1: 4–15, 1957.
53. Robertson, R. D., Sarti, D. A., Brown, W. J., et al. Congenital hydrocephalus in two pregnancies following the birth of a child with neural tube defect: Aetiology and management. *J. Med. Genet.,* 18: 105–107, 1981.
54. Sabbagha, R. E., Tamura, R. K., Dalcompo, S., et al. Fetal cranial and craniocervical masses: Ultrasound characteristics and differential diagnosis. *Am. J. Obstet. Gynecol.,* 138: 511–517, 1980.
55. Sarma, V. Anencephalus of the fetus in obstetric practice. *Clin. Obstet. Gynecol.,* 6: 429–453, 1963.
56. Sever, J. L. Viral infections in pregnancy. *Clin. Obstet. Gynecol.,* 21: 477, 1978.
57. Stroker, E. M., and Harwood Nash, D. C. *Neuroradiology,* Chapter 105.
58. Tal, Y., Freigang, B., Dunn, H., et al. Dandy-Walker Syndrome: Analysis of 21 cases. *Dev. Med. Child Neurol.,* 22:189, 1980.
59. Volpe, J. J. Neonatal periventricular hemorrhage: past, present and future. *J. Pediatr.,* 92: 693–696, 1978.
60. Vraa-Jenses, J. Massive congenital intracranial teratoma. *Acta Neuropathol.,* 30: 271, 1974.
61. Wagner, J. A., Douglass L. H., and Slager, U. T. Dystocia caused by a fetal intracranial teratoma: Report of a case. *Obstet. Gynecol.,* 4: 647, 1954.
62. Wapner, R. J., Jurtz, A. B., Ross, R. D., and Jackson, L. G. Ultrasonographic parameters in the prenatal diagnosis of Meckel Syndrome. *Obstet. Gynecol.,* 57: 388–392, 1981.
63. Warkany, J. *Congenital Malformations,* pp. 189–200, Chicago Year Book, 1971.
64. Warkany, J., and Dignan, P. S. J. Congenital malformations: Microcephaly. *Ment. Retard. Rev.,* 5: 113, 1973.
65. Wenger, F. Venezuelan equine encephalitis. *Teratology,* 16: 359–362, 1977.

*Ultrasound Annual 1983*, edited by R. C.
Sanders and M. Hill. Raven Press, New York
© 1983.

# Ultrasonic Measurement of Human Umbilical Circulation in Various Pregnancy Complications

## P. Kirkinen and P. Jouppila

*Department of Obstetrics, University of Oulu, Oulu, Finland*

Investigation of the circulation in the human fetus has been greatly restricted by methodological difficulties, and consequently our knowledge of this topic is based mainly upon animal experiments, postnatal blood flow measurements, and the examination of aborted fetuses. However, in recent years, ultrasonography has made it possible to study the structure and dynamics of the human fetus *in utero*. It has been used to investigate the circulation in the fetal heart, aorta, and umbilical vessels (3, 5, 6, 8, 9, 19, 26). An important landmark in the investigation of fetal hemodynamics was the application of Doppler ultrasound to the measurement of blood flow in the umbilical circulation. Fitzgerald and Drumm described the use of continuous wave Doppler techniques for recording velocity signals from the umbilical cord (6). More recently, quantitative blood flow measurements in the fetus have been reported using pulsed Doppler ultrasound in combination with B-scan or real-time ultrasound (5, 8, 9, 17).

We have been using pulsed Doppler measurements of blood velocity in the fetal vessels in combination with real-time ultrasonic imaging since early 1980. The following is a summary of our main findings concerning blood flow volume measurements in the umbilical vein in different clinical conditions.

## METHOD

Our equipment comprises a direction-sensitive, single-channel 2 MHz pulsed Doppler instrument (Pedof, Vingmed A/S, Oslo, Norway) and a real-time ultrasonic scanner with a 3.5 MHz linear probe (Toshiba SAL 20). The principles of this system have been described previously by Eik-Nes et al. (4, 5). The fetal vessel of interest is visualized with real-time equipment, and the ultrasonic probe is placed parallel with the vessel being examined. The transducers are attached at a fixed angle of 50 degrees and so the angle between the vessel and the isonating Doppler beam is 50 degrees (Fig. 1).

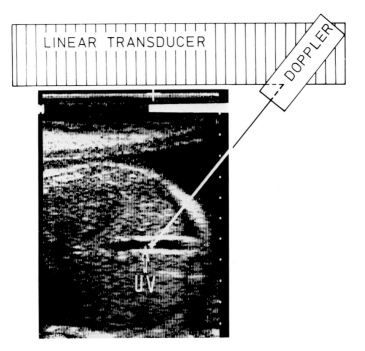

**FIG. 1.** Cross-sectional image at the level of fetal umbilical vein (UV) with a schematic illustration of the measurement of blood velocity. The black/white line represents the direction of the Doppler ultrasound pulse.

The umbilical vein and fetal aorta can be visualized in the third trimester of pregnancy in almost all patients.

Using the sample volume control of the Doppler instrument, it is possible to select the depth for the measurement of the Doppler shift signals so that the measurement is made only in the area of the vessel. Any interaction from other structures is filtered out and a high-pass filter of 150 Hz is used for cutting off signals from slowly moving structures such as vessel walls. On the basis of the mean Doppler shift over the cross section of the vessel ($f_d$), the Doppler instrument calculates the mean blood velocity ($V$), which is also dependent on the angle between the Doppler beam and the direction of the moving red cells inside the vessel ($\alpha$).

$$V = \frac{f_d \cdot c}{2 f_0 \cdot \cos \alpha}$$

where $c$ is the velocity of ultrasound in blood and $f_0$ is the operating frequency.

An audio output giving signals typical of the umbilical vein or fetal aorta is used to check the correct location of the sample volume position in the vessel. A spectrum analyzer (Kranzbuhler S-A 8106) is used to record the typical velocity profiles of these vessels. The diameter of the vessel is measured carefully from the real-time ultrasound image using electronic calipers, and the weight of the fetus is estimated from the biparietal diameter and abdominometry (9). Knowledge of the mean blood flow velocity, cross-sectional area of the vessel, and estimated weight of the fetus enables the blood flow value to be calculated in ml/min/kg of fetal weight.

$$\text{Flow} = \frac{\text{velocity} \times \text{area}}{\text{weight}}$$

## RESULTS OF MEASUREMENTS IN VARIOUS CLINICAL CONDITIONS

### Normal Pregnancy

The mean value for the blood flow volume in the umbilical vein at the beginning of the 3rd trimester of a normal pregnancy was 100 ml/min/kg of fetal weight. This result was based on measurements performed in 101 normal pregnancies (9). Blood velocity remained quite constant during the last trimester, at approximately 10 cm/sec, whereas the vein diameter increased slowly but steadily toward term (Fig. 2). The blood velocity was affected by fetal breathing movements. The flow volume/kg of fetal weight decreased slightly after the 36th gestational week. The distribution of the different velocity components in the velocity spectrum for the umbilical vein remained much the same for the whole of the last trimester and had the typical parabolic flow profile (Fig. 3).

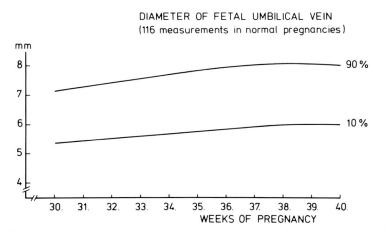

**FIG. 2.** Growth rate (90th and 10th percentiles) of the umbilical vein diameter from the 30th gestational week to term.

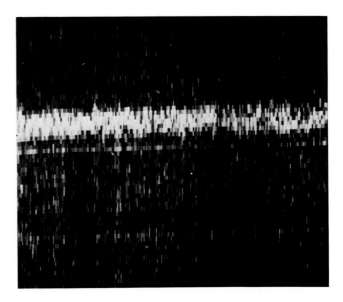

**FIG. 3.** Typical velocity spectrum from the umbilical vein in the last trimester of a normal pregnancy. *Horizontally:* time; *vertically:* Doppler shift frequencies.

### Fetal Growth Retardation

In 60 small-for-date fetuses (birth weight below the 10th percentile), there were 18 (31%) cases where the umbilical vein blood flow values (ml/min/kg) were below the normal range for the gestational week concerned (10). More than half of the severely retarded fetuses (birth weight below the 25th percentile) had a low umbilical vein blood flow. This study did not include growth-retarded fetuses with structural or chromosomal abnormalities. The main factor affecting the blood flow volume in fetal growth retardation was the vein diameter, which was below the normal range for size in 50% of cases. When growth impairment was associated with severe maternal preeclampsia, 69% had low umbilical vein blood flow values.

Eleven of these growth-impaired fetuses developed severe fetal distress before birth. The condition was diagnosed by abnormal findings in the cardiotocographic records. Delivery was by cesarian section and all the neonates had low Apgar scores ($\leq 7$). The umbilical vein blood flow was measured 1 to 12 hr before delivery and all 11 had low blood flow. In 3 cases, the narrowing of the umbilical vein was so extreme that the exact measurement of blood velocity was impossible. Low umbilical vein blood flow was also found in cases of maternal hypertension. When this was associated with severe fetal distress there were alterations in the shape of the velocity spectrum in the descending aorta of the fetus, possibly signifying increased peripheral resistance (Fig. 4).

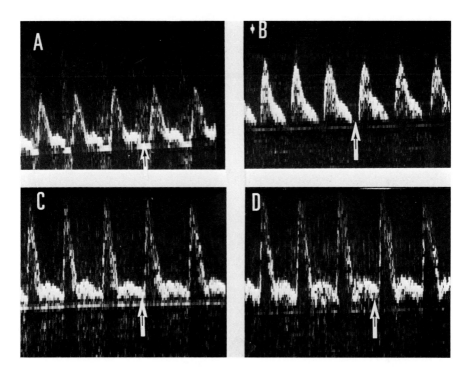

**FIG. 4.** Four different velocity spectrums from the fetal descending aorta at the 32nd to 34th gestational weeks. **A:** Severe preeclampsia with severe fetal growth retardation. **B:** Severe preeclampsia with severe fetal hypoxia and growth retardation; the measurement was made 4 hr before emergency cesarian section. **C:** Mild preeclampsia with incipient fetal growth retardation. **D:** Normal pregnancy with normally growing fetus. In severe preeclampsia the end-diastolic part *(arrows)* and the slope of the systolic part of the spectrum are different from normal pregnancy, probably reflecting the increased peripheral resistance.

## Rhesus-Isoimmunization

Since the publication of our preliminary report concerning alterations in umbilical vein blood flow in rhesus-isoimmunization (14), we have analyzed blood flow measurements in 20 pregnancies complicated by mild to severe fetal erythroblastosis (13). The severely isoimmunized fetuses were all born with a cord hemoglobin level below 140 g/liter and had significantly ($p <$ 0.05) higher umbilical vein blood flow values than the fetuses with mild isoimmunization and normal cord hemoglobins. This difference was mainly due to increased blood velocity; however, the severe cases also had relatively large umbilical vein diameters compared with those with mild isoimmunization.

We evaluated the effect of 8 intrauterine blood transfusions into the fetal peritoneal cavity on the umbilical vein blood flow. The flow increased after the transfusion in 7 cases, and the immediate increase was approximately 30%. Most of the cases demonstrated a gradual decrease in this flow over the next 7 days.

### Uterine Bleeding

Patients with uterine bleeding during the last trimester have an increase in umbilical vein blood flow. Out of 10 pregnancies with placenta previa and 9 with abruptio placentae, 13 had flow values above the normal 90th percentile (13). None of these cases had massive bleeding and in no instance was an emergency cesarian section necessary.

### Diabetes Mellitus and Intrahepatic Cholestasis of Pregnancy

No abnormalities were found in the umbilical vein blood flow in the 18 fetuses of diabetic mothers (White B-F) or in 13 mothers with latent diabetes mellitus (Fig. 5). Those patients with an abnormally high flow did not differ from those with normal flow levels and also did not differ with regard to the clinical severity of their diabetes. All the mothers except one in the group with abnormally low flow values had severe vascular complications of diabetes mellitus. Fourteen of 18 cases with intrahepatic cholestasis of pregnancy had a normal umbilical vein blood flow value. The remaining 4 fetuses had elevated blood flow while none had decreased flow.

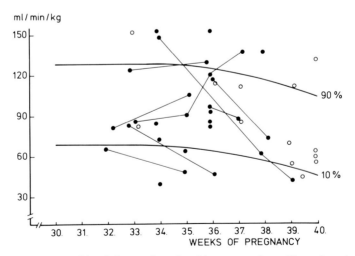

**FIG. 5.** Umbilical vein blood flow values for 31 pregnancies with maternal diabetes mellitus. *Solid circles:* White B-F. *Open circles:* White A. The values for a normal pregnancy are indicated by *dark lines.*

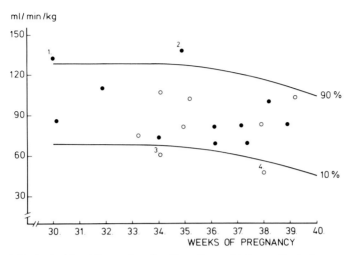

**FIG. 6.** Umbilical vein blood flow values for 19 malformed fetuses. Central nervous system anomalies are indicated by *solid circles*. 1, anencephaly; 2, hydrocephalus; 3, gastrointestinal tract atresia; 4, Muliberic nanismus.

## Fetal Abnormalities

Nineteen fetuses with congenital anomalies had normal umbilical vein blood flow levels (Fig. 6). This group included hydrocephalics (10), anencephalics (1), polycystic kidney disease (1), Potter syndrome (1), gastrointestinal tract atresias (3), cardiac anomaly (1), Muliberic nanismus (1), and 1 fetus with multiple anomalies.

## Effect of Certain Chemical Factors

We have evaluated the effect of certain chemical factors on the fetoplacental circulation. The intervillous flow (examined by a $^{131}$Xe-clearance method) and the umbilical vein blood flow were investigated in 20 pregnant patients before and 30 minutes after the maternal intake of coffee containing 200 mg of caffeine (15, 21). A significant ($p < 0.05$) decrease in the intervillous blood flow was noted, but the umbilical vein blood flow was not impaired. Similarly, short-term oxygen inhalation by the mother resulted in a significant decrease in the intervillous blood circulation ($p < 0.01$) among 22 pregnant women whereas the fetal umbilical vein flow was unchanged (11). The acute effect of one cigarette smoked by the mother upon umbilical vein blood flow was insignificant (12). Preliminary results concerning the effects of the intravenous administration of dihydralazine on the mother seem to show that the hemodynamic response in the placental and fetal circulation is variable with no clear trend in alteration noted.

## Clinical Aspects of Umbilical Blood Flow Measurements

The combination of real-time and pulsed Doppler ultrasound offers a non-invasive and repeatable means of studying the umbilical vein circulation of the human fetus in its physiological environment (4). The results for normal pregnancies obtained by different groups using this method are quite comparable, and conform well with earlier findings from animal and human experiments (1, 5, 8, 17, 23, 25). This confirms that there is a rational basis for applying this methodology to the evaluation of different kinds of complications that can occur in pregnancy. Even though our knowledge of the human umbilical circulation and its regulation is incomplete, one has to be careful when interpreting these early results and one should not attempt to draw any firm conclusions regarding their sensitivity, specificity, or predictive value.

A major finding in our measurements was the association between a low umbilical vein blood flow and poor fetal growth. It has been claimed that 75% of intrauterine growth retardation is connected with a reduced vascular or nutritional supply to the fetus, whereas 25% is due to a reduced growth potential of the fetus itself, e.g., for genetic reasons (16). We demonstrated a clear connection between severe maternal hypertension and reduced blood flow in the umbilical circulation. This reduction in placental blood circulation results in a hypoxic fetal environment, thus slowing its normal rate of growth (18). It has been shown in animal experiments that many alterations in fetal dynamics occur with hypoxia, e.g., redistribution of blood flow between the various organs, alterations in blood pressure, changes in portal and hepatic circulation, and hematological changes (1, 22, 24, 25).

Our cases of growth retardation were mainly severe and represented the extreme effects of this process. It is probable that the fetal response at the beginning of growth retardation, even before it is clinically possible to diagnose this condition, may be different from that noted in the final stages of the process. Knowledge of the changes in fetal hemodynamics that precede growth impairment might be of clinical value in the early diagnosis of high risk cases. Analysis of the velocity spectrum in the umbilical artery or in the fetal aorta may be one early diagnostic possibility, as suggested by McCallum, who noted alterations in the pulsatile index in hypertensive pregnancies (19). Extreme constriction of the umbilical vein lumen is a warning of imminent fetal demise in a fetus with fetal distress and growth retardation associated with material hypertension.

An alteration in the fetal growth profile, without any marked alteration in placental hemodynamics, seems to have little or no affect on the umbilical circulation. The flow values associated with fetal malformations in our series included small-for-date fetuses, which for the most part had a normal umbilical vein blood flow. The reduction in the maternal contribution to the placental circulation in cases of diabetes with vascular complications was reflected in a low umbilical vein blood flow. The chemical environment of the fetus is different in a diabetic pregnancy and may be reflected by changes in fetal hemodynamics, e.g., through alterations in blood viscosity (7). This may account for the great variation in umbilical vein blood flow values in our diabetic patients.

In contrast to growth retardation of the fetus, fetal anemia was associated with an increase in the umbilical blood circulation. In cases with abruptio placentae and placenta previa, uterine bleeding is known to produce a reduction in the amount of fetal blood (2). It may be that the increase in umbilical vein blood flow volume in cases of fetal anemia is a compensatory phenomenon secondary to hemolysis or hypovolemia and that it takes place without any alteration in the fetal pulse rate. Umbilical vein flow measurements can be used to evaluate the fetus with rhesus-isoimmunization after an intraperitoneal blood transfusion. The decrease in flow values after this procedure may reflect a gradual improvement in fetal hemoglobin levels.

Investigation of the effects of pharmacological agents on the fetal hemodynamics *in vivo* is also possible by this method. Routine obstetrical practice, for example, entails the use of many antihypertensive agents but the effects of these drugs on the fetus are largely unknown. We have looked at the effects of dihydralazine, caffeine, smoking, and oxygen inhalation on the umbilical circulation. The umbilical circulation appears fairly resistant to these agents despite some alteration in the maternal and even the placental hemodynamics. We are still in the early stages of investigating the pharmacological aspects of fetal hemodynamics. One example of this is the recent report demonstrating a direct relationship between umbilical vein blood flow and the ability of the umbilical vessels to produce a prostaglandin derivative (prostacyclin) (20).

## REFERENCES

1. Assali, N. S., Rauramo, L., and Peltonen, T. (1960): Measurement of uterine blood flow and uterine metabolism. *Am. J. Obstet. Gynecol.*, 79: 86–98.
2. Clayton, E. M., Pryor, J. A., Wierdsma, J., and Whitacre, F. E. (1964): Fetal and maternal components in third-trimester obstetric hemorrhage. *Obstet. Gynecol.*, 24: 56–60.
3. De Vore, G. R., Donnerstein, R. L., Kleinman, C. S., Platt, L. D., and Hobbins, J. C. (1982): Fetal echocardiography. I. Normal anatomy as determined by real-time-directed M-mode ultrasound. *Am. J. Obstet. Gynecol.*, 144: 249–260.
4. Eik-Nes, S. H., Marsal, K., Kristofferson, K., and Vernersson, E. (1981): Transcutaneous measurement of human fetal blood flow—methodological studies. In: *Recent Advances in Ultrasound Diagnosis*, Vol. 3, edited by A. Kurjak and A. Kratochwil, pp. 209–219. Excerpta Medica, Amsterdam.
5. Eik-Nes, S. H., Marsal, K., Brubakk, A. O., Kristofferson, K., and Ulstein, M. (1982): Ultrasonic measurement of human fetal blood flow. *J. Biomed. Engng.*, 4: 28–36.
6. Fitzgerald, D. E., and Drumm, J. E. (1977): Non-invasive measurement of human fetal circulation using ultrasound: a new method. *Br. Med. J.*, 2: 1450–1451.
7. Foley, M. E., Collins, R., Stronge, J. M., Drury, M. I., and MacDonald, D. (1981): Blood viscosity in umbilical cord blood from babies of diabetic mothers. *J. Obstet. Gynecol.* 2: 93–96.

8. Gill, R. W., Trudinger, B. J., Garrett, W., Kossoff, G., and Warren, P. S. (1981): Fetal umbilical venous flow measured in utero by pulsed Doppler and B-mode ultrasound. *Am. J. Obstet. Gynecol.*, 139: 720–725.

9. Jouppila, P., Kirkinen, P., Eik-Nes, S., and Koivula, A. (1981): Fetal and intervillous blood flow measurements in late pregnancy. In: *Recent Advances in Ultrasound Diagnosis, Vol.* 3, edited by A. Kurjak, and A. Kratochwil, pp. 226–233. Excerpta Medica, Amsterdam.

10. Jouppila, P., and Kirkinen, P. (1982): Human fetal blood flow of the umbilical vein in pregnancy complications. In: *Abstracts of the International Symposium of Dilemmas in Gestosis, Vienna, 1982*, p. 52.

11. Jouppila, P., Kirkinen, P., Koivula, A., and Jouppila, R. (1982): The effect of maternal oxygen inhalation on blood flow in the intervillous space and fetal umbilical vein and descending aorta. *Ultrasound Med. Biol.*, 8(Suppl. 1): 92.

12. Jouppila, P., Kirkinen, P., and Eik-Nes, S. H. (1983): Acute effect of maternal smoking on the human fetal blood flow. *Br. J. Obstet. Gynecol.*, 90: 7–10.

13. Jouppila, P., and Kirkinen, P. (1983): Umbilical vein blood flow in the human fetus in cases of maternal and fetal anemia and uterine bleeding. *Ultrasound Med. Biol. (in press)*.

14. Kirkinen, P., Jouppila, P., and Eik-Nes, S. H. (1981): Umbilical venous flow as indicator of fetal anemia. *Lancet*, 2: 1004–1005.

15. Kirkinen, P., Jouppila, P., and Puukka, M. (1982): Effects of caffeine on fetoplacental circulation in human pregnancy. In: *Abstracts of XXII Kongressen, Nordisk Förening för obstetric och gynecologi, Helsinki, 1982*, No. 130.

16. Kurjak, A., Latin, V., and Polak, J. (1978): Ultrasonic recognition of two types of growth retardation by measurement of four types fetal dimensions. *J. Perinat. Med.*, 6: 102–108.

17. Kurjak, A., and Rajhvajn, B. (1982): Ultrasonic measurements of umbilical blood flow in normal and complicated pregnancies. *J. Perinat. Med.*, 10: 3–16.

18. Käär, K., Luotola, H., and Jouppila, R. (1980): Placental blood flow by an intravenous [133]Xe-method in complicated late pregnancy. *Acta Obstet. Gynecol. Scand.*, 59: 7–14.

19. McCallum, W. D., Williams, C. S., Napel, S., and Daigle, R. E. (1978): Fetal blood velocity waveforms. *Am. J. Obstet. Gynecol.*, 132: 425–429.

20. Mäkilä, U–M., Jouppila, P., Kirkinen, P., Viinikka, L., and Ylikorkala, O. (1983): Umbilical prostacyclin production may determine umbilical blood flow in humans. *Lancet (in press)*.

21. Rekonen, A., Luotola, H., Pitkänen, M., Kuikka, J., and Pyörälä, T. (1976): Measurement of intervillous and myometrial blood flow by an intravenous [133]Xe-method. *Br. J. Obstet. Gynecol.*, 83: 723–728.

22. Reuss, M. L., and Rudolph, A. M. (1980): Distribution and recirculation of umbilical and systemic venous blood flow in fetal lambs during hypoxia. *J. Develop. Physiol.*, 2: 71–84.

23. Rudolph, A. M., Heymann, M., Teramo, K., Barrett, C. T., and Räihä, M. (1971): Studies on the circulation of the previable human fetus. *Pediatr. Res.*, 5: 452–456.

24. Rudolph, A. M., Itskovits, J., Iwamoto, H., Reuss, L. M., and Heymann, M. (1981): Fetal cardiovascular responses to stress. *Semin. Perinatol.*, 5: 109–121.

25. Stembera, Z. K., Hodr, J., and Janda, J. (1968): Umbilical blood flow in newborn infants who suffer intrauterine hypoxia. *Am. J. Obstet. Gynecol.* 101: 546–554.

26. Wladimiroff, J. W., Vosters, K., and McGhie, J. S. (1982): Ultrasonic assessment of fetal cardiovascular geometry and function. *Br. J. Obstet. Gynecol.*, 89: 839–844.

*Ultrasound Annual 1983,* edited by R. C. Sanders and M. Hill. Raven Press, New York © 1983.

# The Uses of Sonography for Monitoring Ovarian Follicular Development

*Arthur C. Fleischer, †Donald E. Pittaway, †Anne Colson Wentz, *Gary A. Thieme, *Albert L. Bundy, †Wayne S. Maxson, †James F. Daniell, †Charles E. Torbit, †John E. Repp, and *A. Everette James, Jr.

*Department of Radiology and Radiological Sciences, Ultrasound Section, and †Department of Obstetrics and Gynecology, Center for Fertility and Reproductive Research, Vanderbilt University Medical Center, Nashville, Tennessee 37232*

The recent births of children conceived by *in vitro* fertilization and embryo transfer (IVF-ET) has generated much public interest in this procedure. It has been estimated that some 500,000 couples in the United States are infertile owing to tubal occlusion, and might benefit from this technique (1, 42). Many patients with ovulation disorders are being treated with a variety of medications for ovulation induction while artificial insemination is being utilized in couples with male infertility disorders. With the recent improvements in resolution of real-time sonographic imaging, this has allowed the sonologist to detect and follow the growth of human ovarian follicles (32). Sonographic information concerning the number, size, and location of these follicles has significant clinical implications in the management and treatment of a variety of infertility disorders that utilize ovulation induction, timed artificial insemination, and IVF-ET. This review will focus on the use of sonography for monitoring follicular development in patients undergoing ovulation induction and on other potential applications of this technique. The information and opinions expressed are based on over 4 years' experience with sonographic evaluation of the ovary in spontaneous cycles, during ovulation induction, and in women undergoing timed insemination. The use of sonography in IVF-ET will be emphasized.

## CLINICAL BACKGROUND

As many as 1 out of every 5 couples in this country experiences some type of fertility disorder (2). A couple is considered to be "infertile" if conception does not occur after 1 year of unprotected intercourse (2). Infertility in the male accounts for one-third of these cases. The commonest female causes for infertility are tubal disease, i.e., adhesions, endometriosis (30 to 40%), an ovulation abnormality (10%), cervical factors (10 to 15%), and luteal phase abnormalities (5%) (44). Sonography can be used in infertile patients to not only monitor follicular development but also to diagnose other causes of infertility, such as hydrosalpinx, uterine fibroid, tubo-ovarian abscess, endometrioma, and polycystic ovarian disease (3, 40, 41).

In ovulatory disorders, either clomiphene citrate (Clomid®, Serophene®)* or human menopausal gonadotropin (HMG) (Pergonal®)† alone or in combination are used for ovulation induction (37). The exact mechanism of action of clomiphene is probably multifactorial but, as a generalization, it promotes follicle stimulating hormone (FSH) release from the pituitary (2). HMG is derived from the urine of postmenopausal women and contains FSH.

The IVF-ET procedure is reserved for patients with totally occluded or absent fallopian tubes or where there is severe oligospermia. Artificial insemination by a donor is used when infertility can be traced to a sperm disorder.

Sonography has an important role in ovulation induction, artificial insemination, and IVF-ET. It can: (a) detect the presence or absence of mature preovulatory follicles and, when present, establish their number, size, and location; (b) monitor the growth of the follicles so that human chorionic gonadotropin (HCG) can be administered at the proper time to induce final maturation and ovulation of the oocyte; (c) determine if the follicles have developed on a particular side when tubal patency is unilateral or when only one ovary is accessible laparoscopically; (d) assess the follicle and cul-de-sac for the presence or absence of ovulation; and (e) direct transabdominal follicular aspiration using real-time sonography in selected patients.

## INSTRUMENTATION AND SCANNING TECHNIQUE

Ever since the first description of sonographic delineation of the ovary, potential applications of this painless, biologically innocuous, and repeatable diagnostic modality have been recognized (4). Although the ovary could be delineated in the majority of patients with articulated arm scanners, real-time sonography has made possible practical, reliable routine delineation of the ovary (Figs. 1A, B, C) (5). We recommend the use of a mechanical real-time sector scanner as it allows rapid adjustment of the scanning plane while, at the same time, having excellent resolution. Its pie-shaped beam optimally delineates the adnexal structures including the ovary and its follicle, along with the iliac vessels and distal ureter in the pelvis (Fig. 1C) (6). Peristalsis can also be identified, thus helping to differentiate fluid-filled loops of bowel from cystic adnexal structures (see Fig. 11F).

---

*Clomid®—Merrill National Inc., Cincinnati, OH. Serophene®—Serono Inc., Braintree, MA.
†Pergonal®—Serono Inc., Braintree, MA.

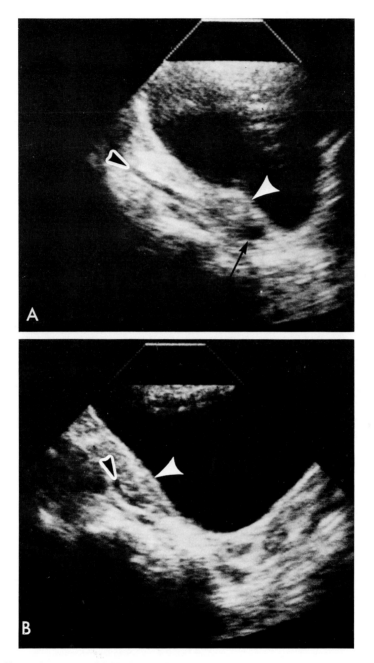

**FIG. 1.** Normal ovary and follicle. **A:** Modified longitudinal real-time sonogram of a patient demonstrating immature follicle *(small black arrow)* within right ovary *(white arrowhead)*. The right ovary *(arrowhead)* can be identified by its position immediately anterior to the distal ureter *(black arrowhead)*, internal iliac artery and vein. **B:** Longitudinal real-time sonogram of same patient demonstrating left ovary *(white arrowhead)*. This ovary does not contain any preovulatory follicles but can also be identified by its proximity to the internal iliac vein *(black arrowhead)*.

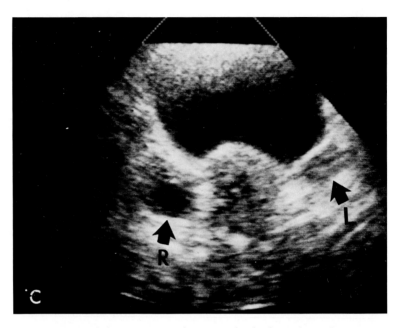

**FIG. 1C.** Transverse real-time sonogram demonstrating both ovaries and uterus. A mature preovulatory follicle is present within the right ovary (R) in this spontaneously ovulating patient (L = left ovary).

A high frequency transducer that has its focal range in the region of the ovary should be used, and we recommend a 3.5- or 5-MHz transducer with a medium or long internal focus. The region of interest should be magnified as this allows accurate measurements of the follicles to be made in three dimensions. The follicles can be measured either with the digital calipers, which can be manipulated on the screen by a joystick, or by manual measurement of the follicles comparing their size to the centimeter gradations along the periphery of the image. Theoretically, the most accurate measurements are obtained using the digital calipers since the centimeter gradations along the periphery of the image are distorted by the camera and by the TV optics. Using the digital calipers does prolong the examination and this is especially true when numerous follicles are present.

The patient must have a fully distended bladder for optimal delineation of the uterus, ovaries, and cul-de-sac. It has been our experience that the ability to visualize the ovary depends upon the amount of bladder distention and accounts for the day-to-day variations in the location of the ovary. A fully distended bladder displaces any intervening structures between the bladder and the ovary and it optimizes the angle at which the ovaries can be visualized, which may be from the side of the bladder opposite to the ovary being examined. We perform our examinations with the greatest degree of bladder distention that can be reasonably tolerated by the patient.

A sonographic examination for follicular development is started in the transverse plane as the ovaries can be identified on both sides of the uterus (Fig. 1A). Finding them on a transverse scan is less dependent upon scan angulation than on a longitudinal scan. Once adequate images of the ovaries are obtained, modified longitudinal or parasagittal scans are performed utilizing a slight angulation to the opposite side (Figs. 1B, C). For example, if the right ovary is examined, it is usually best approached by placing the transducer slightly to the left of midline and angling it to the right side wall. In this longitudinal plane, the pulsations of the internal iliac artery and vein can be identified in most patients along with the distal ureter. These anatomic landmarks typically lie posterior to the ovary (Fig. 1C).

A complete examination can be recorded on one transparent film using a 9 on 1 format. A black background is preferred since this enhances visual perception of the boundaries of the follicles. Two to three images of each ovary in its long and short axis are obtained along with one or two images of the uterus in its long axis to document flexion of the uterus, thickening of the endometrium, and the presence or absence of an endometrial or cul-de-sac fluid collection. Each follicle should be measured carefully in its long, short, and anteroposterior dimensions. Although some have advocated the calculation of intrafollicular volume by assuming that the volume of a follicle is a prolate ellipsoid (length × width × height × 0.523), we feel that an average dimension in millimeters is sufficient (7). Theoretically, calculation of the intrafollicular volume would be helpful to the laparoscopist who could determine whether or not the contents of a particular follicle had been completely aspirated by checking the volume of the aspirate that was collected (Fig. 2B) (7, 33).

Since the ovaries of a patient undergoing ovulation induction often contain two or more preovulatory follicles, we recommend that the same individual scan and interpret the sonogram to decrease intraobserver error. Otherwise, in patients with multiple follicles, it may be difficult to keep straight the location and size of the various follicles. We communicate the results of the sonogram as soon as they are available to the referring clinician. The clinician combines the results of the sonographic data with hormonal and other biochemical and clinical parameters to make appropriate decisions regarding the patient's management.

## NORMAL SPONTANEOUS CYCLES

Before discussing the sonographic findings of follicular development in induced cycles, we will review the findings observed in the normal, spontaneously ovulating woman. The ovaries may be difficult to recognize in the early (follicular phase) of the cycle when the follicles are very small and isoechoic with the ovary and surrounding muscle and fat. The presence of one or more preovulatory follicles facilitates sonographic evaluation of the

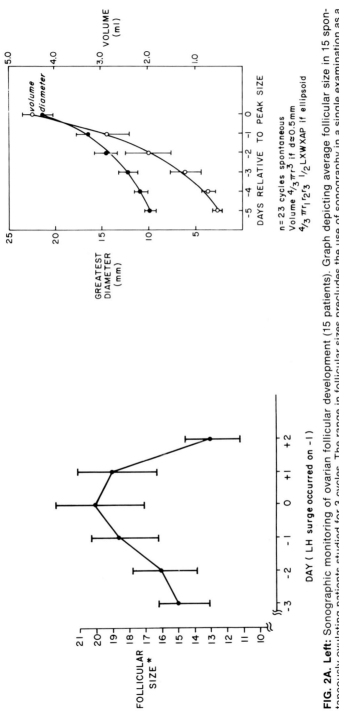

**FIG. 2A. Left:** Sonographic monitoring of ovarian follicular development (15 patients). Graph depicting average follicular size in 15 spontaneously ovulating patients studied for 3 cycles. The range in follicular sizes precludes the use of sonography in a single examination as a means to assess follicular maturation (*average dimension in mm).

**FIG. 2B. Right:** Graph depicting greatest follicular diameter and volume in 23 spontaneously cycling patients. (Reproduced with permission, from ref. 7.)

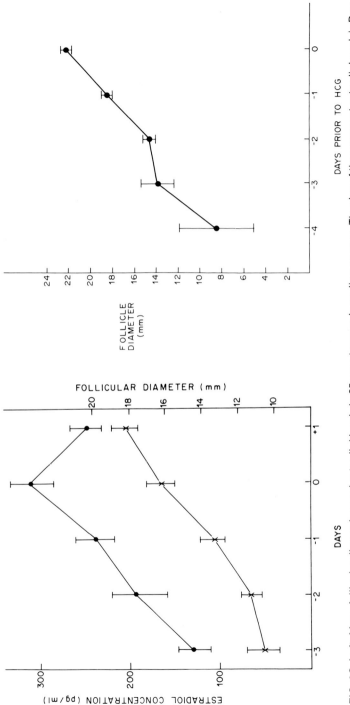

**FIG. 2C. Left:** Mean follicular dimension and estradiol levels in 25 spontaneously cycling women. The day of the apparent estradiol peak is Day 0. Ovulation would be expected to occur on days +1 or +2. The mean and standard deviation are indicated.

**FIG. 2D. Right:** Mean follicular dimension in 28 women who received clomiphene. Day 0 designates when HCG was administered. The follicles were slightly larger and grew faster than in spontaneous cycles (46).

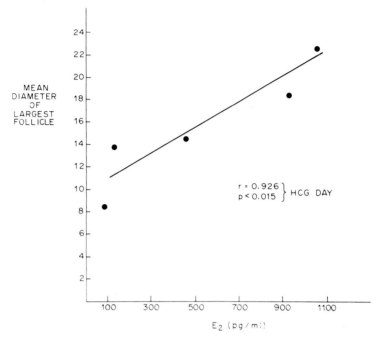

**FIG. 2E.** Correlation between mean follicle dimension and mean $E_2$ according to day of HCG administration. Follicular size and estradiol levels in 28 women who received clomiphene. There is a nearly linear relationship between follicular size and E2 levels.

ovary as the anechoic follicular fluid contrasts sharply with the surrounding ovarian stroma (Figs. 1A, B).

Follicular development occurs in response to two hormones produced by the pituitary—the follicle stimulating hormone (FSH) and luteinizing hormone (LH). A slight increase in FSH prior to menstruation is believed to initiate early follicular development, whereas oocyte maturation and ovulation occur in response to LH. A sharp rise in LH occurs prior to ovulation and detection of this LH "surge" by serial assays is an accurate method of predicting ovulation which usually occurs within 29 hrs (range 22 to 36 hr) (29). The estradiol (E2) produced by the granulosa cells slowly increases as the follicle matures. However, the serum levels of E2 do not correlate with the number and size of the developing follicles. Thus, the sonographic data concerning the number and size of maturing follicles is important in the correct interpretation of E2 levels (46). Progesterone, which is produced primarily by the corpus luteum, increases during the latter half of the menstrual cycle.

Each ovary contains hundreds of oocytes. Although more than one immature follicle may begin to develop in the early follicular phase, usually only one oocyte-containing follicle matures and ovulates in each cycle (Figs. 3A,

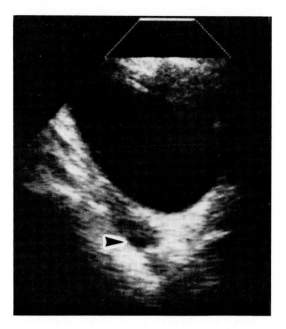

**FIG. 3.** Growth of a preovulatory follicle. **A.** Longitudinal real-time sonogram on cycle day 6 demonstrating a small, immature, preovulatory follicle *(black arrowhead)* in the posterior portion of the left ovary.

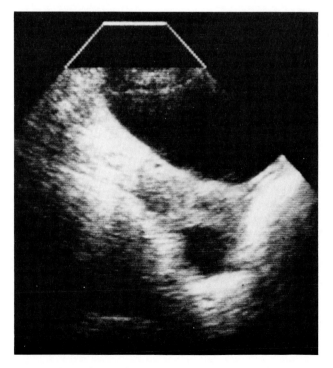

**FIG. 3B.** Same follicle on day 11 demonstrating marked enlargement of the follicle.

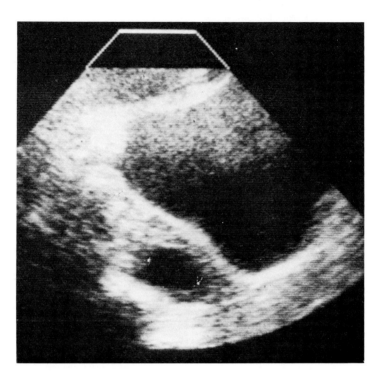

**FIG. 3C.** Same patient on day 14 demonstrating interval enlargement of the preovulatory follicle which now averages 21 mm in diameter. This image is slightly magnified when compared to Figs. 3A and B.

B, C). The typical preovulatory follicle appears as a small anechoic area within the ovary, measuring approximately 10 mm in dimension. As the follicle matures under the influence of FSH and LH it grows by approximately 2 to 3 mm per day and at maturity measures approximately 20 mm in average dimension (Figs. 2A, 3A, B, C) (5, 8).

The data from several studies in which the size of the mature preovulatory follicle was measured has shown a substantial variation ranging from 10 to 27 mm (Table 1) (8–14). Some of this discrepancy is due to the difference in bladder distention, variations in the resolutions of the scanners used, and in the technique by which the follicle was measured. The average follicular size of a mature preovulatory follicle cited in these reports (19.8 mm) is similar to our data (20.0 mm) (5, 7–14, 30). Microscopic and hormonal analysis of the follicle and its fluid agree with this figure and indicate that the mature preovulatory follicle in spontaneously ovulating women ranges from 18–25 mm in average dimension (18). Our study of patients undergoing mid-cycle capture also found that follicular size averaged 18.2 mm when E2 levels peaked (48).

TABLE 1. *Mean values of follicles in normal women[a]*

| Principal investigator (Ref.) | No. of pts (Cycles monitored) | Mean values (mm) |
|---|---|---|
| Hackeloer (8) | 15 (15) | 19.8 |
| Renaud (9) | 10 (18) | 27.0 |
| Ylostalo (10) | 7 (7) | 12.8 |
| Hall (11) | 16 (20) | 10.0 |
| Christie (12) | 6 | 16.0 |
| Kurjak (13) | 25 (25) | 20.6 |
| Smith (14) | 13 (20) | 25.0 |
| Fleischer (5) | 15 (45) | 20.0 |
| O'Herlihy (30) | 17 (28) | 20.1 |
| Queenan (7) | 18 (21) | 23.0[b] |
| Average (mm) | | 19.8 |

[a]Adapted from ref. 13.
[b]Greatest diameter.

The mature 20-mm preovulatory follicle is anechoic, has smooth borders, and is spherical or slightly oval in shape. It is typically located along the periphery of the ovary. Only the most peripheral portion of it may be seen on laparoscopic examination, thus accounting for the minor discrepancy in the estimation of follicular size on sonography versus laparoscopy (15). Occasionally, the cumulus oophorus can be identified as a rounded intrafollicular structure, approximately 1 mm in size, along the border of the follicle (Figs. 4A, B). The oocyte itself measures only one-tenth of a millimeter and is contained within the cumulus and is below the resolution capabilities of present-day sonographic equipment. Just prior to ovulation, a sonolucent line within the wall of the follicle may be detected and is thought to correspond to edema between the theca and granulosa cell layers as they begin to separate (36). As ovulation approaches, the oocyte and its surrounding granulosa cells become free within the follicular fluid. In rare instances, this change in the location of the cumulus can be detected sonographically. Crenation or notching of the wall occurs immediately after ovulation and probably corresponds to the folded and thickened wall of the collapsed follicle (Figs. 5A, B, C). In addition, internal echoes that arise from blood in the follicle may be observed. The ovulated fluid (3 to 5 cc) may initially layer around the follicle but eventually collects in the cul-de-sac (Figs. 5D, E, F) (11). Intraperitoneal blood from a recent ovulation is anechoic, whereas clotted blood is usually moderately echogenic (Figs. 5G, H).

Variations in the sonographic features of follicular maturation, ovulation, and corpus luteum formation have been reported (7). In some patients, after ovulation the follicle may remain anechoic and smooth-walled and may actually appear larger due to the accumulation of blood (Fig. 6). This sonographic appearance might be expected in women in whom the follicle fails to

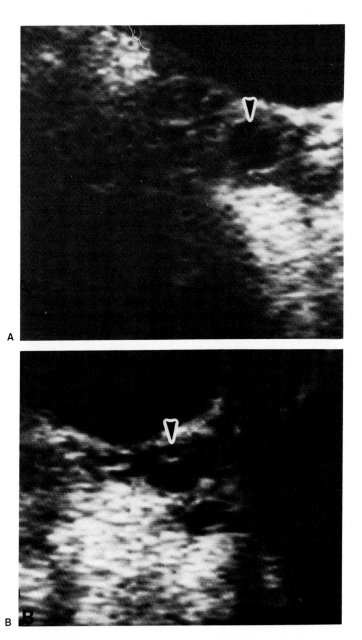

**FIG. 4.** Mature, preovulatory follicle. **A:** Magnified, longitudinal real-time sonogram demonstrating a mature preovulatory follicle. Within the follicle, the cumulous oophorus can be identified *(arrowhead)*. **B:** Transverse image of same follicle demonstrating cumulous *(arrowhead)*.

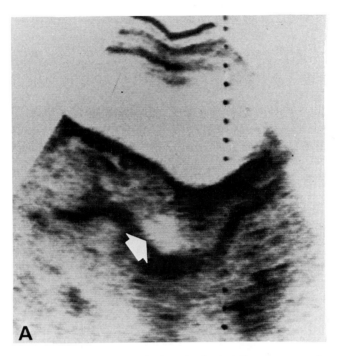

FIG. 5. Sonographic findings in ovulation. A: Longitudinal static sonogram of mature, preovulatory follicle *(arrowhead)*.

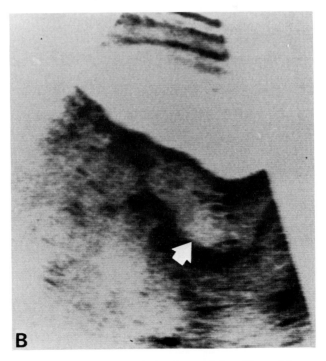

FIG. 5B. Same follicle *(arrow)*, approximately 24 hr after ovulation. The wall is crenated or notched and low level echoes can be identified within the follicle.

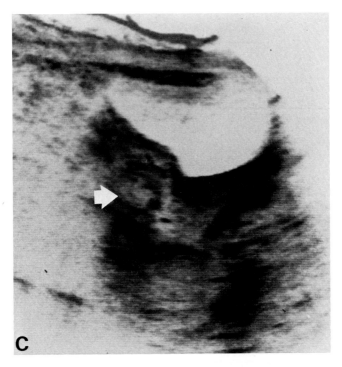

**FIG. 5C.** Same follicle *(arrow)* approximately 3 days after ovulation. The wall of the follicle is thickened, a sign of luteinization.

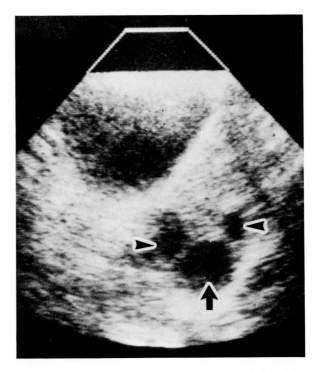

**FIG. 5D.** Transverse real-time sonogram of left ovary prior to ovulation. A mature preovulatory follicle is present *(large arrow)* with two smaller immature follicles *(arrowheads)*.

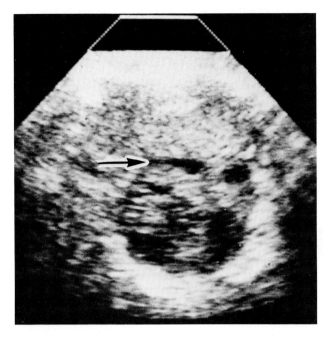

**FIG. 5E.** Immediately prior to laparoscopy, this sonographic study demonstrated the interval development of internal echoes within two follicles as well as a sliver of fluid anterior to one of the ovulated follicles *(arrow)*.

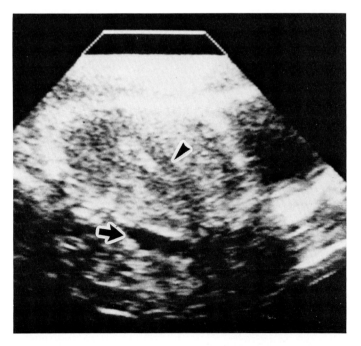

**FIG. 5F.** Transverse sonogram of same patient demonstrating small collection of blood *(large arrow)* between the ovary and uterus resulting from ovulation of one of the follicles. The endometrium *(arrowhead)* is thickened and hypoechoic when compared to the myometrium. The endometrial surface appears as a thin, echogenic interface.

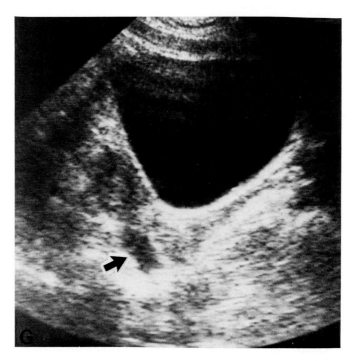

**FIG. 5G.** Longitudinal real-time sonogram demonstrating a moderately echogenic collection posterior to the uterus *(arrow)*. At laparoscopy, clotted blood probably from an ovulation during a previous cycle was found.

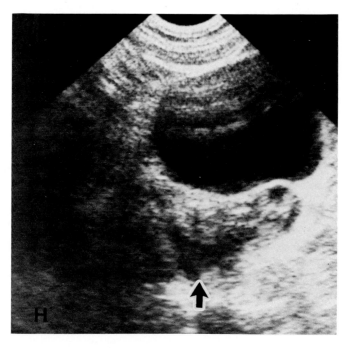

**FIG. 5H.** Transverse sonogram of patient depicted in Fig. 5G demonstrating the sonographic appearance of clotted blood in the cul-de-sac.

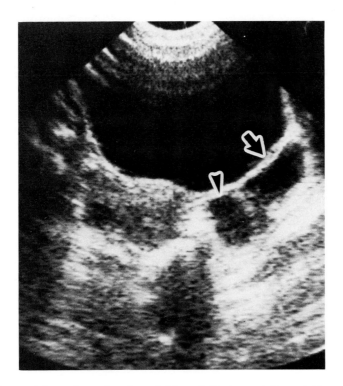

**FIG. 6.** Corpus luteum *(arrowhead)* medial to a follicular cyst *(arrow).* The wall of the follicle is thickened and notched ("crenated"). A "fresh" corpus luteum was found at laparoscopy.

rupture after the oocyte is mature (the so-called luteinized unruptured ovum syndrome) (26, 45). In other patients the follicle may be difficult to identify after ovulation as it may be isoechoic with the remainder of the ovary.

In a spontaneously ovulating patient, usually only one follicle matures and ovulates in each cycle. It is not known whether follicular development occurs within the same ovary or alternates between the ovaries. It has been suggested that the presence of a corpus luteum in one ovary may inhibit follicular development in that ovary during the next menstrual cycle. We believe that follicular development alternates from one ovary to the other, and establishing this sequence by sonography may be advantageous in the woman with a unilaterally patent Fallopian tube.

Serial examinations of spontaneously cycling women with sonographic and hormonal assays have shown that there is a significant variation in follicular growth and LH levels among the patients studied (29). In one study as many as 35% of the cycles had a significantly reduced estradiol and progesterone level and abnormal follicular development despite a biphasic basal body temperature curve and normal cycle length. In those patients who were studied for several cycles, each patient exhibited a similar pattern of follicular development (29). Thus, sonography seems to have the potential to detect subtle abnormalities in patients with ovulation disorders and may have a role in assessing the efficacy of certain treatment regimens (28).

## OVULATION INDUCTION

Ovulation disorders account for approximately 10% of gynecological infertility. At present in this country, the number of patients undergoing ovulation induction for ovulation disorders is greater than the number of patients that undergo ovulation induction in IVF-ET protocols. Therefore, the use of sonography in evaluating patients undergoing ovulation induction is potentially more extensive than its use in IVF-ET programs.

The two most widely utilized medications for ovulation induction are clomiphene citrate and human menopausal gonadotropin (HMG). Clomiphene citrate promotes the development of multiple mature preovulatory follicles whereas HMG tends to accelerate maturation of several oocytes which may be contained within several relatively small follicles (37). In patients undergoing ovulation induction, usually more than one follicle develops and reaches maturity. Sonography has an important role in detecting the number of follicles that are maturing, as well as localizing which ovary contains mature follicles (Figs. 7A, B, C, D). This information is important

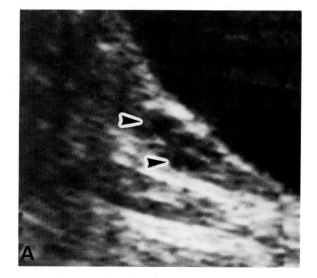

**FIG. 7.** Ovulation induction. **A:** Longitudinal real-time sonogram of the left ovary in a patient with polycystic ovaries who received ovulation induction medications. Only a few small immature follicles *(arrowheads)* are present after induction.

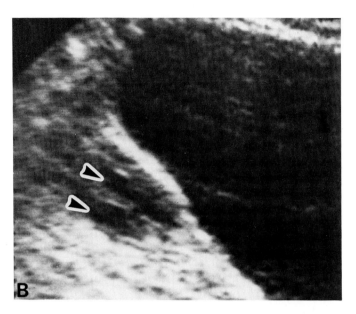

**FIG. 7B.** Real-time sonogram of same patient, 4 days later. The follicles *(arrowheads)* have not enlarged and have remained immature. Estradiol levels also failed to increase.

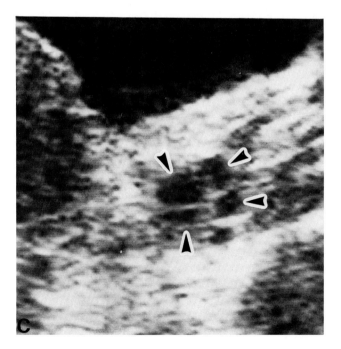

**FIG. 7C.** Transverse real-time sonogram of patient undergoing ovulation induction demonstrating a 10-mm follicle and 3 immature follicles *(arrowheads)* within the right ovary.

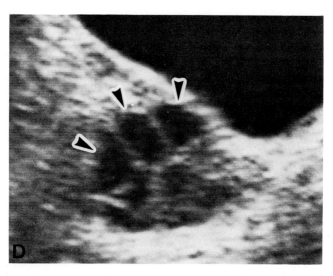

**FIG. 7D.** Same patient as in Fig. 7C, 4 days later, demonstrating interval enlargement of three follicles *(arrowheads)*.

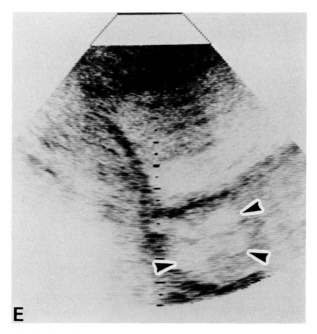

**FIG. 7E.** Poor stimulation in a patient with polycystic ovaries as demonstrated by the presence of multiple small, immature follicles *(arrowheads)* after 10 days of medication.

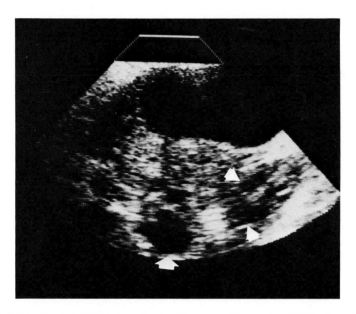

**FIG. 7F.** Adequate stimulation in patient with polycystic ovaries. Within the left ovary, multiple immature follicles *(small arrows)* are present. Within the right ovary, a mature preovulatory "dominate" follicle *(large arrow)* is present.

since, if a follicle is within an ovary on the side of an absent or diseased tube, the cycle in which conception is attempted may be postponed. Serial sonographic studies can also detect the adequacy of the follicular response to stimulation, especially in patients with polycystic ovaries. In these patients, multiple immature follicles may be present prior to induction. Optimally, only one or two dominant follicles should develop since these follicles are most likely to contain a mature oocyte (Figs. 7E, F, G). Failure of adequate follicular development can be depicted by sonography and usually correlates with a deficiency in the rise of the estradiol levels (Figs. 7E, F).

Although a few investigators have reported that the size of preovulatory follicle in stimulated patients is larger than those encountered in spontaneously ovulating women, the majority of recent studies have found no significant difference (Figs. 2A, 2C) (Table 2). The apparent reported discrepancy in follicular size is most likely related to the differences in measurements and scanning techniques. The rate at which follicular dimensions increase, however, appears to be greater in stimulated patients than in spontaneously ovulating women (Fig. 2B) (30, 47). Daily sonographic examinations in these patients is recommended since marked enlargement of the follicle can occur from day to day. We have seen patients in whom an earlier examination had shown a follicle no greater than 5 mm while 24 hr later this follicle had grown to 12 to 15 mm (Figs. 8A, B). Furthermore, in patients

TABLE 2. Average dimension (mm) of follicles in ovulation induction[a]

| Principal investigator (Ref.) | No. pts[b] | Mean follicular size (mm) | | |
|---|---|---|---|---|
| | | Type of Stimulation | | |
| | | Clomiphene | HMG | Bromocryptine |
| Ylostalo (10) | 12(C); 5(H) | 15.4 | 15.6 | |
| Renuard (11) | 29(C); 37(H) | 24.9 | 24.3 | |
| Christie (12) | 10(C); 4(B) | 18.0 | | 22.0 |
| Kurjak (13) | 70(C); 28(H); 2(B) | 22.4 | 22.8 | 23.0 |
| Nitschke— Dabelstein (24) | 20(C); 5(H); 10(B) | 22.6 | 22.0 | 21.0 |
| Picker (14) | 5(C) | 30.0 | | |
| Terinde (23) | 65(H) | | 22.0 | |
| O'Herlihy (30) | 17(C) | 21.4 | | |
| Vargyas (16) | 38(C) | 22.1 | | |
| | Average (mm) | 22.2 | 22.5 | 18.9 |

[a]Adapted from ref. 13.
[b]C = Clomiphene pts; H = HMG pts; B = Bromocryptine pts.

receiving HMG and HCG, a mature oocyte may be retrieved from follicles between 13 and 15 mm in dimension.

As opposed to the IVF patient who may require daily sonograms, patients who are undergoing ovulation induction may require only 1 or 2 sonographic examinations prior to the expected time of ovulation. Sonography is used to assess the number and size of the follicles since this cannot be assessed by estradiol levels alone. Since follicular size does not always correlate with the physiologic maturity of the follicle, the combined use of sonography with hormonal assays is necessary in determining follicular development. Sonography can be used to avoid ovarian hyperstimulation, which is likely to occur when ovulation induction with HCG is continued when multiple, small, immature follicles are present. As discussed previously, sonography can also be used in combination with other clinical and laboratory parameters to confirm the presence or absence of ovulation in patients undergoing ovulation induction in combination with timed artificial insemination.

When multiple follicles develop with ovulation induction, the ultrasound findings may be helpful in postponing insemination in cycles where 3 or more follicles are present. It is thought that the chance of developing a multiple pregnancy is increased when more than 3 follicles are delineated by ultrasound (34). In one study, ovulation was induced in three patients in whom 2 mature follicles were present; one developed a single intrauterine pregnancy, another a dizygotic twin pregnancy, while the final patient had a combined extrauterine pregnancy along with an intrauterine pregnancy that aborted (34).

Although the information gained from sonographic examination of the ovary is considerable, how much this data contributes to improved pregnan-

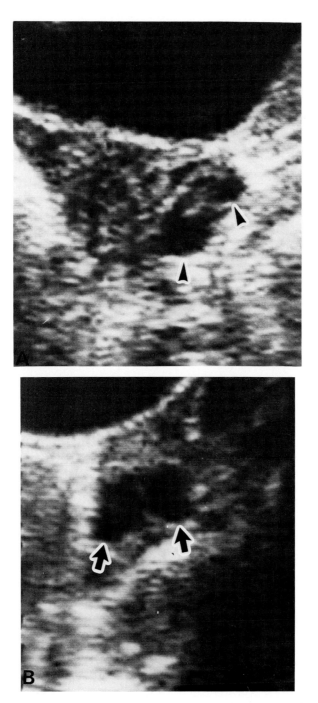

**FIG. 8A.** Transverse real-time sonogram of the left ovary in a patient undergoing ovulation induction showing a 5-mm and 10-mm follicle *(arrowheads).* **B:** Same patient next day demonstrating the presence of two mature follicles *(arrows).*

cy rates and which patients will benefit the most from this information is largely unknown.

## IVF-ET: The Procedure

*In vitro* fertilization and embryo transfer (IVF-ET) was first successfully performed by Edwards and Steptoe in England (31). Their initial protocol involved serial hormonal assays of patients in a noninduced cycle and did not utilize sonographic monitoring which is now used in most IVF-ET programs (31).

IVF-ET is presently reserved primarily for patients who have absent or totally occluded fallopian tubes. However, it can be used for infertility secondary to antisperm antibodies, deficient cervical mucous, severe oligospermia, or where the causes are known. Presently it is performed at only a small number of medical centers in England, Australia, and the United States. The cost to the patient varies but averages between $3,000 and $5,000 per attempt. It requires the expertise and close cooperation of several medical specialists including a gynecological endocrinologist and laparoscopist, a sonologist, embryologist, and numerous laboratory and nursing personnel. In the United States a successful pregnancy occurs in 17 to 22% of the cycles attempted and so patients may have to participate in the protocol several times to achieve a viable pregnancy (49, 50, 51). The seemingly low success rate of IVF-ET should be considered relative to the probability of a fertilized oocyte in a spontaneous cycle becoming a viable pregnancy. It has been estimated that only 30% of all fertilizations result in the production of viable offspring. As of January 1983, there have been 115 live births reported, and all of these children have been normal except for one with transposition of the great vessels while one abortus was found to be triploid (37). Thus, the initial results do not indicate that IVF-ET is associated with a higher rate of fetal anomalies or miscarriages although concern still remains (37).

The success of any IVF-ET protocol is dependent on the carefully timed recovery of the preovulatory oocyte. In Australia and the United States, clomiphene and HMG are used to stimulate ovarian follicular development and indirectly assist in timing laparoscopic oocyte recovery. These medications also increase the number of follicles and so improve the chance that one or more will fertilize, cleave, and be successfully implanted to produce a viable pregnancy. Unexpected side-effects, such as accelerated maturation of the endometrium, however, may reduce the chance of successful implantation (38). Clomiphine is usually administered orally for 5 days between days 3 and 7 or 5 through 9 of the menstrual cycle. HMG is administered over a longer period, usually between 7 and 10 days. Daily sonographic examinations for assessment of follicular development are initiated after completion of clomiphene and 3 to 4 days after initiation of HMG administration.

The sonographic findings are correlated with the serial estradiol levels and the quality of cervical mucus. As stated previously, the absolute value of the estradiol level must be interpreted in light of the number of maturing preovulatory follicles that are present. In those patients treated with clomiphene, between 400 and 500 pg/ml/day is produced by one mature preovulatory follicle (46). The consistency and quantity of the cervical mucous changes as the midcycle approaches and becomes thinner, more copious, and has good stretchability *(Spinnbarkheit)*. All of the parameters used to monitor follicular development have a certain range of normal values and associated measurement errors. Sonographic assessment of follicular size seems to be one of the more objective anatomic parameters of follicular development (17, 34). A follicle between 15 and 18 mm in average dimension should contain a mature oocyte after HCG administration. Similar figures for patients treated with HMG are 12 to 15 mm. One fairly accurate method of determining imminent ovulation in clomiphene cycles is serial assay of LH levels. Although specific levels are not reported with the "rapid assay" of LH, a general trend can be ascertained. The LH levels begin to rise between 22 and 38 hr prior to ovulation and tend to peak within 14 hr of ovulation. Rapid LH assays are of no value in HMG stimulated cycles because this hormone contains LH.

Once the sonographic, laboratory, and clinical data suggest follicular maturation, an intramuscular injection of HCG is given to initiate the final maturation of the oocyte. This occurs between 36 and 38 hr after the HCG injection while the oocyte recovery is performed at about 36 hr. Most follicles greater than 13 to 18 mm in size potentially contain a mature oocyte and are aspirated under laparoscopic visualization (17). At our institution, laparoscopic aspiration is performed utilizing a 14 gauge needle (see Fig. 10A) (47). The needle is placed directly into the follicle during laparoscopy and the follicular fluid is aspirated (Fig. 9A). Sonographically guided percutaneous needle aspiration of the follicle has been performed through the full bladder (18). Real-time sonography allows continuous monitoring and positioning of the needle; however, the success rate of oocyte retrieval with this technique (52%) is lower than laparoscopy (80 to 90%) (1, 18). In patients in whom laparoscopy cannot be performed (owing to adhesions), ultrasound guided aspiration may be the only way to retrieve the oocyte and, unlike laparoscopy, general anesthesia is not needed.

The oocyte can be identified within a clump of cumulus cells in the aspirated follicular fluid. The cumulus mass with the embedded oocyte can be seen without magnification under a microscope (Fig. 9C). After one or more mature oocytes have been recovered, they are transferred immediately to a petri dish containing the medium that will be used for the insemination. The

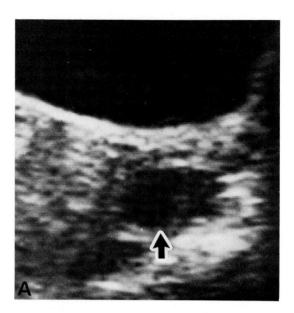

**FIG. 9.** IVF-ET. **A:** Sonographic depiction of a mature preovulatory follicle immediately prior to laparoscopy.

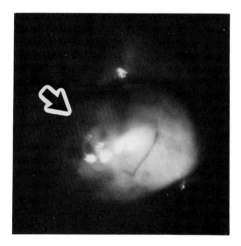

**FIG. 9B.** At laparoscopy the follicle is identified as a bulge in the ovary *(arrow).*

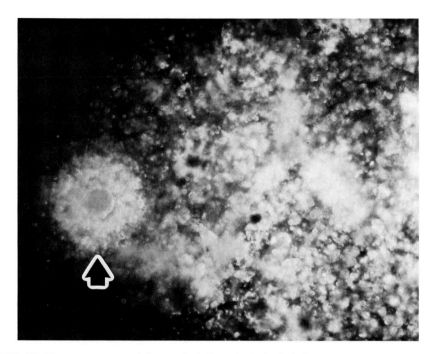

**FIG. 9C.** The appearance of the aspirated contents included an oocyte with a corona *(arrow)* and granulosa cells mixed in mucus (phase contrast microscopy, magnification ×270).

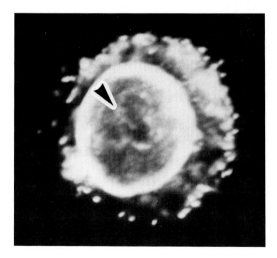

**FIG. 9D.** Photomicrograph of fertilized one cell oocyte, taken 12 hr after insemination. The rounded structures in the nucleus are pronuclei *(arrowhead)*. Their presence indicates that fertilization has occurred. (Magnification ×1200.)

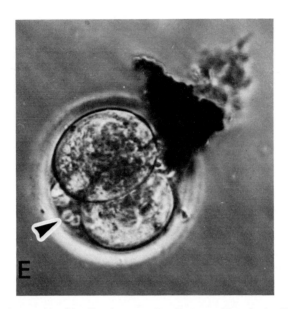

**FIG. 9E.** Photomicrograph of fertilized oocyte, 2-cell stage with polar bodies *(arrowhead)*. This form of the conceptus should be observed 42 hr after insemination and is ready for transfer into the uterus. (Magnification × 1200.)

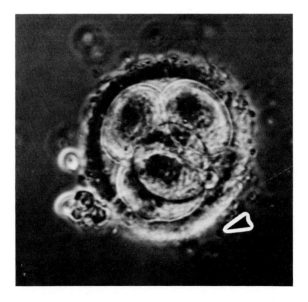

**FIG. 9F.** Photomicrograph of 4-cell embryo. Sperm *(arrowhead)* can be seen at the periphery of the corona. (Magnification × 1200.)

oocyte is left undisturbed for approximately 7 hr and is then mixed with the husband's sperm. At approximately 14 hr, the egg is removed and examined for the presence of a pronucleus. The appearance of two distinct pronuclei is evidence that fertilization has occurred (Fig. 9D). In order for cleavage to be considered normal, a minimum of a two-cell embryo must be observed after a 40-hr period (Figs. 9E, F). In this country, all oocytes that demonstrate normal fertilization and cleavage are transferred back into the uterus. Those that demonstrate absent or abnormal cleavage are not transferred.

The actual procedure for embryo transfer is relatively simple. Once observation of normal embryonic development is documented, the embryos are placed in a catheter and its tip is inserted into the uterine cavity. With gentle pressure, the embryo is placed within the lumen of the upper portion of the uterus. In some centers, the patient is routinely given antibiotics prior to transfer to decrease the possibility of a transient inflammatory reaction in the endometrium. The maternal serum is tested for Beta HCG 10 to 14 days after the embryo transfer to determine if pregnancy has been achieved. The developing embryo from a patient without a uterus could be transferred into the uterus of a surrogate mother. The ethical aspects of this continue to be discussed (43).

### IVF-ET: The Role of Sonography

Sonography is utilized to monitor follicular development by assessing the size, number, and location of mature follicles and the presence or absence of ovulation (8, 17). It is also used to monitor the location of the needle tip during transcutaneous follicular aspiration (19).

The size of the follicle correlates closely with the maturation of the oocyte, particularly in clomiphene cycles. In histologic studies of spontaneously ovulating patients, follicles greater than 18 to 25 mm in dimension contain several layers of granulosa cells, high levels of steroids within the follicular fluid, and most importantly a mature oocyte (18). In our experience, sonography can reliably detect follicles greater than 10 mm in dimension. Follicles less than this size usually do not contain mature oocytes and therefore are not clinically significant. Typically, 2 to 3 follicles ranging from 12 to 20 mm in average dimension will be seen in patients receiving clomiphene and/or HMG. Clomiphene promotes the concomitant development of multiple codominant preovulatory follicles, whereas, with HMG, one large (15 to 18 mm) dominant follicle and several smaller follicles, which may contain mature oocytes, develop. Occasionally, one may encounter abnormal patterns of follicular development in patients whose ovaries contain several small immature follicles that fail to grow. Such patients do not have the expected increase in estradiol levels (Figs. 7E, F).

Because of the necessity to closely monitor follicular growth, daily sonograms are necessary in most patients. The results of the serial sonograms are

combined with data concerning hormonal and clinical evaluation to determine the optimal time for HCG administration as well as laparoscopy. Some
believe that the sonographic assessment of follicle size is a sufficiently accurate predictor of follicular maturation to be used alone (17, 20, 32). Others
combine the results of sonography with E2 levels so as to assess both the
anatomic and physiologic maturity of the follicle. It may be helpful to the
laparoscopist for the sonographer to comment upon the location of the mature follicles within an ovary since a mature follicle may be located within
the substance of the ovary and not be visible from its surface. The actual
location of the follicle relative to the edges of the ovary is not important since
the laparoscopist will typically position and immobolize the ovary within the
pelvis in order to obtain the best view of its surface prior to aspiration.

Sonography may be performed immediately before laparoscopy to see
whether ovulation has occurred (19). In patients with more than 2 follicles,
this finding is not as important as in the patient with only 1 or 2 mature
follicles. If signs of ovulation can be conclusively documented by sonography, laparoscopy can be postponed until another cycle since there is a
diminished chance of successful oocyte recovery (48). The chance of retrieving a mature oocyte that will fertilize and cleave normally after ovulation has
occurred is low. Laparoscopy might also be postponed if the mature follicles
are in an inaccessible ovary.

Sonography may detect unsuspected adnexal lesions in patients being
examined for the IVF-ET program. We have encountered several patients
who had cystic adnexal masses either separate from or within the ovary
(Figs. 10A, B, C, D, E). The sonographic differential diagnosis of cystic
masses includes follicular cysts, paraovarian cysts, endometriomas, cysts of
Morgagni, and epithelial tumors, to name but a few. In most cases, these
adnexal cysts can be moved aside during laparoscopy allowing successful
follicular aspiration. It is helpful to the laparoscopist, however, for the
sonographer to report on the location of the follicle-bearing ovary in relation
to the adnexal mass. We have encountered cystic adnexal masses that enlarge during the menstrual cycle and these most frequently represent a hydrosalpinx (Figs. 10C, D). The fluid within a hydrosalpinx arises from
secretions from the tubal epithelium and can be confused with a normally
developing follicle. Another sonographic misdiagnosis involves a follicle
that contains fresh blood, as it may still appear as an anechoic follicle (Fig.
6C). It is difficult to distinguish sonographically between clotted blood within a follicle and the normal preovulatory follicular fluid. Hemorrhage may
also be encountered in luteinized unruptured follicles, a subtle and sup-
posedly rare cause of infertility (26).

Sonographic identification of the ovary that contains the mature follicle is
of help to the laparoscopist since efforts to aspirate follicles can be directed
toward the ovary that contains the follicle. This decreases the time necessary for laparoscopic aspiration. Identification of the follicle-containing ova-

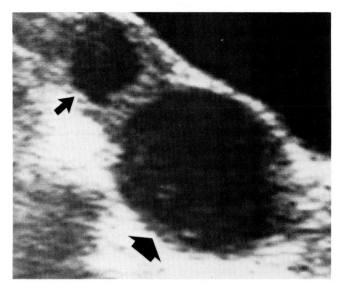

**FIG. 10.** Adnexal masses in ovulation induction patients. **A:** Magnified longitudinal sonogram demonstrating 4 × 5 cm cyst *(large arrow)* inferior to a follicle containing left ovary *(small arrow)*.This cyst was aspirated prior to aspirating the follicular contents.

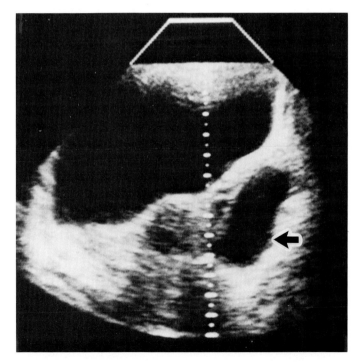

**FIG. 10B.** Transverse real-time sonogram depicting fusiform cystic left adnexal mass *(arrow)* thought to represent a hydrosalpinx. At laparoscopy, this mass was a physiologic ovarian cyst and was successfully aspirated prior to oocyte retrieval.

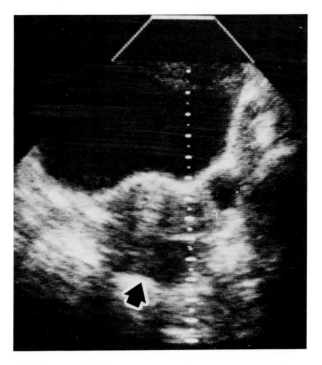

**FIG. 10C.** Transverse sonogram demonstrating a cystic mass *(arrow)* posterior to the uterus thought to represent a preovulatory follicle. An immature preovulatory follicle is present within the left ovary.

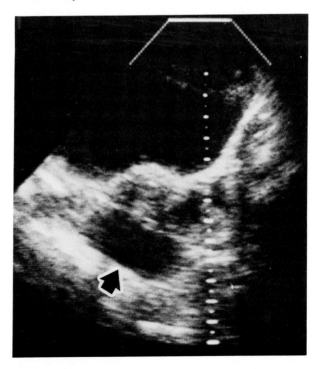

**FIG. 10D.** Transverse sonogram of patient in Fig. 10C 2 days later demonstrating apparent enlargement of the retrouterine cystic mass. At laparoscopy, this mass represented a hydrosalpinx of the right fallopian tube.

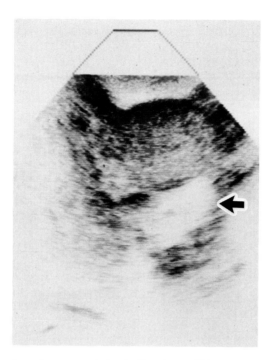

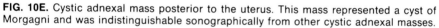

**FIG. 10E.** Cystic adnexal mass posterior to the uterus. This mass represented a cyst of Morgagni and was indistinguishable sonographically from other cystic adnexal masses.

ry may be difficult sonographically when it is located in the cul-de-sac or when there is a retroflexed uterus (Fig. 11B). We have also encountered difficulty where the patient has undergone an ovarian suspension with placement of the ovary directly beneath the uterine fundus or corpus (Fig. 11A).

The presence of fluid within the cul-de-sac is not always an indication that ovulation has occurred as small amounts of fluid or blood may be encountered in the preovulatory period or in patients with peritonitis (Fig. 11C). This fluid may represent serous effusions from the bowel or peritoneal surface. Fluid-filled loops of bowels can be confused with cystic adnexal masses; however, peristalsis will be apparent on real-time with loops of bowel (Figs. 11E, F).

## HYPERSTIMULATION SYNDROME

The ovarian hyperstimulation syndrome is a complex of symptoms and signs in patients receiving ovulation medication, especially HCG, and its incidence is fortunately low (20). Most commonly it results in a mild degree of abdominal discomfort and has a limited course, although some patients suffer nausea, severe abdominal pain, and acites and there is a predisposition to thromboembolic disorders. This syndrome is thought to be the result

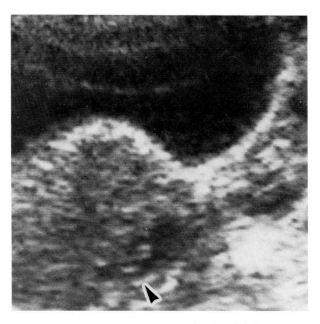

**FIG. 11.** Problem situations. **A:** Transverse magnified sonogram of uterus and ovary in a patient who underwent ovarian suspension. It is difficult to completely delineate the ovary in these patients since the ovary *(arrowhead)* is sutured to the posterior aspect of the uterine fundus.

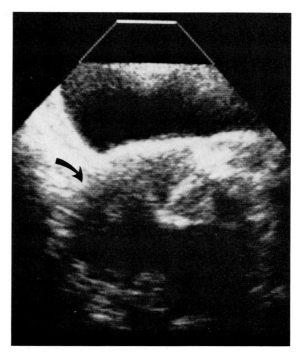

**FIG. 11B.** Longitudinal midline sonogram of retroflexed uterus *(curved arrow)* prohibiting adequate delineation of adnexal structures.

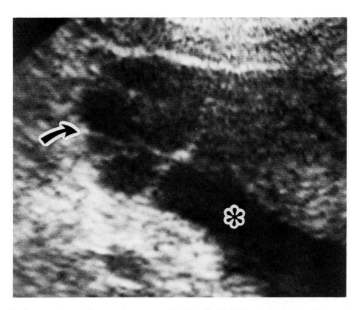

**FIG. 11C.** Ovary *(curved arrow)* surrounded by fluid (*) in a patient with peritonitis.

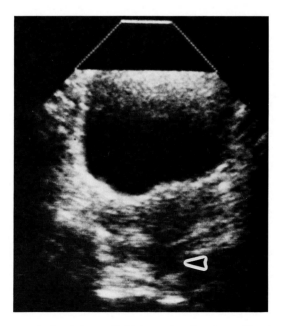

**FIG. 11D.** Small amount of cul-de-sac fluid *(arrowhead)* not resulting from ovulation. At laparoscopy, 5 cc of serous fluid was found.

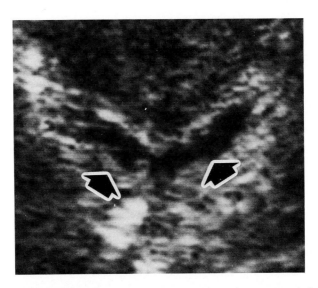

**FIG. 11E.** Fusiform cystic structure *(arrows)* posterior to the uterus mimicking a cystic adnexal lesion on this transverse real-time sonogram.

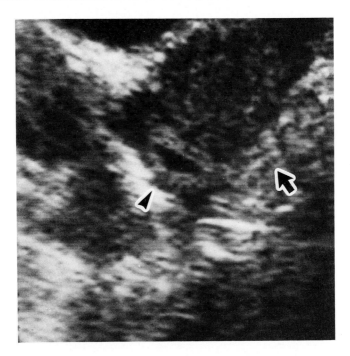

**FIG. 11F.** Same patient, approximately 2 sec later demonstrating contraction of the bowel segment on the left of the midline *(arrow)*. A short segment of bowel remain distended *(arrowhead)*.

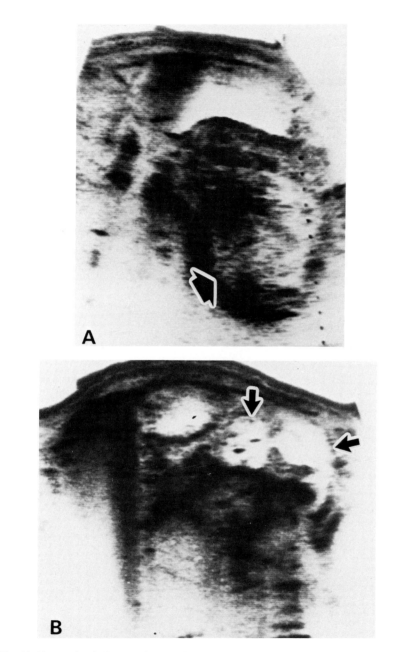

**FIG. 12.** Hyperstimulation syndrome. **A:** Longitudinal static sonogram demonstrating a markedly enlarged ovary *(arrow)* posterior to the uterus. **B:** Transverse static sonogram of same patient demonstrating multiple follicular cysts *(arrows)* within the enlarged left ovary.

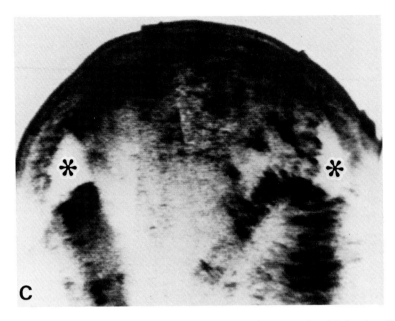

**FIG. 12C.** Transverse static sonogram of same patient demonstrating bilateral peritoneal effusions (*).

of increased capillary permeability resulting in the accumulation of peritoneal and pleural fluid leading to hemoconcentration. Massive edema of the
stroma of the ovary occurs, resulting in marked enlargement. The ovaries
may contain large cysts that can undergo torsion. Sonographically, the
marked enlargement of the ovaries (10 to 12 cm) is due to the presence of
multiple cysts that range in size from a few millimeters to several centimeters (Figs. 12A, B, C) (21, 22). Peritoneal fluid can also be identified. The
signs and symptoms of this syndrome usually improve after the medications
are discontinued.

## IVF-ET: Future Developments

The removal of the fertilization process from the natural milieu of the
fallopian tube and endometrium into an artificial environment introduces
factors which diminish the success rate of IVF-ET. Much of the current
research is aimed at optimizing ovulation induction and improving implantation techniques, and potential alternatives are also being investigated (42).
The success rate of IVF-ET can only be expected to approximate the 30%
rate of successful conception that is encountered in spontaneously ovulating
women. At present, with the use of sonographic, hormonal, and clinical
assessment, an 80 to 90% success rate in retrieving mature oocytes from
preovulatory follicles is being achieved (42). Significant problems remain in

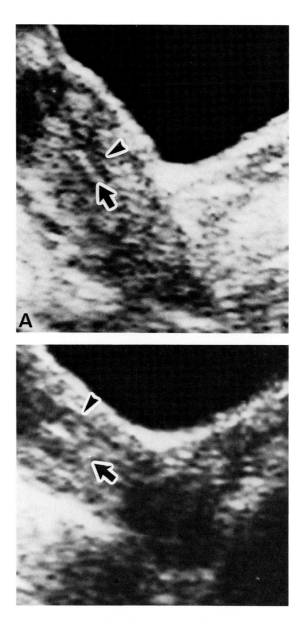

**FIG. 13.** Endometrial changes. **A:** Real-time sonogram through the long axis of the uterus demonstrates a thin (1 to 2 mm) endometrium *(arrowhead)*. Arrow points to endometrial surface. **B:** Real-time sonogram of a patient on clomiphene demonstrating a markedly thickened endometrium *(arrowhead)*. Arrow denotes endometrial surface.

the areas of successful fertilization and implantation, and alternatives to transcervical embryo transfer are being studied (37, 42).

The possibility that the treatment of patients with ovulation induction with certain drugs may produce a dyschrony between the changes in the endometrium and the implanted embryo, thus reducing the chance of a successful implantation, is being investigated. Changes in the endometrial thickness occur in patients on clomiphene and HMG and sonography can be used to evaluate these changes (Figs. 13A, B) (38). Attempts are being made to diminish the possible inflammatory response that occurs in the endometrium secondary to insertion of the transcervical catheter during embryo transfer. Real-time monitoring of the embryo transfer might also allow optimal placement of the developing embryo within the uterus.

### SUMMARY

Sonography has, and will continue to have, a significant role in the monitoring of follicular development (25). This sonographic data can be utilized in several areas of infertility therapy including timed artificial insemination, ovulation induction, and in *in vitro* fertilization and embryo transfer protocols. Although serial sonographic examinations are essential in IVF-ET, their contribution to improving pregnancy rates with timed insemination and ovulation induction is as yet unknown. With greater utilization and investigation of techniques to treat gynecological infertility, the role of sonography in monitoring follicular development will become better defined and improved.

### ACKNOWLEDGMENTS

The authors would like to express their appreciation to the many health care professionals at the Center for Fertility and Reproductive Research (CFARR) for their referral of their patients for sonographic study. We acknowledge the pioneering work of the late Pierre Soupart, MD, PhD, formerly of this institution, in establishing that human oocytes could be fertilized *in vitro*. Annie M. Lindsey, RT RDMS, Charlotte M. Grace, RT RDMS, and James T. Haynes, RT, RDMS are acknowledged for their assistance in the sonographic examination of these patients. Cathy Garner, RN and Betsy Brach, RN contributed to the clinical management of these patients. Sarah Clark, Georgia Pilszak, and John Bobbitt are thanked for their efforts in preparing this text and figures of this review.

### REFERENCES

1.  Marrs, R. P. Update: *In-vitro* fertilization: A reality. *Endocrine & Fertility Forum*, Vol. IV, Number IV, October 1981.

2.  Evans, T. Infertility and other office gynecologic problems. In *Textbook of Obstetrics and Gynecology*, edited by W. Danforth, pp. 768–769. Harper & Row, New York, 1981.
3.  Swanson, M., Sauerbrei, E., and Coopersburg, P. Medical implications of ultrasonically detected polycystic ovaries. *J. Clin. Ultrasound*, 9:219–222, 1982.
4.  Kratochwil, A., Urban, G., and Friedrick, F. Ultrasonic tomography of the ovary. *Ann. Chir. Gynecol. (Fenn)*, 61:211–214, 1972.
5.  Fleischer, A. C., Daniell, J. F., Rodier, J., Lindsay, A. M., and James, A. E. Sonographic monitoring of ovarian follicular development. *J. Clin. Ultrasound*, 9:275–280, 1981.
6.  Fleischer, A. C., Wentz, A., Jones, H., and James, A. E. Sonography of the ovary. In: *Ultrasonography in Obstetrics and Gynecology*, edited by P. Callen. W. B. Saunders, Philadelphia, 1983.
7.  Queenan, J. T., O'Brien, G. D., Bains, L. M., Simpson, J., Collins, W. P., and Campbell, S. Ultrasound scanning of ovaries to detect ovulation in women. *Fertil. Steril.*, 34(2): 99–105, 1980.
8.  Nitschke-Dabelstein, S., Hackeloer, B. J., and Sturm, G. Ovulation and corpus luteum formation observed by ultrasonography. *Ultrasound Med. Biol.*, Vol. 7, pp. 33–39, 1981.
9.  Renaud, R. L., Maclere, J., and Dervain, I. Echographic study of follicular maturation and ovulation during the normal menstrual cycle. *Fertil. Steril.*, 33:272, 1980.
10. Ylostalo, P., Ronnberg, L., and Jouppila, P. Measurement of ovarian follicle by ultrasound in ovulation induction. *Fertil. Steril.*, 31:61, 1979.
11. Hall, D. A., Hann, L. E., Ferruci, J. T., and Black, E. B. Sonographic morphology of the normal menstrual cycle. *Radiology*, 133:185, 1979.
12. Christie, A. D. Ultrasound diagnosis of follicular growth in hormone stimulated ovaries. In *Recent Advances in Ultrasound Diagnosis*, edited by A. Kurjak, p. 389. *Excerpta Medica*, Amsterdam-Oxford, 1980.
13. Funduk-Kurjak B., and Kurjak, A. Ultrasound monitoring of follicular maturation and ovulation in normal menstrual cycle and in ovulation induction. *Acta Obstet. Gynecol. Scand*, 61:329–335, 1982.
14. Smith, D., Picker, R. H., Sinosich, M., and Sanders, D. The assessment of ovulation by ultrasound and estradiol levels during spontaneous and induced cycles. *Fertil. Steril.*, 33(4):387–390, 1980.
15. O'Herlihy, C., DeCrespigny, L., Lopata, A., Johnston, I., Hoult, I., and Robinson, H. Preovulatory follicular size: A comparison of ultrasound and laparoscopic measurements. *Fertil. Steril.*, Vol. 34, No. 1, July, 1980.
16. Vargyas, J. M., Marrs, R. P., Kletzky, O. A., and Mishell, D. R. Correlation of ultrasonic measurement of ovarian follicle and serum estradiol levels in ovulatory patients following clomiphene citrate for *in vitro* fertilization. *Am. J. Obstet. Gynecol.*, 144(5):569, 1982.
17. Sallam, H. N., Marinho, A. O., Collins, W. P., Rodeck, C. H., and Campbell, S. Monitoring gonadotrophin therapy by real-time ultrasonic scanning of ovarian follicles. *Br. J. Obstet. Gynaecol.*, 89:155–159, 1982.
18. McNathy, K., Smith, D., and Makvins, A. The micro environment of the human antral follicle: Interrelationships among steroid levels in antral fluid, the population of granulosa cells, and the status of the oocyte *in vivo* and *in vitro*. *J. Clin. Endocrinol. Metab.*, 49:851–870, 1980.
19. Lenz, S., and Cauritsen, J. Ultrasonogically guided percutaneous aspiration of human follicles under local anesthesia: A new method of collecting oocytes for *in vitro* fertilization. *Fertil. Steril.*, 38(6):673–697, 1982.
20. Wetzels, L. C. G., and Hoogland, H. J. Relation between ultrasonographic evidence of ovulation and hormonal parameters: Luteinizing hormone surge and initial progesterone rise. *Fertil. Steril.*, 37(3):336–341, 1982.
21. Scenker, J. G., and Weinstein, D. Ovarian hyperstimulation syndrome: A current survey. *Fertil. Steril.*, 30(3):255–268, 1978.
22. Rankin, R. N., and Hutton, L. C. Ultrasound in the ovarian hyperstimulation syndrome. *J. Clin. Ultrasound*, 9:473–476, 1981.
23. Terinde, R. Monitoring of human ovulation by ultrasound compared to biochemical and clinical findings. In: *Recent Advances in Ultrasound Diagnosis, II*, p. 409, edited by A. Kurjak. *Excerpta Medica*, Amsterdam, 1980.
24. Nitschke-Dabelstein, S. Comparison of ultrasonic and hormonal monitoring of follicular

growth in patients receiving ovarian stimulating therapy. In: *Recent Advances in Ultrasound Diagnosis, II*, p. 397, edited by A. Kurjak. *Excerpta Medica*, Amsterdam, 1980.

25. Cadkin, A. Follicular ultrasound: Ovarian and follicular monitoring during spontaneous and induced ovulatory cycles. *Dia -Log*, 1(1):2–3, 1982.

26. Marik, J., and Hulka, J. Luteinized unruptured follicle syndrome: A subtle cause of infertility. *Fertil. Steril.*, 29(3):270–274, 1978.

27. Hackloer, B., Fleming, R., Robinson, H., Adam, A., and Coults, R. Correlation of ultrasonic and endocrinologic assessment of human follicular development. *Am. J. Obstet. Gynecol.*, 135:122–126, 1979.

28. Polon, M., Totora, M., Caldwell, B., et al. Abnormal ovarian cycles as diagnosed by ultrasound and serum estradiol levels. *Fertil. Steril.*, 37(3):342–347, 1982.

29. Lemay, A., Bastide, A., Lambert, R., and Rioux, J. Prediction of human ovulation by rapid luteinizing hormone (LH) radioimmunoassay and ovarian ultrasonography. *Fertil. Steril.*, 38(2):194–201, 1982.

30. O'Herlihy, C., Pepperell, R., and Robinson, H. Ultrasound timing of human chorionic gonadotropin administration in clomiphene—Stimulated cycles. *Obstet. Gynecol.*, 59(1): 40–45, 1982.

31. Edwards, R., Steptoe, P., and Purdy, N. Establishing full-term human pregnancies using cleaving embryos grown *in vitro*. *Br. J. Obstet. Gynecol.* 87:737–740, 1980.

32. deCrespigny, L., O'Herlihy, C., Hoult, L., and Robinson, H. Ultrasound in an *in vitro* fertilization program. *Fertil Steril.*, 35(1):25–28, 1981.

33. Hill, L., Breckle, R., and Coulam C. Assessment of human follicular development by ultrasound. *Mayo Clin. Proc.*, 57:176–180, 1982.

34. Cahau, A., and Bessis, R. Monitoring of ovulation induction with human menopausal gonadotropin and human chorionic gonadotropin by ultrasound. *Fertil. Steril.*, 36(2): 178–182, 1981.

35. Bryce, R., Shuter, B., Sinosich, M., et al. The value of ultrasound, gonadotropin, and estradiol measurements for precise ovulation prediction. *Fertil. Steril.*, 37(1):42–45, 1982.

36. Picker, R., Smith D., Tucker M., and Saunders D. Ultrasonic signs of imminent ovulation. *J. Clin Ultrasound*, 11:1–2, 1983.

37. Trounson, A., and Conti, A. Research in human *in vitro* fertilization and embryo transfer: A review. *Br. Med. J*, 285:244–248, 1982.

38. Fleischer, A., Pittaway, D., and Wentz, A. Sonography of the endometrium in ovulation induction *(in preparation)*.

39. Glass, R. *Infertility In Reproductive Endocrinology Physiology and Pathophysiology and Clinical Management*, p. 401, edited by S. Yen and R. Jaffee, Saunders Co., Philadelphia, 1978.

40. Berland, L., Lawson, T., Foley, W., and Albarelli, T. Ultrasound evaluation of pelvic infections. *Radiol. Clin. North Am.*, 20(12):367–382, 1982.

41. Fleischer, A., Porath, S., Entman, S., and James, A. E. Sonography of uterine malformations and disorders. In: *Principles and Practice of Ultrasonography in Obstetrics and Gynecology*, edited by R. Sanders and A. E. James, 3rd ed. Appleton-Century-Crofts, New York *(in press)*.

42. Hodgen, G. *In vitro* fertilization and alternatives. *JAMA*, 246(6):590–597, 1981.

43. Tiefel, H. Human *in vitro* fertilization: A conservative view. *JAMA*, 247(23):3235–3242, 1982.

44. Hammond, M., and Talbert L. *Infertility: A Practical Guide for the Physician*, p. 2. Health Sciences Consortium, Chapel Hill, 1981.

45. Coulam, C., Hill, L., Breckle, R. Ultrasonic evidence of luteinization of unruptured preovulatory follicles. *Fertil. Steril.* 37(4):524–527, 1982.

46. Maxson, W., Wentz, A., Daniell, J., Garven C., Torbit C., Fleischer, A., and Pittaway, I. Initial experience with clomiphene stimulated cycles for *in vitro* fertilization attempts. *Obstet. Gynecol. (in press)*.

47. Jones, A., Acosta, A., and Garcia, J. A technique for aspiration of oocytes from human ovarian follicles. *Fertil. Steril.*, 37:26–29, 1982.

48. Wentz, A., Torbit, C., Daniell, J., and Fleischer, A. Combined laparoscopy and timed follicle aspiration for human *in vitro* fertilization. *Fertil. Steril.*, 1983.

49. Garcia, J., Jones, G., Acosta A., and Wright G. Human menopausal gonadotropin/human

chorionic gonadotropin follicular maturation for oocyte aspiration: Phase I, 1981. *Fertil. Steril.,* 39(2):167–173, 1983.

50. Garcia, J., Jones, G., Acosta, A., and Wright, G. Human menopausal gonadotropin/human chorionic gonadotropin follicular maturation for oocyte aspiration: Phase II, 1981. *Fertil. Steril.,* 39(2):167–173, 1983.

51. Jones, H., Acosta, A., Garcia, J., Sandow, B., and Veeck, L. On the transfer of conceptuses from oocytes fertilized *in vitro. Fertil. Steril.,* 39(2):241–243, 1983.

52. Biggers, J. *In vitro* fertilization and embryo transfer in human beings. *N. Engl. J. Med.,* 304(6):336–342, 1982.

Ultrasound Annual 1983, edited by R. C. Sanders and M. Hill. Raven Press, New York © 1983.

# Scrotal Ultrasonography

*Gail Phillips, †Henry J. Abrams, and *Sheila Kumari-Subaiya

*Department of Radiology and †Department of Urology, Long Island Jewish Hospital-Hillside Medical Center, New Hyde Park, New York 11042

During the last five years, gray scale ultrasonography has become increasingly important as a diagnostic modality in the assessment of scrotal pathology. This is because of its improving resolution and absence of harmful biological effects, along with the superficial location of the scrotal contents (5, 10, 31, 47, 54). On the basis of physical examination alone, it is often difficult to determine whether a palpable abnormality arises from the testicle itself or from extratesticular elements. Cystic and solid masses are not always easily differentiated by transillumination while tenderness and swelling may limit the examination. Sonography can determine the true nature (cystic, solid, complex) of a scrotal mass. It can also differentiate testicular torsion from inflammatory conditions of the scrotum in conjunction with nuclear scanning, Doppler ultrasound, and thermographic techniques (17, 46, 60). The cryptorchid testis can also be sonographically located (35).

## NORMAL ANATOMY

The normal testis is an ovoid mass, with a homogeneous granular texture of medium gray scale echoes (Figs. 1, 2). Occasionally, scattered specular echoes may be seen within the otherwise homogeneous testis (31). The size of the normal testis ranges from 1.0 cm in length in infants to 3.5–4.0 cm in length in adults (47). The body of the epididymis is seen as one or two strongly echogenic parallel lines posterior and lateral to the testis. The epididymal tail is poorly visualized because of its anatomic position, and when an abnormality exists in this region it can be confused with intratesticular pathology (see Fig. 30). The broadest portions of the epididymis are the head and body which are easily seen using high frequency transducers in most patients, particularly those with a hydrocele. The mediastinum testis is a fibrous band arising from the tunica albuginea and is identified as an echogenic stripe extending in a cephalo-caudad direction along the lateral aspect of the testis and extending to a variable degree into the testis. It is infrequently seen using contact scanners; however, Wilson has been able to identify it in 90% of patients, using an automated water path scanner (69).

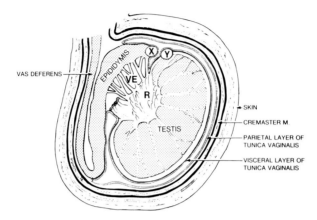

**FIG. 1.** Diagram. Normal anatomy. X, appendix epididymis; Y, appendix testis; R, rete testis; VE, vasa efferentes (efferent ducts).

In the normal scrotum, the membrane surrounding the testicle is known as the tunica vaginalis. The cavity of the tunica vaginalis contains a thin fluid which can be visualized using high frequency transducers (47). When an abnormal collection of fluid occurs in this space it is known as a hydrocele.

The rete testis is infrequently seen. When it is seen, it appears as a small rounded anechoic area along the posterior aspect of the testis adjacent to the body of the epididymis, which can be confused with an intratesticular neoplasm. Two small vestigial remnants, the appendix testis and appendix epididymis, are present along the upper pole of the testis and epididymis, respectively, and are not normally visualized (Fig. 1). Although these structures are functionally inert, they may be involved by infarction, inflammation, or neoplastic disease of the scrotum.

## TECHNIQUE

The usual method of ultrasonic examination is contact scanning using a high frequency 7.5 mHz transducer. This technique is slightly limited by the extremely deformable nature of the scrotum and the mobility of the testes, particularly in small children. Water path scanning methods have been used to obtain a more panoramic view of the scrotum (26) and to alleviate the discomfort in patients with painful scrotal conditions. Naser has achieved this by placing a small water bag on top of the supported scrotum, similar to the method used in thyroid and eye scanning (42). Using the automated water path method, compound scanning is performed by suspending the scrotum on a polyethylene membrane which is then immersed in a tank of water (69). High frequency real-time scanners are being used with greater frequency in testicular diagnosis; however, the small field of view limits their ability to distinguish anatomical relationships within the scrotal contents, especially when testicular torsion or large scrotal masses are present. The advantages of higher frequency real-time scanners, however, are that they afford much greater resolution and opportunity for quick scanning of the scrotum, and particularly for localization of small intratesticular tumors.

Because the examination is of an extremely personal nature, it is important to explain the procedure, demonstrate the equipment, and allay the fears of the patient in order to facilitate the examination. A history should be obtained and the scrotum must be palpated by the examiner to locate areas of focal abnormality. In adolescents and adults, the scrotum is suspended by

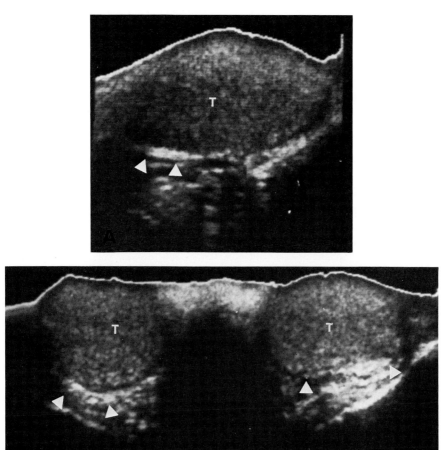

**FIG. 2.** Longitudinal **(A)** and transverse **(B)** scans demonstrate the normal sonographic relationship of testis (T) and epididymis *(arrowheads).*

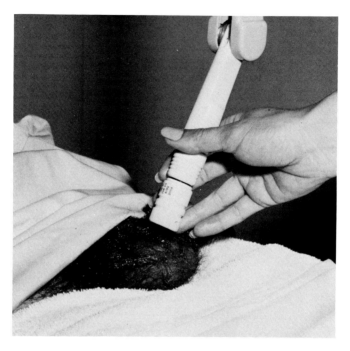

**FIG. 3.** Technique. See text.

a support device or by a towel placed under the scrotum and wrapped tightly around the patient's thighs (Fig. 3). In infants and young children, scrotal immobilization is obtained by holding the scrotum in the examiner's hand. This is particularly important because of the increased mobility of the testes in young patients. The penis is covered with a sheet or drape to hold it off the scanning field. Patients are scanned either by a physician or by other experienced technical personnel and warm mineral oil or jelly is applied to the scrotal skin as a couplant. Real-time equipment may be used initially to quickly scan the scrotum and localize focal pathology. Direct contact scans are then performed using high frequency transducers with short focal lengths (Fig. 3). Near field suppression is not recommended so that the testicular tunics and entire testes are visualized. The time-gain-compensation curve is adjusted by scanning the asymptomatic hemiscrotum first so as to give the normal testis a uniform parenchymal texture of moderate gray scale echogenicity. Transverse, longitudinal, and oblique scans are performed over both testes to obtain their precise length, width, and height. The epididymis should also be examined in its entirety.

## THE NONACUTE SCROTUM

The value of scrotal ultrasonography in evaluating the nonacute scrotum has been well established (5, 10, 31, 47, 54). High resolution quality imaging of intrascrotal contents has provided the clinician with a method for resolving the following clinical problems:

1. Differentiating testicular from extratesticular masses when the clinical evaluation is difficult.
2. Determining whether the testis alone, or both testis and epididymis are involved in a pathologic process. This is important in differentiating neoplastic from inflammatory and vascular processes.
3. Evaluating the cystic or solid nature of a mass, i.e., hydrocele versus tumor.
4. Determining the unilateral or bilateral nature of testicular inolvement as this may ultimately affect both therapeutic and surgical management.
5. Searching for primary testicular neoplasms in patients with known metastatic disease of undetermined etiology, i.e., para-aortic adenopathy at the level of the kidney.
6. Localizing a cryptorchid testis.
7. Visualizing the nonpalpable testis in the presence of a large hydrocele to rule out potential pathology.
8. Differentiating a hernia from a hydrocele.

## INTRATESTICULAR MASSES

Testicular tumors are the most common solid tumors in men between the ages of 20 and 35. Seminoma accounts for 30 to 40% of all testicular tumors and so is the most common tumor experienced sonographically (44). Other germinal neoplasms, including embryonal carcinoma and teratocarcinoma, have a 25% incidence while adult teratoma and choriocarcinoma make up 10% (44). Like other testicular tumors, seminoma presents as a gradual symmetric testicular enlargement and is painful in about 10 to 15% of cases owing to hemorrhage into the tumor (36). Initial symptoms may occur as a result of distant metastasis although this is less common with seminoma than with the other tumors (38). The predominant mode of dissemination is by the lymphatic route, and CT of the abdomen and pelvis should be performed to evaluate the extent of disease for staging and management (11, 50).

Patients with a previous undescended testis or who have undergone an orchiopexy have an increased incidence of malignancy. The probability of malignant degeneration occurring in an undescended testis is 20 to 30 times greater than that of the normally descended organ (7). Although seminoma is most likely, any of the other malignant tumors may occur. There is also a higher incidence of malignancy in the contralateral normally descended testis (51). Orchiopexy does not appear to influence the risk of neoplasia or the age of onset of the subsequent tumor (51). Sonographic follow-up is important in these patients as small nonpalpable tumors can be detected.

Testicular tumors in infants and children are uncommon. They represent

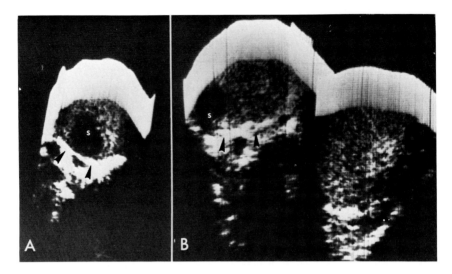

**FIG. 4.** Seminoma. Twenty-three-year-old presented with acute pain to rule out testicular torsion. Longitudinal **(A)** and transverse **(B)** scans demonstrate a small anechoic mass (S) in lateral portion of testis. The epididymis *(arrowheads)* is normal.

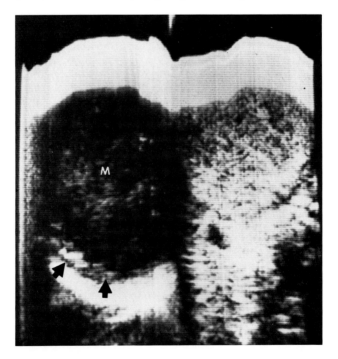

**FIG. 4C.** Transverse scan demonstrates a normal left testis. The right testis is replaced by a mass (M) of low echogenicity. The epididymis *(arrows)* is clearly seen to be normal, but compressed around the tumor.

the seventh most common neoplasm in this age group and 1% of all cases of malignant disease in childhood (6, 59). Sixty percent of these patients are younger than 2½ years, and 80% of these tumors are malignant. Any scrotal mass found in an infant or child other than hydrocele or hernia should be considered malignant until proven otherwise (12). Very little has been written on the sonography of malignant testicular tumors in children. One must interpolate from parallel conditions in the adult that the sonographic patterns of these malignancies are similar.

The sonographic patterns of seminoma and other testicular tumors are indistinguishable from one another. Patients with palpable masses will demonstrate an enlarged testis with an area of decreased echogenicity which is either focal and well-defined or diffuse, ill-defined, and occupying most of the testis (Figs. 4, 5). A rim of normal testicular parenchyma may be visualized around or interspersed between areas of focal abnormality. Hemorrhagic foci within tumors are seen as well-defined anechoic areas with increased through transmission either in the central or peripheral portions of the mass. The epididymis is usually spared in seminoma and is easily identi-

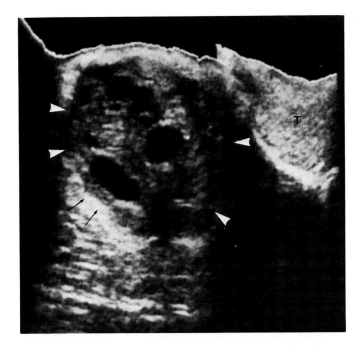

**FIG. 5.** Malignant tumor, mixed type. Transverse scan demonstrates a normal left testis (T). The right testis is replaced by a mass of mixed echogenicity with multiple anechoic areas of hemorrhage. The epididymis can be seen to be normal *(arrows)* and compressed around the tumor *(arrowheads)*.

fied by ultrasound examination. More aggressive tumors may invade portions of the epididymis, but usually some normal epididymal elements can be found.

Infrequently, seminomas and other testicular masses are more echogenic or isoechoic with the normal testicular parenchyma (10). There may be only a subtle disorganization of the usual homogeneity of the testis and comparison with the opposite testis is especially important. When the entire testis is replaced by tumor the testicular contour becomes "lumpy." In patients with a solitary testicle, this may be the only clue to the presence of the neoplasm, as the echo texture of the opposite testis is not available for comparison (Fig. 6). In patients presenting with acute scrotal pain, in the presence of an echogenic testicular mass, the identification of normal epididymis will differentiate a tumor from a testicular torsion.

Teratomas are composed of tissue from the three germ cell layers (44). The childhood form is considered benign and represents 25% of testicular masses in this age group. It most commonly occurs between the ages of 3 months and 5 years (12). The adult form is potentially malignant. The pres-

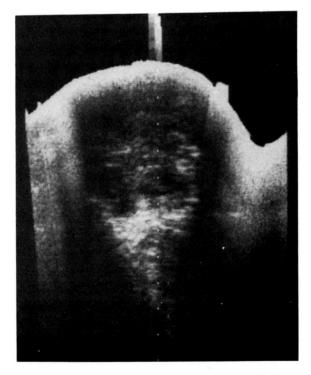

**FIG. 6.** Seminoma. Inguinal testis. Scan demonstrates a mass with "lumpy" borders and with a slightly heterogeneous echo pattern. Epididymis not present.

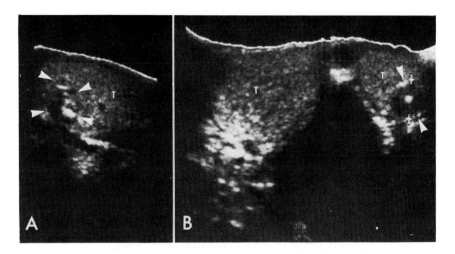

**FIG. 7.** Testicular teratoma. Longitudinal **(A)** and transverse **(B)** scans demonstrate a well-defined mass *(arrowheads)* in the upper pole of the left testis. Strong echoes are identified within the mass with acoustic shadowing due to calcifications. The opposite testis is normal (T).

ence of cartilage in these lesions is common (51). We have seen one adult patient with teratoma. The mass was small and extremely well demarcated from normal testicular tissue, although no capsule was identified. The echo texture was decreased with several focal echogenic areas with acoustic shadowing suggestive of calcifications (Fig. 7). A radiograph confirmed the presence of multiple small areas of calcifications.

Testicular cysts are benign epidermoid cysts that are lined by squamous epithelium (73). They are extremely rare and occur in children; however, their growth ceases at puberty.

## LEUKEMIA, LYMPHOMA

Leukemic and lymphomatous infiltration of the testis is uncommon (33). Clinical recognition is important as testicular involvement may be the first manifestation of extramedullary disease in the absence of bone marrow involvement (61). Clinically evident disease is reported to be as low as 8% in acute lymphocytic leukemia (53) whereas the autopsy incidence of testicular leukemia is as high as 92% (16). All ultrasonic work to date in this area has been done retrospectively. No prospective studies have been done to evaluate the use of ultrasound in detecting disease that is clinically nonpalpable at the time of initial diagnosis, during the course of therapy, and while the patient is in remission. This is important as chemotherapy may not be effective in treating testicular involvement.

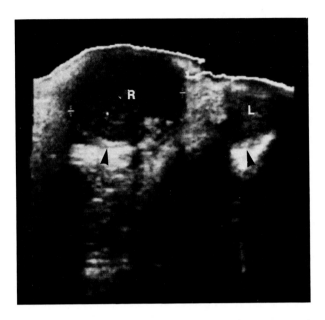

**FIG. 8.** Leukemic infiltration. Six-year-old. Transverse scan demonstrates the right (R) and left (L) testis to be of decreased echogenicity. The right testis is markedly larger than the left. The right and left epididymis *(arrowheads)* are normal. Testicular biopsy was positive bilaterally.

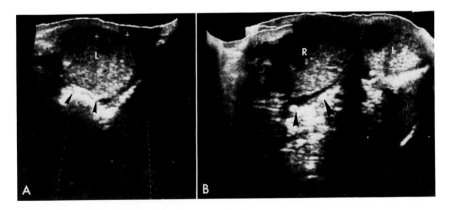

**FIG. 9.** Diffuse lymphocytic lymphoma. Fifty-seven-year-old male noticed an increase in size of the right testis. Ultrasound demonstrates the right testis (R) to be larger than the left (L); however, the echo pattern is relatively homogeneous. A lesion of low echogenicity is seen in the left testis. Right and left epididymis are normal *(arrowheads)*.

Two sonographic patterns have been reported in testicular leukemia and lymphoma (33). In children with acute leukemia, the testis is usually enlarged with focal or diffuse areas of decreased echogenicity (Fig. 8). Testicular enlargement without obvious abnormality of testicular echo pattern is usually indicative of leukemic infiltration if disease has been documented elsewhere. Testicular biopsy is required, however, before therapeutic regimens can be instituted. In contrast, in adults, sharply defined septated anechoic masses within the testis are present, which are frequently bilateral (Fig. 9). The epididymis is normal and hydroceles may be present secondary to lymphatic obstruction. In adults over 50 years of age presenting with a unilateral palpable mass, where sonography demonstrates bilateral disease and the testicular adnexae are spared, leukemia or lymphoma should be the primary diagnostic consideration.

## GRANULOMATOUS DISEASE

Granulomatous orchitis as a primary infection is extremely rare and is usually secondary to epididymal involvement (37). It has been estimated that the testis is infected in 60% of cases within 6 months and in 85% of patients within 12 months after the onset of tuberculous (TB) epididymitis (36). The disease occurs more commonly in young men with a history of renal tuberculosis, or primary genital tract TB involving the prostate or seminal vesicles. Genital sarcoidosis has been reported in less than 5% of postmortem cases. Clinically apparent sarcoidosis most commonly affects the epididymis whereas involvement of the testis has been reported in only two cases (45).

There are few sonographic reports of genital granulomatous disease. When the testis alone is involved, the testicular echo pattern may be decreased (Fig. 10) (34) or increased and it may be indistinguishable from a malignancy (10). We have seen one patient with unilateral scrotal tuberculosis. The testicular echo pattern was distorted, with a mixed sonographic pattern. The entire epidiymis, however, was markedly enlarged, solid, and easily separable from the testis. The combination of testicular and epididymal involvement suggests inflammatory rather than neoplastic disease (Fig. 11).

## THE UNDESCENDED TESTIS

Management of the nonpalpable undescended testis has always been an important clinical problem. Undescended testes occurs in 0.1 to 0.8% of all children, of which 20% are nonpalpable (58). Of these, most are located either intraabdominally or within the inguinal canal, while in 0.4% the testes are absent (64). Orchiopexy is advised prior to age 5 (58). Although the risk of malignant degeneration (7) is unchanged by orchiopexy, exteriorization of the testis makes it more accessible to frequent examination, and earlier

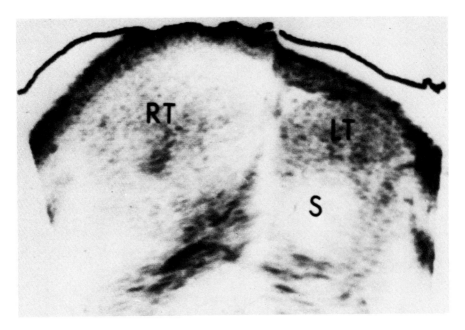

**FIG. 10.** Testicular sarcoid. Anechoic nodules seen in both right (RT) and left testis (S). A small rim of normal left testicular parenchyma is identified (LT). (Courtesy Dr. Anthony Lupetin, Allegheny General Hospital.)

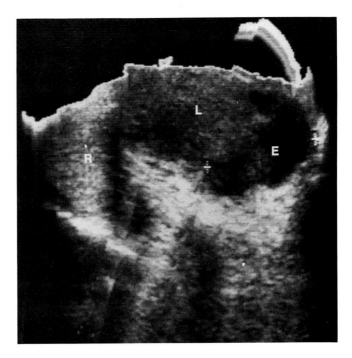

**FIG. 11.** Scrotal tuberculosis. Transverse scan demonstrates the right testis (R) to be normal. The left testis (L) is enlarged, and of decreased echogenicity. The epididymis (E) is markedly enlarged, lobulated, and separable from the testis.

detection of neoplastic change. Early surgical correction of cryptorchidism enhances the fertility potential of the patient and, most importantly, helps to avoid the psychologic and cosmetic sequelae of an empty scrotum or hemiscrotum (32). The undescended testes brought into the scrotum are usually small or hypoplastic (27).

Preoperative demonstration of the presence and location of the nonpalpable testis is important to limit the extent of surgical exploration. Herniography (68), gonadal venography (67), angiography (66), CT(71), and ultrasound (35) have all been used for this purpose. Angiography is not frequently used as it is technically difficult, requires anesthesia, and the quantity of ionizing radiation is high. Gonadal venography has a higher success rate in localizing impalpable testes and is technically less difficult, rarely requires anesthesia, and produces less radiation exposure. CT is quick, simple, accurate, noninvasive and rarely requires anesthesia. The testis is easily localized in the inguinal ring, canal, or superficial inguinal pouch. The greatest problem is differentiating the testis from surrounding soft tissues in patients with little fat (72).

Sonographic evaluation is easily performed with real-time scanners. Longitudinal scanning along the orientation of the inguinal ring, and abdominal scanning through a distended bladder from the umbilicus to the symphysis pubis is recommended. The anterior superior iliac spine should be used as a landmark as this structure is several centimeters cephalad to the internal inguinal ring. Madrazo successfully localized 8 of 9 undescended inguinal testes, but was unsuccessful in visualizing the undescended abdominal testis (34). Associated inguinal hernias create difficulty in localizing undescended testes which are posteriorly located. Scanning in the Trendelenberg position is helpful when this occurs. The sonographic pattern of an undescended testis is similar to that of a normal scrotal testis though it is usually small, and the epididymis is not present.

At this time in most institutions, sonography is the primary screening modality for cryptorchid testis. As most impalpable testes are inguinal in location, it is felt that more invasive studies should be performed only in patients in whom sonography has excluded an inguinal gonad or in whom the study has been inconclusive (72).

## ASYMPTOMATIC ENLARGED TESTIS

Asymptomatic enlargement of the testes in children is rare and should alert the physician to the possibility of a neoplastic or metabolic condition. The common causes of testicular enlargement include congenital adrenal hypoplasia and metastatic tumors (43). Other less frequent causes include juvenile hypothyroidism with precocious puberty, megalotestis syndrome (with X-linked mental deficiency), and benign idopathic testicular

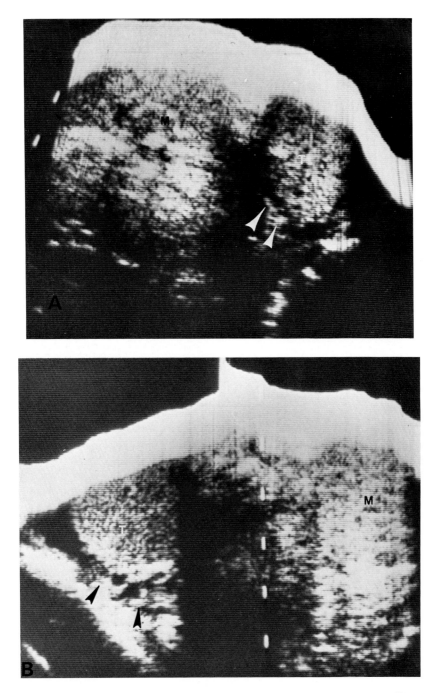

**FIG. 12.** Spermatic cord myxoliposarcoma. Longitudinal **(A)** and transverse **(B)** scans demonstrate a normal testis (T). A highly echogenic elongated mass is present cephalad to the testis with acoustic shadowing. The area of the epididymis *(white arrowheads)* is not well defined. The opposite testis (T) and epididymis *(black arrowheads)* is normal.

enlargement (30). Compensatory hypertrophy of a solitary testis also occurs in cases of contralateral undescended testis (29). In all these cases, regardless of etiology, the testicular echo pattern is normal. Following a herniorraphy in infancy, there may be infarction of the testis on the side of the surgery owing to interruption of the testicular artery. The atrophic testis is clinically softer and smaller that its fellow on the opposite side while sonographically it is more hypoechoic.

## PARATESTICULAR SOLID TUMORS

Primary neoplasms of the testicular adnexa are rare, although these structures may be involved by extension from primary testicular tumors (39). Spermatic cord tumors comprise the vast majority of paratesticular tumors, of which 70% are benign (21). Fibrosarcoma and liposarcoma are the most common malignant tumors in adults whereas rhabdomyosarcoma is the most common in children (19). Fibroma, fibrosarcoma, hemangioma (14), leiomyoma, and leiomyosarcoma are known to occur, but only rarely. Most epididymal tumors are benign and approximately 30% are of the adenomatoid variety (39).

It is difficult to ascribe a particular sonographic pattern to paratesticular tumors as few have been reported. Rhabdomyosarcoma (19) and myxoliposarcoma (20) are predominantly echogenic and focal anechoic areas of necrosis may be found within them. When calcifications or fat are present, areas of increased echogenicity with or without acoustic shadowing are seen (Fig. 12). Invasion of the testis by paratesticular tumors can be misleading as it makes it difficult to define the primary site (40).

## CYSTIC EXTRATESTICULAR MASSES

### Hydrocele

A hydrocele is a fluid collection within the tunica vaginalis that totally surrounds the testis and epididymis anteriorly. It may be congenital or acquired (13, 65) and is the most common cause of scrotal masses in infants and children (13, 54, 65). Acquired hydroceles usually accompany (or are the result of) inflammation, intermittent torsion, or neoplasm. Forty percent of testicular tumors in children and adults are associated with a secondary hydrocele (10, 40).

The clinical diagnosis of hydrocele is difficult if transillumination is nondiagnostic. The painless "rock hard" mass of a chronic hydrocele with thickening of the tunica vaginalis may not transilluminate and can be confused with a neoplasm. Scrotal hernias, on the other hand, may transilluminate

and lead to an incorrect diagnosis. Ultrasound is very useful in these circum-
stances as it can delineate the testis when it cannot be palpated due to the
presence of a large amount of fluid.

As more detailed sonographic evaluation of the fetus is being performed
routinely, the visualization of male genitalia and the presence of hydrocele is
being reported with increasing frequency (Fig. 13) (13, 65). Fetal hydroceles
are the consequence of a persistent processus vaginalis which normally
closes late in fetal life and may not close until 1 year of age (4). In fact, it has
been reported that a patent processus vaginalis is identified in 94% of children at birth and in 57% at 1 year of age (57). It follows, therefore, that in

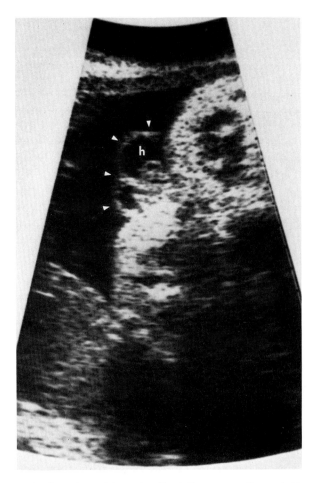

**FIG. 13.** *In utero* hydrocele at 34 weeks. Real-time scans through the scrotum *(arrowheads)* demonstrate fluid in both scrotal sacs (h). Right and left testes are visualized.

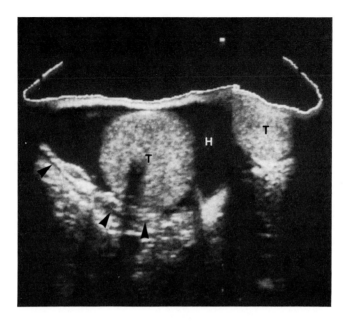

**FIG. 14.** Simple idiopathic hydrocele. Transverse scan demonstrates a normal right and left testis (T). The epididymis is clearly defined *(arrowheads)* and is normal. Fluid (H) surrounds the testis.

children who are seen for a scrotal examination from birth to 1 year, the finding of a hydrocele is not clinically significant. The finding of a hydrocele beyond 1 year of age, however, is suspicious, and an etiologic factor should be sought.

Hydrocele is seen sonographically as a totally echo-free collection surrounding the testis (Fig. 14). Septations or dependent echoes within the fluid suggest previous hemorrhage (hematocele) or infection (pyocele), and the testis and epididymis should be carefully examined for associated pathology. In the presence of hydrocele, the appendix testis may be visualized (Fig. 15). One should be aware of this anatomic structure and not confuse it with a testicular neoplasm. If hydroceles are large, they can be confused clinically with a hernia and ultrasound is helpful in distinguishing one from the other. Echogenic foci with shadowing may represent air within the scrotal sac whereas peristaltic activity, seen with real-time ultrasound, will confirm the presence of a hernia (62).

Although rare, a hydrocele may extend along the spermatic cord into the groin or even into the abdomen. Abdominal-scrotal hydrocele may in fact be the cause of an abdominal mass in children, and ultrasonography can confirm its presence (9).

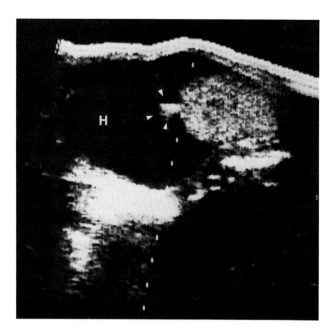

**FIG. 15.** Simple hydrocele. Normal appendix testis. Occasionally the appendix testis *(arrowheads)* can be visualized in the presence of a hydrocele (H). It should not be mistaken for a testicular tumor.


## SPERMATOCELE

A spermatocele or epididymal cyst is a confluence of small cysts of the efferent ducts of the testis and is filled with seminal plasma. When the masses are very large and present in a position cephalad to the testis they are referred to as spermatoceles; when they are small and present within the body or head of the epididymis they are considered epididymal cysts (40). Usually they occur secondary to chronic epididymitis in the adult whereas in children they are due to trauma. Diagnosis of a spermatocele is easily made by palpation or transillumination and aspiration. When they are very large, however, they are difficult to distinguish from a hydrocele. Ultrasound helps in distinguishing these fluid collections by localizing the fluid either within the tunica vaginalis (hydrocele) or separate from it (spermatocele). Treatment for a hydrocele is usually surgical, whereas a spermatocele can be treated medically.

Sonographic patterns in simple spermatocele are diagnostic. The masses are cephalad to the testis, are anechoic, and are round or oval depending on their size. Normal epididymis can be seen surrounding the mass either posteriorly or laterally (Fig. 16). Masses appear septated if multiple cysts are

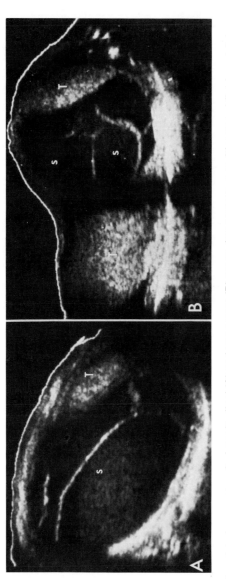

**FIG. 16.** Multiloculated spermatocele. Longitudinal **(A)** and transverse **(B)** scans demonstrate a multiseptated fluid-containing mass cephalad to the testis (T). Several cystic spaces are filled with echoes (s) secondary to an old infectious process.

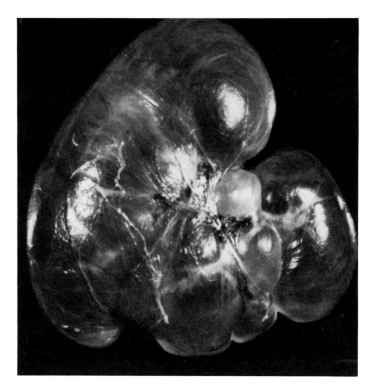

**FIG. 16C.** Surgical specimen. Multiloculated spermatocele.

adjacent to one another. If the spermatocele becomes infected, scattered echoes can be identified within it. We have seen epididymal cysts as small as 5 mm in diameter usually within the body of the epididymis itself (Fig. 17). The testicular echo pattern is always homogeneous and the area of the tunica vaginalis is free of fluid. Should the testicular echo pattern be disturbed, associated intratesticular pathology should be suspected.

## VARICOCELE

Varicocele refers to any abnormal dilatation and tortuosity of the veins of the pampiniform plexus within the scrotum. They may be of the primary or secondary type.

The primary type usually occurs between the ages of 15 to 25, is idiopathic, and 99% are left-sided owing to the entry of the left spermatic vein into the left renal vein. In the standing position the diagnosis is readily made by palpating a mass of tortuous veins (40). Sonographic examination of these patients is usually nondiagnostic as the mass promptly disappears in the supine position. This limits the usefulness of ultrasound in the diagnosis of

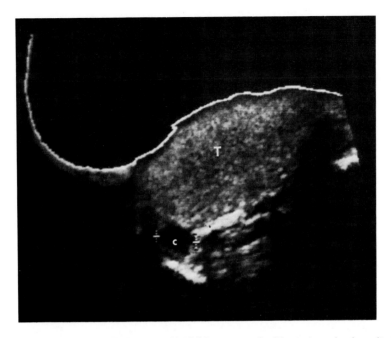

**FIG. 17.** Epididymal cyst. Eight-year-old child presented with acute pain. Longitudinal scan demonstrates a normal testis (T). A small cyst is present in the body of the epididymis (c).

varicocele in patients with infertility. The only sonographic clue may be that the ipsilateral testis can be smaller than the contralateral testis, presumably owing to increased scrotal heat (41).

Secondary varicoceles do not disappear on recumbency. In these patients, retroperitoneal disease or an intraabdominal mass is obstructing the spermatic vein (39). Ultrasound is more successful in visualizing the varicocele in these instances. Examination of the abdomen and pelvis should be performed at the time of scrotal examination. Sonographic findings depend on the size of the varicocele. Small varicoceles are seen as an area of high amplitude linear echoes cephalad to the testis with a serpiginous "bag of worms" appearance (69). The lumina of the veins may not be visualized. Testicular measurement should be performed in these cases to determine whether ipsilateral testicular atrophy is present. In larger varicoceles (Fig. 18), the same "bag of worms" persists, and is identified by highly echogenic and tubular serpiginous structures representing dilated vessels. The testis in these patients is usually small and atrophic and often difficult to identify. It is sometimes helpful to scan the patients with a tilt table to evaluate changes in varicocele size.

Thermography (17), retrograde phlebography (1), pampiniform Doppler

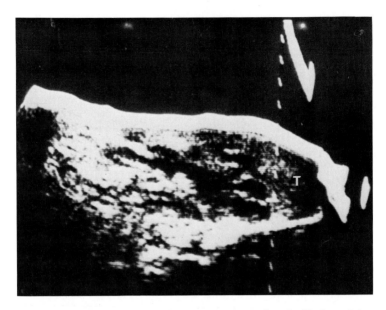

**FIG. 18.** Varicocele. Longitudinal scan demonstrates a small testis (T). A serpiginous fluid-containing mass is identified cephalad to the testis.

stethoscopy (22), and $^{99m}$Tc scanning (41) have been used in an attempt to increase diagnostic accuracy with small varicoceles. Results have not been rewarding.

## ACUTE SCROTAL PATHOLOGY

More and more children are being referred for ultrasonography with the major complaint of scrotal pain with or without scrotal enlargement. In all situations in which the clinical diagnosis is confusing, adjunctive diagnostic modalities must be used to exclude the diagnosis of testicular torsion. This condition, which compromises the viability of the testis, must be separated from other entities that mimic this condition, such as inflammatory disease, torsion of the scrotal appendages, trauma, epididymal cystic masses, and, less commonly, hemorrhage into a testicular tumor. Institutions vary as to the diagnostic modality that is most readily available in an emergency situation. Ultrasonic and isotopic scanning procedures complement one another. Where both are not available the initial procedure of choice should provide the most cost-effective and expeditious evaluation of the patient.

Doppler studies and radioisotope studies have been the conventional modalities of choice in distinguishing those conditions that are acute surgical emergencies, i.e., testicular torsion, scrotal abscess, or testicular rupture. Doppler ultrasound is noninvasive, quick and easy to perform, and particularly lends itself to repeated examinations. The arterial pulse over the testis will indicate a lack of perfusion in the presence of torsion. False positive findings may occur with this method. If the patient is examined immediately after the onset of torsion, faint arterial pulsations may still be present as venous congestion predominates early. Also, in missed torsion, scrotal hyperemia may falsely indicate positive arterial pulsations (46). Rodriquez reports only 79% accuracy in differentiating torsion from other acute conditions using Doppler ultrasound (52).

Accuracy rates with $^{99m}$Tc scanning have been reported between 94 and 99% (52). This method is preferable when it is available on an emergency basis; however, it is more expensive and requires highly trained personnel. In acute torsion, nuclear scanning reveals decreased perfusion to the testis. By 6 hr after the onset of torsion, blood flow through the pudendal artery to the surrounding dartos muscle will result in a halo-like effect (23). This is in contrast to inflammation and testicular trauma, in which there is a relatively increased uptake of tracer to the hemiscrotum. Like Doppler, the radionuclide scan in missed torsion may be confusing, with a perceptible increase in vascular perfusion noted on the affected side (15).

Ultrasound is a nonphysiologic modality and the evaluation of intrascrotal contents is based solely on anatomic structure and echo texture. The accuracy of high frequency real-time and contact scanning in excluding the clinical diagnosis of torsion testis has been 98% in our experience (49).

## TESTICULAR TORSION

Torsion of the testis is possible at any age although it is most common in the adolescent age group from 12 to 18 years. Few cases occur in newborns and occasionally this condition occurs in infancy and childhood. When present, testicular torsion is a surgical emergency. The decision must be made rapidly as spermatogenic cells are damaged after 2 hr and destroyed after 6 hr (3). Testicular salvage rates of 60 to 70% are reported for surgery performed less than 24 hr after the onset of pain, and is less than 20% if the delay is greater than 24 hr (3). When there is any question as to the clinical diagnosis, adjunctive diagnostic modalities must be performed without delay. The most common presentation is that of a boy who is awakened at night by groin pain, only to discover later that the testis is swollen and tender. Redness of the scrotum occurs within a few hours after the onset of torsion. Urinary symptoms are absent and the urine is clear of bacteria and/ or cells (4). The differential diagnosis includes torsion of an intrascrotal hernial sac, acute idiopathic scrotal edema, and hemorrhage into intra-

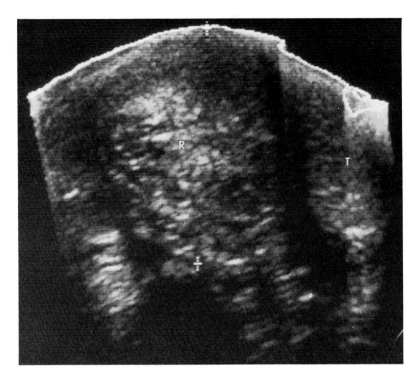

**FIG. 19.** Testicular torsion, 6 hr. Transverse scan demonstrates the right testis (R) to be enlarged compared to the left, with focally increased echos. Epididymis is not identified.

testicular tumors (28). In this latter group of patients, there is frequently a history of previous recurrent unilateral scrotal pain which has resolved spontaneously in the presence of a normal sized testis. In such patients, the diagnosis of a malignancy should be strongly suspected.

Torsion results when a spermatic cord twists upon itself and the primary blood supply to the testis and epididymis is compromised. In experimentally induced torsion in dogs, Hricak reported that there was an increase in the size of the testis, epididymis, and cord along with decreased echogenicity of the testis and epididymis. These findings were present prior to the demonstration of any histological changes in the testis (25).

In our institution, a series of 75 children presented with an "acute scrotum." Twelve children were surgically proven to have testicular torsion. None presented with less than a 4-hr history of pain and all children had changes of ischemic necrosis by the time of the sonographic examination (49). We encountered little difficulty in examining the patients with a tender scrotum. Proper and adequate support of the scrotum and the use of a thick

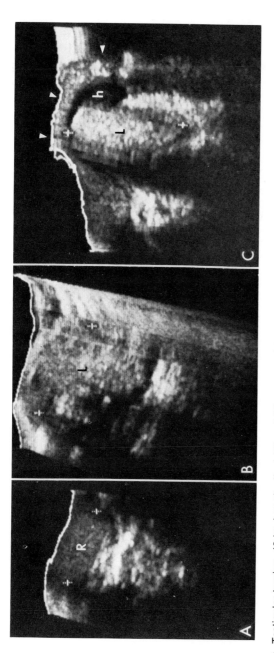

**FIG. 20.** Testicular torsion, 48 hr. Longitudinal (**A**) and (**B**) scans and transverse (**C**) scan demonstrate a large, lobulated echogenic mass in the left hemiscrotum. Testis and epididymis not identified. The wall of the hemiscrotum is thickened (*arrowheads*). A small hydrocele (h) is present.

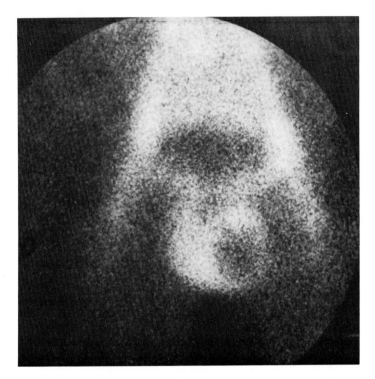

**FIG. 20D continued:** Technetium-99m scan demonstrates decreased profusion in the left hemiscrotum compatible with vascular ischemia.

gel as a couplant in most instances was adequate to prevent patient discomfort during the examination.

After adjusting the time–gain compensation curve for the normal testis, several short quick sweeps are performed over the abnormal hemiscrotum. In the presence of torsion of greater than 4 hr duration, the sonographic testicular echo pattern is abnormal. The testis is enlarged and the homogeneous echotexture is disrupted, with multiple areas of increased echogenicity secondary to necrosis and infarction. Surgery is recommended in any patient who has this sonographic pattern (Figs. 19,20).

In the early phase of torsion (<4 hr), the testis and epididymis are enlarged and have a homogeneously decreased echo pattern (25). In patients who have endured more than 4 hr of pain, the epididymis is consistently enlarged, echogenic, and inseparable from the testicular "mass." The overall sonographic pattern is that of a large heterogeneously echogenic mass within the scrotal sac, involving both testis and epididymis (49).

The scrotal wall in the ipsilateral scrotal sac becomes thickened after 24 to 48 hr and is an indication of the chronicity of the process. Hydrocele may or may not be present. In our series, 2 of 16 patients had a reactive hydrocele. Twelve of our 16 patients underwent surgery for confirmation of infarction and the testicle was removed in 8. Sonographic follow-up of these patients demonstrated a small atrophic testis 2 months after operation with a generally decreased echo pattern compared to the contralateral normal testis. In patients with missed testicular torsion, in whom surgery was not performed, sonographic follow-up revealed the testis to enlarge for 48 hr and then begin to decrease in size after 14 days.

In patients presenting with acute pain of over 4 hr duration, if the testicular echo pattern was homogeneously decreased in the presence of enlargement, testicular torsion was correctly excluded in 98% of patients. Other etiologies for acute pain were found.

## TORSION OF THE TESTICULAR APPENDAGES

These structures are vestiges of the mullerian and mesonephric duct systems and have no clinical significance (4). They may become involved in pathologic conditions of the scrotum and may be the cause of acute scrotal pathology if they become twisted. A single episode of appendiceal torsion, which may be recurrent, simulates the acute symptomatology of torsion of the testis and must be promptly differentiated from the latter. As the viability of the testis is not compromised in this condition, surgical intervention is not indicated except for the relief of pain (24).

Torsion of the testicular appendages occurs most commonly in children between the ages of 6 and 12 years, a younger age group than seen with torsion of the testis. The onset of pain in this condition is more commonly during activity or exercise, although it can also occur during sleep. Pain may be localized to the supratesticular area, a small pea-sized mass may be palpated, or a "blue dot" may be visualized through an accompanying hydrocele (4). Immediately after the onset of symptoms, pain and redness are localized to this area, but after several hours the reactive edema and swelling become generalized and the condition is clinically inseparable from torsion of the testis (4). If $^{99m}$Tc radionuclide scans are performed in patients with torsion of the appendix testis or epididymis, uptake is usually normal, but increased perfusion may be present in the affected hemiscrotum (63).

When sonographic evaluation is performed, the normal testis is examined first. In the presence of torsion of the appendix testis or epididymis, the testicular echo pattern is almost always homogeneously decreased and the abnormal testis is enlarged secondary to edema (Fig. 21). The testis is well-defined and easily separable from the epididymis. The infarcted appendix, though palpable, is not always visible on ultrasound. In infants and small children, in whom the size of the mass is large relative to the size of the testis, the infarcted appendix is seen with greater frequency (Fig. 22). In

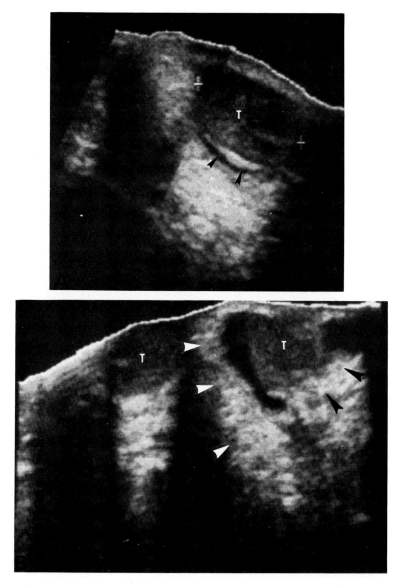

**FIG. 21.** Torsion of the appendix testis. Six-year-old with acute pain. Longitudinal **(A)** and transverse **(B)** scans demonstrate an enlarged left testis (T) with a homogeneously decreased echo pattern. The epididymis is normal *(black arrowheads)*. The testicular tunics are thickened *(white arrowheads)*. A small hydrocele is present.

**FIG. 22. A:** Torsion of the appendix testis. Three-month-old. Transverse scan demonstrates an echogenic mass *(black arrowheads)* adjacent to a normal right testis (t). The testis is clearly defined. The opposite testis (t) is normal. **B:** Surgical specimen. Torsion appendix testis (M).

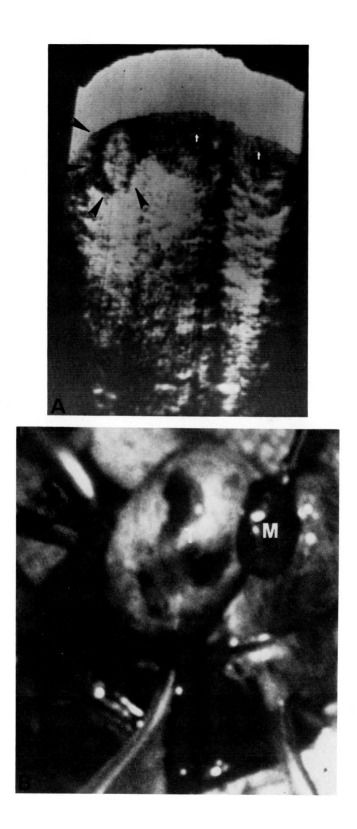

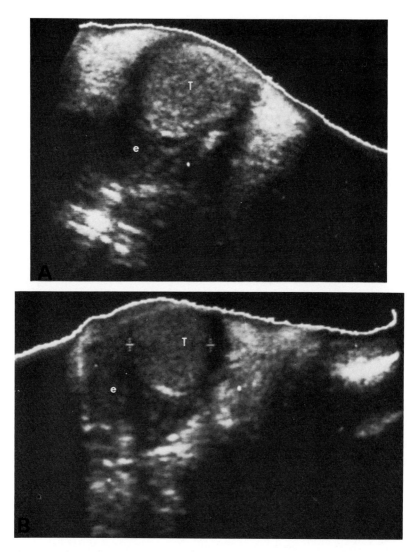

**FIG. 23.** Torsion of the appendix epididymis. Seven-year-old with acute pain. Longitudinal **(A)** and transverse **(B)** scans demonstrate a normal testis (T). The epididymis (e) is markedly enlarged and decreased in echogenicity secondary to edema. This pattern is indistinguishable from epididymitis; however, testicular torsion is excluded.

these instances, it is seen as a predominantly echogenic mass with anechoic areas representing hemorrhage and necrotic infarction.

Other sonographic findings that we have seen in our patients include early ipsilateral echogenic thickening of the testicular tunics and the presence of a small hydrocele. Epididymal swelling was seen in all patients with torsion of the appendix testis. The epididymal swelling seen in torsion of the appendix epididymis is much greater and out of proportion to the amount of testicular edema (Fig. 23). The presence of this finding tends to favor the diagnosis of torsion of the appendix epididymis, although this cannot be differentiated sonographically from epididymitis, and clinical evaluation is necessary. Thickening of the testicular tunics is rarely seen in inflammatory disease of a relatively simple uncomplicated nature.

In the acute setting we feel it is not important to be able to make the diagnosis of torsion of the appendix testis or appendix epididymis. Rather, by establishing a homogeneous testicular echo pattern, testicular torsion can be safely excluded.

## SPERMATOCELE, EPIDIDYMAL CYST

It has been demonstrated that spermatocele or epididymal cyst may cause acute scrotal pain in the pediatric patient (49). Ultrasonic scanning of these patients demonstrates a normal testicular and epididymal echo pattern with no evidence of a hydrocele. It is not known why epididymal masses in children are painful. It is presumed that increased masturbatory activity or trauma in the young age group is causal. Surgical resection of these masses completely eliminates the pain in all children and there is no recurrence. At surgery there is no evidence of trauma, torsion, or hemorrhage into the cyst (49).

Sonography is particularly helpful in those patients with supratesticular pain. A palpable mass such as spermatocele can be differentiated from torsion of the appendix testis or epididymis.

## INFLAMMATORY DISEASE OF THE SCROTUM

Epididymitis is the most common of all intrascrotal inflammations. It is a disease of adults and rarely affects the prepubertal child. In adults, epididymitis is usually bacterial in origin, whereas in children viral etiologies are cited (70). Orchitis rarely occurs alone and is usually the result of infection extending from the epididymis. Orchitis, epididymitis, and/or epididymoorchitis may or may not be accompanied by a hydrocele. Untreated bacterial epididymitis usually progresses to abscess formation with concomitant pyocele formation and involvement of the other intrascrotal contents (37). When viral epididymitis occurs in the absence of fever or pyuria, the condition may be confused with torsion of the testis. When the diagnosis cannot be established with certainty by clinical examination, nuclear scanning will demonstrate increased flow in the affected scrotum (18).

Ultrasound can define precise anatomic structures involved by inflammatory processes when nuclear scans are positive, and lends itself well to serial follow-up examinations. The sonographic findings in the presence of epididymitis are similar in both the child and the adult. We have been able to diagnose simple epididymitis in an infant as early as 3 months of age. The degree of epididymal enlargement is best evaluated on transverse scans where the body and head of both the right and left epididymis can be compared. In early mild epididymitis there is a slight increase in size of the entire epididymis, with prominence of the epididymal head (25). The echo texture of the epididymis is dependent on the severity of the infection and the amount of edema present. Pyogenic epididymitis with the formation of a small abscess tends to be more echogenic, although it has not always been possible to obtain confirmation by bacterial culture. In the presence of a reactive hydrocele, the portion of the epididymis in contact with the fluid may be slightly more echogenic than the remainder of the epididymis owing to increased through sound transmission. This area of increased echoes should not be confused with the presence of an abscess or necrosis. In patients with recurrent bouts of epididymitis and with a recurrent or persistent hydrocele, thickening of the testicular tunics will be present, seen as an echogenic line surrounding the testis and lining the scrotal sac (27). In addition, small calcific echogenic foci are frequently identified within the epididymis or related to the tunics. In patients with recurrent epididymitis,

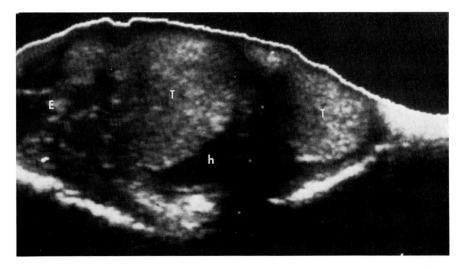

**FIG. 24.** Simple epididymitis. Right and left testis (T) are similar in echo pattern. The epididymis is markedly enlarged and irregular and in configuration (E). A small hydrocele (h) is present.

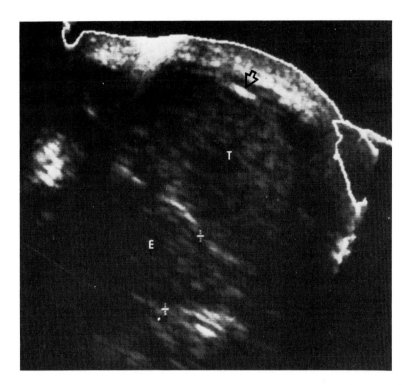

**FIG. 25.** Epididymo-orchitis. Both testis (T) and epididymis (E) are enlarged and anechoic. Testicular tunics are thickened *(arrow)*.

we have seen soft tissue tags arising from the body and head of the epididymis. At surgery these tags represent small epididymal appendages filled with inflammatory tissue.

In the presence of epididymo-orchitis, the primary findings are enlarged testis and epididymis, both of which have a homogeneously decreased echo texture (Figs. 24–26). The testicular echo pattern and size are best compared on transverse scans. A pyocele when present is seen as a complex fluid collection filled with septations or scattered low level echos due to pus and cellular debris. When a pyocele is present, it is important to scan the testis entirely at 5-mm intervals. If the echo pattern is focally or diffusely heterogeneous or if areas of increased echogenicity are identified, then an abscess with necrosis should be suspected (Fig. 27). We have been able to detect this sonographically prior to the clinical evidence of abscess formation, and surgery is indicated in such cases.

When the entire scrotal contents are involved by an abscess of the testis and epididymis, the sonographic pattern is often indistinguishable from a torsion or severe testicular trauma, and can only be distinguished by the

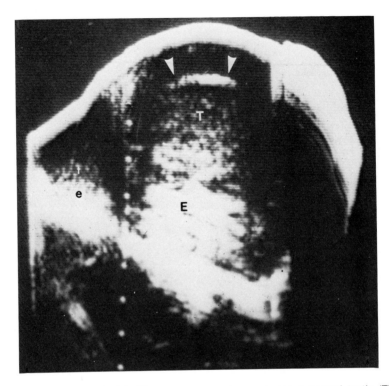

**FIG. 26.** Chronic epididymitis. Transverse scan demonstrates a normal testis (T). The epididymis (E) is markedly enlarged and echogenic. Testicular tunics are thickened *(arrowheads).* The opposite testis (t) and epididymis (e) are normal.

clinical history. A large echogenic mass is present, which has anechoic areas within it. There may be shadowing secondary to the presence of gas and this can be confirmed by coned radiographs of the scrotal area. The testis and epididymis may not be identifiable in the presence of extensive necrotic disease and there may be diffuse thickening of the scrotum.

## SCROTAL TRAUMA

Blunt trauma to the scrotum uncommonly results in testicular rupture. When this occurs, the tunica albuginea is torn with subsequent extrusion of testicular contents into the scrotal sac. Hydrocele is a frequent accompaniment of this process. Early surgical intervention for both the diagnosis of testicular rupture and for testicular salvage is advocated (56). Prior to the use of ultrasound and radionuclide imaging, surgery was the only diagnostic modality available and was frequently delayed. Radionuclide scanning demonstrates increased scrotal heat while ultrasound localizes and delineates the extent of intrascrotal damage (60).

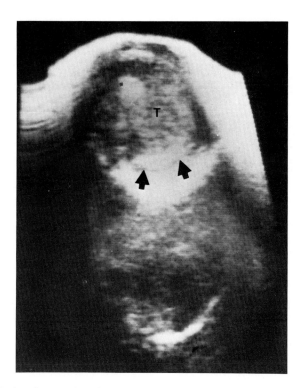

**FIG. 27.** Testicular abscess. Longitudinal scan demonstrates an enlarged heterogeneous testis (T) with areas of increased echogenicity. The epididymis is normal *(arrows).*

Hematomas and hematoceles of the scrotum have sonographic patterns similar to collections of blood elsewhere in the body. Highly echogenic textures are seen early, which become more anechoic with time (8). Scrotal wall and epididymal hematomas are seen as echogenic masses separate from the testis (Fig. 28).

Sonography will clearly indicate the presence or absence of testicular rupture (2). When rupture of the testis has occurred, the homogeneity of testicular echo pattern is disrupted (Fig. 29). Acute intratesticular hematomas are seen as one or more areas of increased or decreased echogenicity within the testis. The testis may be partially or totally ill-defined. Hematoceles are usually seen in the presence of testicular rupture due to a tear of the tunica. These appear as complex fluid collection surrounding the testis.

Again, the principle that we postulated earlier holds true in the presence of trauma. That is, if the homogeneity of the testicular echo pattern is in any way interrupted, prompt surgical intervention is suggested for testicular salvage. Sonographic evidence of a hematocele in the absence of testicular rupture does not require surgery.

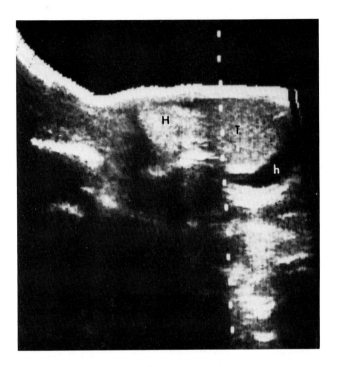

**FIG. 28.** Hematoma of the epididymal head. Longitudinal scan demonstrates an echogenic mass (H) cephalad to the testis (T) which is completely normal. A small hematocele (h) is present.


## PITFALLS IN DIAGNOSIS

Several difficulties are consistently encountered in ultrasonic scanning of the scrotum:

1. No distinguishable ultrasonic patterns have emerged to differentiate benign from malignant testicular tumors. Since benign tumors are rare, all testicular tumors, with the exception of testicular cysts, should be considered malignant until proven otherwise.

2. Pathology of the epididymal tail is often mistaken for an intratesticular neoplasm (Fig. 30) (31, 54). Clinical palpation of the region is difficult. We have unsuccessfully attempted pinhole $^{99m}$Tc scanning to demonstrate an intratesticular defect. Water path sonography may have a better diagnostic yield in this regard.

3. In patients in whom testicular torsion can be confidently excluded, the etiology of the testicular pain cannot always be determined. Torsion of the appendix epididymis is difficult to differentiate sonographically from epididymitis except by history.

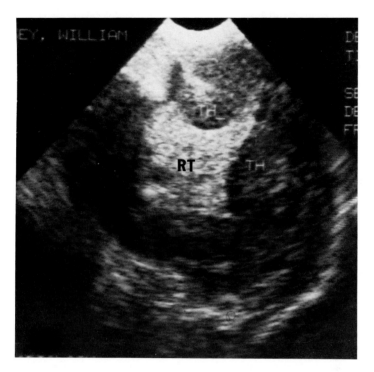

**FIG. 29.** Testicular rupture. Longitudinal scan through a markedly abnormal right testis (RT). Multiple anechoic areas (TH) are seen within the area of the testis representing hematoma secondary to rupture. (Courtesy Dr. Anthony Lupetin, Allegheny General Hospital.)

4. A theoretical difficulty may occur in the patient with acute torsion who presents with pain of less than four hours' duration. If, as Hricak predicts (25), the testis is enlarged and exhibits a homogeneously decreased echo pattern, then torsion of the testis would be incorrectly excluded by our methods. Following ultrasonic examination, these patients should routinely undergo radionuclide examination to evaluate testicular perfusion.

## SUMMARY

Although we have described in great detail the sonographic patterns of multiple pathologies of the scrotum, two important concepts emerge. They are:

1. Regardless of the history or presenting symptoms, if the testicular echo pattern alone is disrupted and the testicular adnexae are normal, the presence of an intratesticular neoplasm should be suspected until proven otherwise.

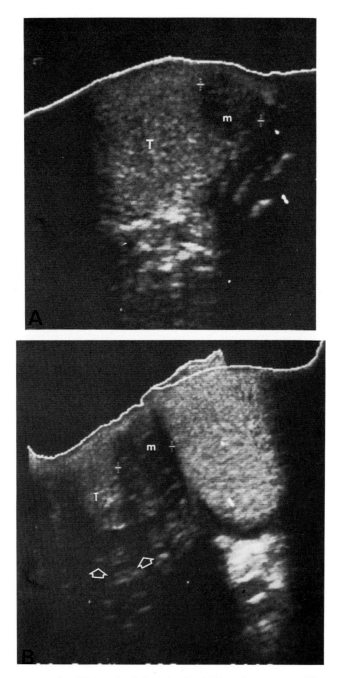

**FIG. 30.** Hematoma of epididymal tail. Longitudinal **(A)** and transverse **(B)** scans demonstrate an "intratesticular mass" (M) with a decreased echo texture. The overall echogenicity of the testis (T) and epididymis *(arrows)* is decreased.

2. In any patient presenting with an "acute scrotum," if there is no disruption of the testicular echo pattern, even in the presence of testicular enlargement or overall decreased echogenicity, testicular torsion can be safely excluded in 98% of patients.

## ACKNOWLEDGMENTS

We wish to thank Mr. Fred Liebman for the preparation of photographic materials, and Mrs. Sandra Bamonte and Ms. Janice Viccora for typing the manuscript.

## REFERENCES

1. Ahlberg, N. E., Bartley, O., Chidekel, N., and Fritjofsson, A. Phlebography in varicocele scroti. *Acta Radiol. [Diagn]*, 4:517, 1966.
2. Albert, N. E. Testicular ultrasound for trauma. *J. Urol.*, 124:558–559, 1980.
3. Allan, W. R., and Brown, R. B. Torsion of the testis: A review of 68 cases. *Br. Med. J.*, 1:1396–1397, 1966.
4. Allen, T. D. Disorders of the male external genitalia. In: *Clinical Pediatric Urology*, edited by P. P. Kelalis, L. R., Kenig, and A. B. Belman, pp. 636–668. W. B. Saunders, Philadelphia, 1976.
5. Arger, P. H., Mulhern, C. B., Coleman, B. G., Pollack, C. B., Wein, A., Koss, J., Arenson, R., and Banner, M. Prospective analysis of the value of scrotal ultrasound, *Radiology*, 141:763–766, 1981.
6. Barzell, W. E. I., and Whitmore, W. F. Neoplasms of the testis. In: *Campbell's Urology*, edited by J. W. Harrison, R. F. Gittes, A. D. Perlmutter, T. A. Stamey, and P. C. Walsh, pp. 1162. W. B. Saunders, Philadelphia, 1979.
7. Batata, M. A. Whitmore, W. F., and Hilaus, B. S. Cancer of the undescended or maldescended testis. *AJR*, 126:302, 1976.
8. Bird, K. I. Emergency testicular scanning. In: *Ultrasound in Emergency Medicine*, edited by K. J. W. Taylor and G. N. Viscomi, pp. 55–70. Churchill Livingstone, New York, 1981.
9. Black, R. E., Cox, J. A., Ahn, B., and Babcock, B. S. Abdominoscrotal hydrocele in children. *Pediatrics*, 67:420–422, 1981.
10. Blei, L., Sihelnik, S., Bloom, D., Stutzman, R., and Chiadis, J. Ultrasonic analysis of chronic intratesticular pathology. *J. Ultrasound Med.*, 2:17–23, 1983.
11. Burney, B. T., and Klatte, E. C. Ultrasound and computed tomography of the abdomen in the staging and management of testicular carcinoma. *Radiology*, 132:415–419, 1979.
12. Colodny, A. H., and Hopkins, T. B. Testicular tumors in infants and children. In: *Urologic Clinics of North America*, edited by E. E. Fraley, pp., 347–358. W. B. Saunders, Philadelphia, 1977.
13. Conrad, A. R., Sheshagiri, A. S. and Rao, Ultrasound diagnosis of fetal hydrocele. *Radiology*, 127:232, 1978.
14. Cooper, T. P., Anderson, R. G., and Chapman, W. H. Hemangioma of the scrotum: A case report. Review and comparison with hydrocele. *J. Urol.*, 112: 623–626, 1974.
15. Dunn, E. K., Macchia, R. J., and Solomon, N. A. Scintigraphic pattern in missed testicular torsion. *Radiology*, 139: 175–180, 1981.
16. Givler, R. L. Testicular involvement in leukemia and lymphoma. *Cancer*, 23:1290–1295, 1969.
17. Gold, R. H., Ehrlich, R. M., Samuels, B., Dowdy, A., and Young, R. T. Scrotal thermography. *Radiology*, 122:129–132, 1977.
18. Goldstein, H. A., and Treves, S. Scintigraphic demonstration of epididymo-orchitis and a hydrocele. *Radiology*, 125:738, 1977.

19. Goodman, J. D., and Haller, J. O The scrotum. In: *Ultrasound in Pediatrics*, edited by J. O. Haller and A. Shkolnik, p. 226. Churchill Livingstone, New York, 1981.
20. Gould. L., Klein, K., and Patel, N. Ultrasound evaluation of a spermatic cord myx-oliposarcoma. *J. Med. Soc. N.J.*, 76:203–204, 1979.
21. Graf, R. A. Malignant tumors of the spermatic cord: A brief review and presentation of a lipofibro-myxosarcoma of the spermatic cord. *J. Urol.*, 93:74, 1965.
22. Greenberg, S. H., Lipshultz, L. I., Morganroth, J., and Wein, A. J. The use of the doppler stethoscope in the evaluation of varicoceles. *J. Urol.*, 117:296, 1977.
23. Holder, L. E., Martire, J. R., Holmes, E. R., and Wagner, H. N. Testicular radionuclide angiography and static imaging: anatomy, scintigraphic interpretation, and clinical indications. *Radiology*, 125:739–752, 1977.
24. Holland, J. M., Graham, J. B., and Ignatoff, J. M. Conservative management of twisted testicular appendages. *J. Urol.*, 125:312–314, 1981.
25. Hricak, H., Lue, T , Filly, R. A., Alpers, C. E., Zeineh, S. J., and Tanagho, E. E. The role of sonography in diagnosing testicular torsion—experimental study. *J. Ultrasound Med. (in press)*, 1983.
26. Jellins, J., and Barraclough, B. H. Ultrasonic imaging of the scrotum. In: *Ultrasound in Medicine*, pp. 151–152. Plenum Press, New York, 1978.
27. Jones, P. G. Undescended testes. *Aust. Paediatr. J.*, 2:36–38, 1966.
28. Kaplan, G. W. Acute idiopathic scrotal edema. *J. Pediatr. Surg.*, 12:647, 1977.
29. Laron, Z., and Zilka, E. Compensatory hypertrophy of the testicle in unilateral cryptorchidism. *J. Clin. Endocr.*, 29:1409–1413, 1969.
30. Laron, Z., Carp, M., and Dolberg, L., Juvenile hypothyroidism with testicular enlargement. *Acta. Ped. Scand.*, 59:317, 1970.
31. Leopold, G. R., Woo, V. L., Scheible, F. W., Nachtsheim, D., and Gosink, B. B. High-resolution ultrasonography of scrotal pathology. *Radiology*, 131:719–722, 1979.
32. Levitt, S. B., Kogan, S. J., and Engel, R. M. The impalpable testis: A rational approach to management. *J. Urol.*, 120:515–520, 1978.
33. Lupetin, A. R., King, W., Rich, P., and Lederman, R. B. Ultrasound diagnosis of testicular leukemia. *Radiology*, 146:171–172, 1983.
34. Lupetin, A. Testicular sarcoid. *Sem. Ultras*, March, 1983.
35. Madrazo, B. L., Klugo, R. C., Parks, J. A., and DiLoreto, R. Ultrasonographic demonstration of undescended testes. *Radiology*, 133:181–183, 1979.
36. Markland, C., Special problems in managing patients with testicular cancer. In: *Urologic Clinics of N. America*, edited by E. E. Fraleg, pp. 421–431. W. B. Saunders, Philadelphia, 1977.
37. Meares, E. M. Urinary tract infections in men. In: *Campbell's Urology*, edited by J. W. Harrison, R. F. Gittes, A. D. Perlmutter, T. A. Stamey, and P. C. Walsh , pp. 512–522. W. B. Saunders, Philadelphia, 1979.
38. Merrin, C. Seminoma. In: *Urologic Clinics of North America*, edited by E. E. Fraleg, pp. 379–392. W. B. Saunders, Philadelphia, 1977.
39. Murphy, G. P., and Gaeta, J. F. Tumors of testicular adnexal structures and seminal vesicles. In: *Campbell's Urology*, edited by J. W. Harrison, R. F. Gittes, A. D. Perlmutter, T. A. Stamey, and P. C. Walsh, pp. 1200–1215. W. B. Saunders, Philadelphia, 1979.
40. Myers, R. P. Male genital tract. In: *Clinical Pediatric Urology*, edited by P. P. Kelalis, L. R. King, and A. B. Belman, p. 937. W. B. Saunders, Philadelphia, 1976.
41. Nahoum, C. R. D., De Almeida, A. S., and Flores, E. Scrotal scan in the diagnosis of varicocele. *Fertil. Steril.*, 34:287–288, 1980.
42. Naser, V., and Ikinger, U. Echographie des scrotums und der testes mit hilfe einer nueen untersuchungstechnik. *Urologe*, A18:321–325, 1979.
43. Nisula, B. C. Benign bilateral testicular enlargement. *J. Clin. Endocrinol. Metab.*, 38:440, 1974.
44. Nochomovitz, L. E., De La Torrer, F. E., and Rosai, J. Pathology of germ cell tumors of the testis. In: *Urologic Clinics of North America*, edited by E. E. Fraley, pp. 359–369. W. B. Saunders, Philadelphia, 1977.
45. Opal, S. M., Pittman, D. L., and Hofeldt, F. D. Testicular sarcoidosis. *Am. J. Med.*, 67:147, 1979.

46. Pedersen, J. F., Holm, H. H., and Hald, T. Torsion of the testis diagnosed by ultrasound. *J. Urol.*, 113:66–68, 1975.
47. Phillips, G. N., Schneider, M., Goodman, J. D., and Macchia, R. J. Ultrasound evaluation of the scrotum. *Urol. Radiol.*, 1:157–163, 1980.
48. Phillips, G., Kumari, S., and Abrams, H. The acute scrotum. Presented RSNA, 1981.
49. Phillips, G., Kumari, S., and Abrams, H. Sonographic exclusion of torsion testis. Presented RSNA, paper 332, 1982 *Radiology*, (submitted).
50. Pillari, G., Rubenstein, W. A., and Siess, J. Seminoma: Improved imaging and tumor characterization with computed tomography. *J. Urol.*, 123:41–43, 1980.
51. Pugh, R. C. B. (Ed.). *Pathology of the Testis*. Blackwell Scientific Publications, Oxford, 1976.
52. Rodriques, D. D., and Rodriques, W. C. Doppler ultrasound versus testicular scanning in the evaluation of the acute scrotum. *J. Urol.*, 125:343–347, 1981.
53. Saiontz, H. I., Gilchrist, G. S., and Smithson, W. A. Testicular relapse in childhood leukemia. *Mayo Clin. Proc.*, 53:212–216, 1978.
54. Sample, W. F., Gottesman, J. E., Skinner, D. G., and Ehrlich, R. M. Gray scale ultrasound of the scrotum. *Radiology*, 127:225–228, 1978.
55. Sample, W. F. Renal, adrenal and scrotal ultrasonography. In: *Diagnostic Ultrasound, Text and Cases*, edited by D. A. Sarti, and W. F. Sample. G. K. Hall, Boston, 1980.
56. Schuster, G. Traumatic rupture of the testicle and a review of the literature. *J. Urol.*, 127:1194–1196, 1982.
57. Scorer, C. G., and Farrington, G. H. *Congenital Deformities of the Testis and Epididymis*. Appleton-Century-Crofts, New York, 1971.
58. Scorer, C. G., and Farrington, G. H. Congenital anomolies of the testis. In: *Campbell's Urology*, edited by J. W. Harrison, R. F. Gittes, A. D. Perlmutter, T. A. Stamey, and P. C. Walsh, pp. 1549–1563. W. B. Saunders, Philadelphia, 1979.
59. Smith, J. P. Testicular tumors in infants and children. *Urology*, 2:353, 1973.
60. Stage, K. H., Schlenvogel, R., and Lewis, S. Testicular scanning: Clinical experience with 72 patients. *J. Urol.*, 125:334–335, 1981.
61. Stoffel, T. J., Nesbit, M. E., and Levitt, S. H. Extramedullary involvement of the testis in childhood leukemia. *Cancer*, 35:1203–1211, 1975.
62. Subramanyam, B. R., Balthazar, E. J., Raghavendra, B. N., Horii, S. C., and Hilton, S. Sonographic diagnosis of scrotal hernia. *AJR*, 139:535–538, 1982.
63. Thomas, W. E. G., and Cooke, P. H. Dynamic radionuclide scanning of the testis in acute scrotal conditions. *Br. J. Surg.*, 68:621–624, 1981.
64. Tibbs, D. J. Unilateral absence of the testis: Eight cases of true monorchism. *Br. J. Surg.*, 48:601, 1961.
65. Vanesian, R., Grossman, M., Metherell, A., Flynn, J. J., and Louschr, S. Antepartum ultrasonic diagnosis of congenital hydrocele. *Radiology*, 126:765–766, 1978.
66. Vitale, P. J., Khademi, M., and Seebode, J. J. Selective gonadal angiography for testicular localization in patients with cryptorchidism. *Surg. Forum*, 25:538–540, 1974.
67. Weiss, R. M., Glickman, M. G., and Lytton, B. Venographic localization of the nonpalpable undescended testis in children. *J. Urol.*, 117:513–515, 1977.
68. White, J. J., Shaker, I. J., and Oh, K. S. Herniography: a diagnostic refinement in the management of cryptorchidism. *Am. Surg.*, 39:624–629, 1973.
69. Wilson, P. C., Day, D. L., Valvo, J. R., and Gramiak, R. Scrotal ultrasound with an octason. *Radiography*, 2:24–39, 1982.
70. Winberg, J. Urinary tract infections in infants and children. In: *Campbell's Urology*, edited by J. W. Harrison, R. F. Gittes, A. D. Perlmutter, T. A. Stamey, and P. C. Walsh, pp. 480–491. W. B. Saunders, Philadelphia, 1979.
71. Wolverson, M. K., Jagannadharao, B., and Sundaram, M. CT in localization of impalpable cryptorchid testes. *AJR*, 134:725–729, 1980.
72. Wolverson, M. K., Houttuin, E., Heiberg, E., Murali, S., and Shields, J. B. Comparison of computed tomography with high-resolution real-time ultrasound in the localization of the impalpable undescended testis. *Radiology*, 146:133–136, 1983.
73. Price, E. B., and Mostofi, F. K. Epidermoid Cysts of the Testes in Children. *J. Pediatr.*, 77:676–679, 1970.

*Ultrasound Annual 1983*, edited by R. C.
Sanders and M. Hill. Raven Press, New York
© 1983.

# Ophthalmic Ultrasonography

Stanley Chang, D. Jackson Coleman, and Mary E. Smith

*Cornell University Medical College, New York, New York 10021*

Continued advances in the management of ocular and orbital diseases have demanded accurate and reliable diagnostic modalities to assess and characterize the pathologic condition prior to treatment. Ultrasonography, because of its ability to depict ocular and orbital tissues with high resolution, is an indispensible diagnostic tool for the clinical ophthalmologist. The development of compact, portable, and convenient-to-use instrumentation has made this modality available to all ophthalmologists whether general or subspecialist.

The ultrasonographic examination is performed in real-time with interpretation of both A- and B-scan images. Spontaneous and induced movements of structures are evaluated to aid in differential diagnosis. Comprehensive texts are available concerning these techniques (6, 8). More recently spectral analysis techniques have been used to characterize tissues acoustically, as well as to enhance image displays (11). These developments offer promise of new dimensions in the diagnostic approach. In clinical usage, ophthalmic ultrasonography includes three broad categories—ocular biometry, ocular diagnosis, and orbital diagnosis. These topics will be discussed individually below.

## TECHNIQUES AND INSTRUMENTATION

Both immersion and contact techniques are used in ophthalmic ultrasound. The immersion technique uses an adhesive small aperture drape sealed around the periorbital structures holding a small volume of saline over the globe. The lids are separated using a lid speculum. The transducer, mounted on a mechanical stage, is lowered into the saline and the eye and orbit are scanned in serial tomographic sections. This technique offers high resolution of the entire eye and orbit in one scan plane. Both B- and A-scans are displayed simultaneously. Examining transducers can be changed to enhance resolution. Ocular examination is usually performed using frequencies of 10 MHz and 15 MHz; the orbit is examined at 10 MHz and 5 MHz. Choroidal and retinal lesions of 0.5 mm can be detected. Real-time examination can be performed by rapid sector scanning to evaluate kinetic activity within the eye and differentiate vitreous hemorrhage from retinal detachment.

In contact ultrasound systems, the transducer (usually 8 to 10 MHz) is mechanically sector-scanned at a rate of 20 to 30 frames/second. The probe is completely enclosed, and coupling to the ocular structures is achieved by applying a small amount of methylcellulose. Using this technique, the anterior ocular structures—cornea, iris, and lens—are usually obscured by the "main bang" of the transducer. However, this method is most popular in office practice because of the convenience and portability of available instrumentation. B-scan resolution is less good when compared with immersion ultrasonography but is adequate for most clinical situations. In complex ocular trauma cases or in orbital disease the improved immersion B-scan resolution may be more useful.

Quantitative A-scan techniques developed by Ossoinig are often used in conjunction with contact B-scan instruments (13). Using this combined technique, Ossoinig has simplified interpretation of A-scan patterns and contributed to the understanding of tissue differentiation in ophthalmic ultrasound. While we prefer a combined system of A- and B-scan in one instrument because of ease of lesion localization, the quantitative technique also provides accurate results.

Recently linear array scanning systems have been introduced in ophthalmology (23). This instrument contains an array of 35 transducers and scans at a rate of 60 frames per second. It is used with either the immersion or contact method. The fast scanning rate allows observation of dynamic vascular changes in the eye and orbit, such as ophthalmic artery pulsations. This generation of linear array scanners is compromised by poor resolution when compared with sector scanners. Future generations may offer improved resolution.

The rapid growth in number of manufacturers in ophthalmic ultrasound instrumentation has not been met by measures to standardize equipment parameters. In addition to differences resulting from design philosophy between manufacturers, there also may be variation in parameters from one unit to another in equipment from the same manufacturer (17). Measures are needed to establish minimum standards within the industry.

## OCULAR BIOMETRY

Ultrasound is the most accurate means of measuring the axial length of the eye to determine intraocular lens power prior to cataract surgery. Using axial length, corneal keratometry measurements, and predicted postoperative anterior chamber depth, the postoperative refractive error can be calculated from a formula based on optical considerations in a model eye. Predictions based on ultrasound have been more accurate than when estimated clinically, and large errors in postoperative refraction can be avoided.

In ultrasound examination of the eye with advanced cataract, B-scan ultrasonography is helpful in ruling out coexisting abnormalities prior to surgery. The cataractous lens often contains internal echoes in contrast to the clear lens which is homogeneous and acoustically clear (Fig. 1). In advanced cases the nucleus of the lens can often be separated from the cortical layers. The posterior structures are evaluated carefully with B-scan. For A-scan measurement of axial length, the alignment must be coaxial with the visual axis and a fixation light within the transducer can be used. Along the optical or visual axis, the surfaces of the cornea, lens, and vitreoretinal interface present highly reflective echoes (Fig. 1). When echoes from the lens surfaces and vitreoretinal interface are maximal, alignment is axial and electronic gates are used to perform the measurements. Ultrasound velocity is faster through the lens and therefore measurement and addition of the separate components—anterior chamber, lens thickness, and vitreous length—is advised. The use of an average velocity for the entire axial length can also be used but is less accurate. Recently the introduction of digital scan converters has facilitated measurement by allowing storage of an optimal A-scan pattern.

The accuracy of predicting postoperative refractive error is good, despite the fact that several variables in the calculation may be affected by the surgical procedure. In several reported series, accuracy is ± 2D in almost 90% or more of patients (1, 10, 12, 18). However, it was noted that eyes with shorter axial lengths tended to have greater errors. As a result, regression formulas were developed based on previous surgical experience (16). These formulas are available for each style of intraocular lens and appear to improve the accuracy of intraocular lens power determination.

Another application of ultrasonic biometry is in the measurement of corneal thickness (pachymetry). Radial keratotomy is a type of refractive surgery used to correct myopia by the placement of radial partial-thickness incisions into the cornea, which reduces the optical power of the cornea. The deeper the incisions, the greater the effect on myopia. The ultrasonic pachymeter has been used to map corneal thickness over its surface in the hope that the depth of the incision can be more carefully controlled. This surgical procedure is currently undergoing controlled clinical trials and the role of ultrasound measurement will be studied.

Computer analysis of digitized A-scan signals has allowed *in vivo* measurement of choroidal thickness (4). The potential for studying choroidal physiology and diseases using this technique appears great since there are few existing methods of studying this layer of the eye *in vivo*.

## OCULAR DIAGNOSIS

Ultrasound has a most valuable role in the clinical evaluation of vitreoretinal disease, ocular tumors, and foreign body localization. The characterization of the abnormal ocular morphology has resulted in greater success in the management of these diseases using new surgical techniques, developed

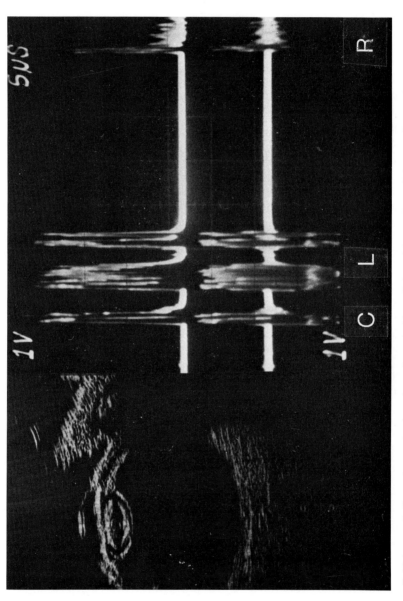

**FIG. 1.** B-scan (*left*) demonstrating advanced cataractous change with outlining of the nucleus of the lens. A-scan demonstrates both surfaces of the cornea (C), internal echoes within the lens (L), and the vitreoretinal interface (R).

over the last decade. With trends toward conservative management of ocular tumors, ultrasonography has a vital role in following patients with choroidal tumors.

The normal vitreous cavity is usually acoustically clear. Fresh vitreous hemorrhage is low in reflectivity with diffuse scattered echoes within the vitreous cavity (Fig. 2). Frequently these echoes exhibit swirling aftermovement, as the patient is instructed to move his eye in different directions. The A-scan reveals echoes lower in amplitude, compared with the retinal reflectivity. Combined A- and B-scan information can be presented in the isometric mode, which allows the image to be rotated and tilted in different perspectives to appreciate the relative A-scan amplitudes of structures within the eye.

Asteroid hyalosis is a vitreous opacity that may be confused with vitreous hemorrhage (Fig. 3). It consists of particles of calcium soaps in the vitreous, which usually do not reduce the visual acuity. These opacities can be differentiated from vitreous hemorrhage by their high reflectivity from individual small particles in the vitreous space. The isometric mode demonstrates the high reflectivity of these opacities compared with vitreous hemorrhage.

Vitreous hemorrhage may be associated with retinal detachment, in which the retina appears as thin, continuous membranes, extending in either direction from the optic nerve toward the ora serrata (Fig. 4). The retina exhibits less aftermovement than hemorrhage in the vitreous. On A-scan the retina is highly reflective, exhibiting a single, high amplitude echo, almost as high as the scleral amplitude. The extent, duration, and degree of organization of the retinal detachment can be determined by ultrasound, providing information concerning surgical prognosis (2). Recent retinal detachment appears as thin, continuous membranes with undulating mobility (Fig. 5). As retinal detachment becomes more organized, it becomes thickened with fibroglial membrane proliferation on the surface of the retina and the development of fixed folds. On B-scan the retina appears straightened and thicker, with closure of the funnel in late stages (Fig. 6). The aftermovement is markedly diminished or absent. This latter configuration offers poor surgical prognosis.

In ocular trauma, damage to any of the ocular structures may appear. Abnormalities in the depth of the anterior chamber, changes in location of the lens, or vitreoretinal abnormalities may be present (Fig. 7). Severe injuries may result in marked disorganization of the globe, and differentiation of intraocular structures may be quite difficult. With intraocular foreign bodies, both computerized axial tomography (CT) and ultrasound should be performed. CT scan offers great accuracy in the detection and location of foreign bodies. Ultrasound offers supplemental information concerning secondary ocular changes as a result of the trauma, such as retinal detachment or vitreous hemorrhage (Fig. 8). Ultrasound is probably more accurate in determining whether a foreign body, which is located near the posterior ocular coats has perforated the globe or is contained within the globe.

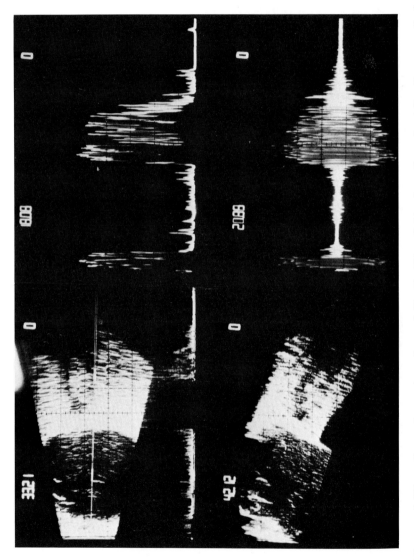

**FIG. 2.** Contact B-scan of diffuse vitreous hemorrhage (*upper left*) with diffuse light echoes throughout the vitreous cavity. Isometric scan (*lower left*) combining A- and B-scan echoes of the lower reflective echoes within the vitreous space. Upper A-scan (*right*) reveals low amplitude echo from vitreous hemorrhage.

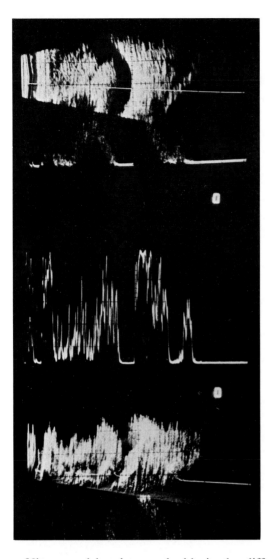

**FIG. 3.** Contact B-scan of asteroid hyalosis reveals right echoes within the vitreous space. The echoes appear to be suspended in the cortical vitreous and are of moderately strong reflectivity on A-scan *(middle)*. Isometric scan combines both A- and B-scan information in one image *(bottom)*.

Ultrasound has been valuable in the differentiation and management of ocular tumors. Choroidal melanoma can be differentiated from metastatic carcinoma, choroidal hemangioma, and subretinal hemorrhage, with high accuracy (Figs. 9–11). In more recent years the trend has shifted to more conservative management of choroidal melanoma by measures such as cobalt plaque or proton beam radiation. In both these methods, ultrasound is the best way to measure tumor thickness for calculation of depth–dose curves. Following treatment serial ultrasound examinations may be used to follow the response to therapy.

Spectral analysis techniques for ocular tumors offer promise in differentiating ocular tumor types with greater accuracy and may provide further

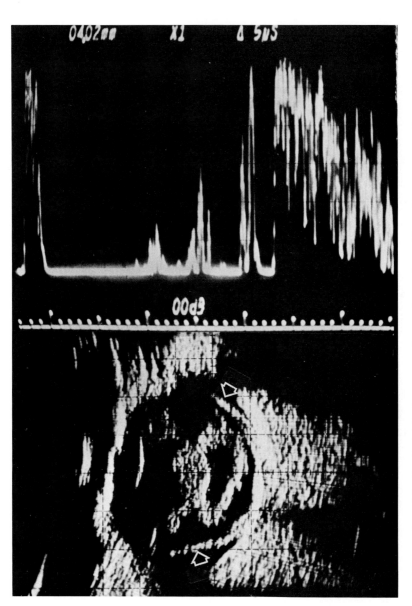

**FIG. 4.** Immersion B-scan of combined retinal detachment and vitreous hemorrhage. The retina appears as thin continuous lines, extending from the optic disc toward the ora serrata (*arrows*). On A-scan it demonstrates a highly reflective single echo, almost as high as the scleral echo.

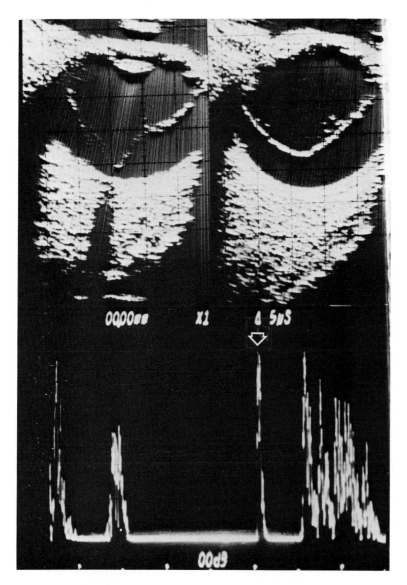

**FIG. 5.** Immersion B-scan *(top)* revealing cataractous lens and total retinal detachment. Two scan planes are demonstrated. A-scan demonstrates a high amplitude, single echo of high reflectivity *(arrow)*.

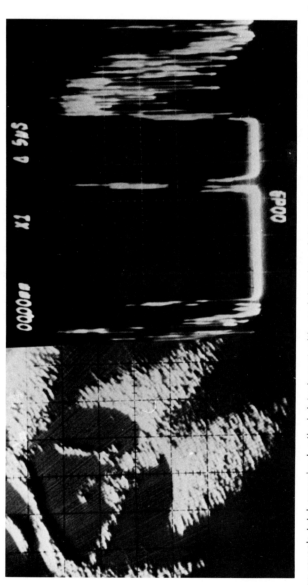

**FIG. 6.** B-scan reveals total organized retinal detachment with straightening of the retina and closing of the funnel. The retina exhibits extremely low mobility in this configuration.

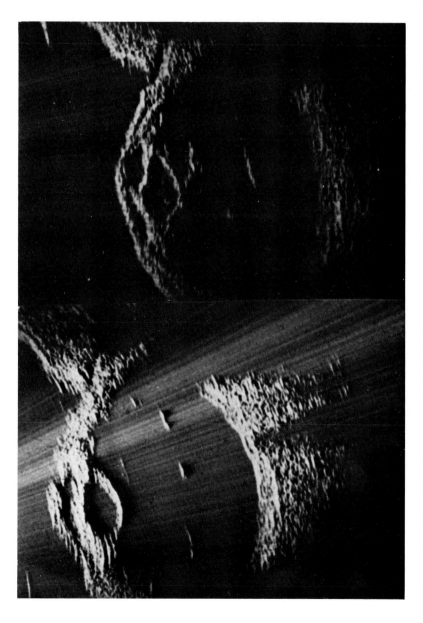

**FIG. 7.** Traumatic subluxation of the lens, associated with shallow anterior chamber and vitreous hemorrhage. The lens is subluxated temporally with a shallow anterior chamber. With loss of zonular attachments the lens exhibits a more globular configuration. There are light diffuse echoes within the vitreous cavity, suggestive of vitreous hemorrhage.

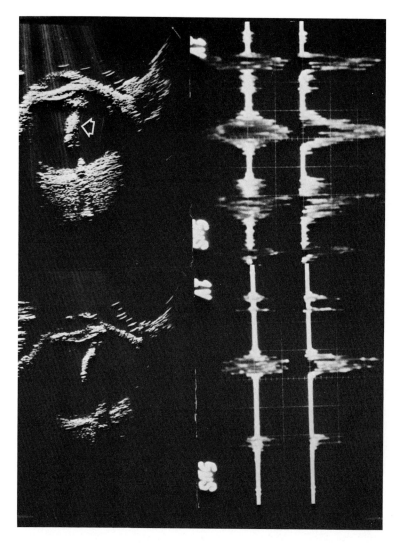

**FIG. 8.** A metallic foreign body *(arrow)* within the eye exhibits a cluster of highly reflective echoes within the vitreous cavity. The absorption of sound by the foreign body results in acoustic shadowing in the image posterior to it. As the sensitivity is reduced *(lower)*, the foreign body reflectivity remains bright as scleral amplitudes begin to disappear.

information concerning cellular histology in choroidal melanomas. Coleman, et al. (5, 7), using spectral parameters, have separated melanoma into two groups—spindle melanomas and mixed cell/epithelioid types, based on computer classification. These findings may offer predictors in the natural course of the tumor, as well as its response to various modes of therapy.

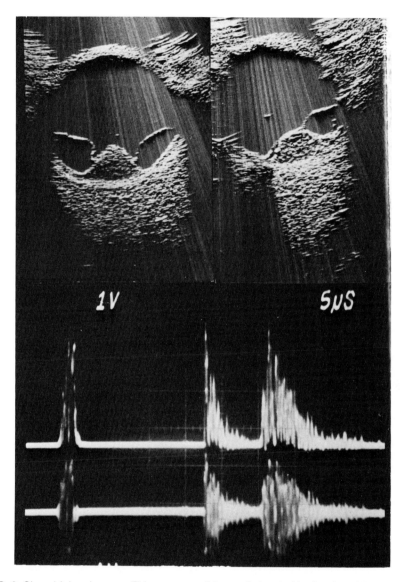

**FIG. 9.** Choroidal melanoma. This convex solid mass is located in the choroid and has an associated retinal detachment. On A-scan there is an exponential decay in the envelope of echoes as the sound is absorbed through this relatively homogenous mass.

## ORBITAL DIAGNOSIS

The development of the CT scan has overshadowed the importance of ultrasound in the diagnosis of orbital disease. Ultrasound is still important in the detection and tissue differentiation for orbital disease, and combined

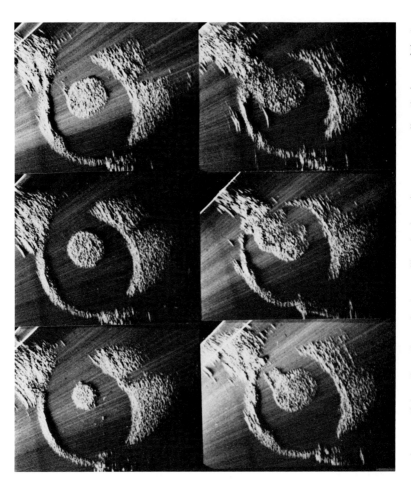

**FIG. 10.** Serial B-scans reveal sequential sections through a large ciliary body melanoma, revealing the base of the tumor located in the region of the ciliary body.

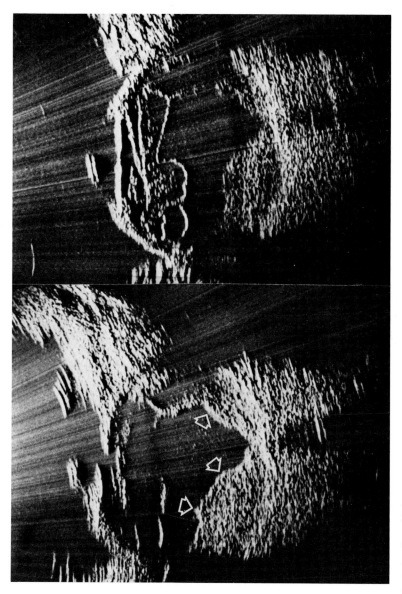

**FIG. 11.** Metastatic choroidal tumor associated with vitreous hemorrhage. There is a large choroidal mass replacing most of the posterior globe (*arrows*) and light scattered vitreous hemorrhage with membrane formation anteriorly in the vitreous.

with a CT scan, a high degree of accuracy in orbital diagnosis can be achieved. The major causes of exophthalmos can be separated into four broad categories: pseudo-proptosis or unusual enlargement of the globe in the orbit, mass lesions, inflammatory changes, and traumatic abnormalities.

In Graves' disease the extraocular muscles are usually diffusely enlarged with accentuation of the muscle sheath (Fig. 12). Changes in the texture of the orbital fat may also be present. While some have emphasized measurement of muscle thickness (14, 20), we have generally felt that this technique is unreliable since orbital anatomy varies from patient to patient and it may not be possible to aim the ultrasonic beam perpendicular to the muscle sheath in all muscles.

Inflammatory changes of the orbit are best detected by ultrasound (Fig. 13). Orbital pseudo-tumor appears ultrasonically as areas of sonolucency in subTenon's space and the region where the optic nerve inserts into the globe. Orbital myositis may appear as diffuse or focal enlargement of one or more muscles (21). This entity can be differentiated from Graves' disease by its response to steroids.

Orbital tumors can be detected and characterized accurately with ultrasound. Cavernous hemangioma of the orbit has a characteristic A- and B-scan appearance of a well-outlined encapsulated tumor with moderate to high internal reflectivity (Fig. 14). The cavernous spaces within the tumor provide strong reflective interfaces and the blood within the tumor allows good sound transmission. Whereas CT scan can often detect these lesions, ultrasonographic tissue characterization is more accurate in establishing tissue diagnosis. Hemangiopericytoma, lymphangioma, orbital varix, meningioma, and mixed cell tumor of the lacrimal gland have also been reported to give a hemangioma-like pattern on the B-scan (3).

Optic nerve tumors appear as alterations in the usual inverted-V pattern of the optic nerve. Optic nerve sheath meningiomas usually demonstrate broadening and irregularity of the optic nerve pattern (Fig. 15). Optic nerve measurements have also been reported and appear to have some clinical application (15, 19). It must be remembered that only the anterior portion of the optic nerve can be measured using these techniques.

Ultrasonically guided needle biopsy of orbital lesions has been described (22). This technique appears to be safe and feasible. However, there are a number of orbital conditions that should not undergo needle biopsy. Experience with this technique is continuing to grow and other forms of interventional ultrasound may be developed.

## CONCLUSIONS

Ultrasound remains valuable in diagnosis of ocular and orbital diseases and is essential in the determination of intraocular lens power. New techniques for tissue characterization are currently under investigation and offer exciting new approaches to improving diagnostic accuracy.

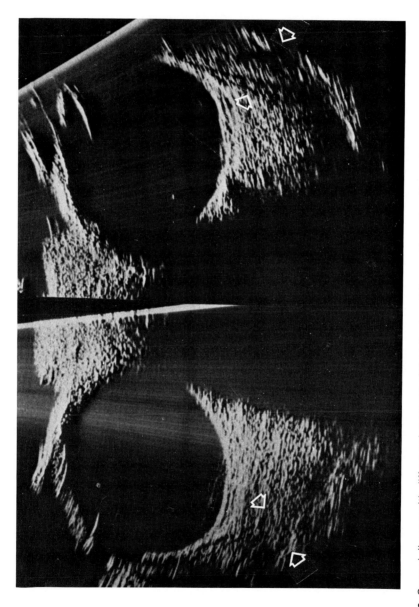

**FIG. 12.** Graves' disease with diffuse enlargement of the lateral recti (*arrows*) in both orbits and accentuation of the muscle sheath.

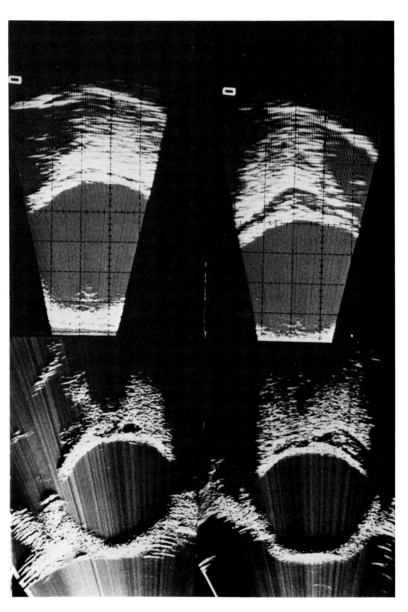

**FIG. 13.** Orbital pseudo-tumor demonstrating areas of the sonolucency in the orbital fat posterior to the globe. The muscles are enlarged. Both immersion technique *(left)* and contact technique *(right)* are demonstrated.

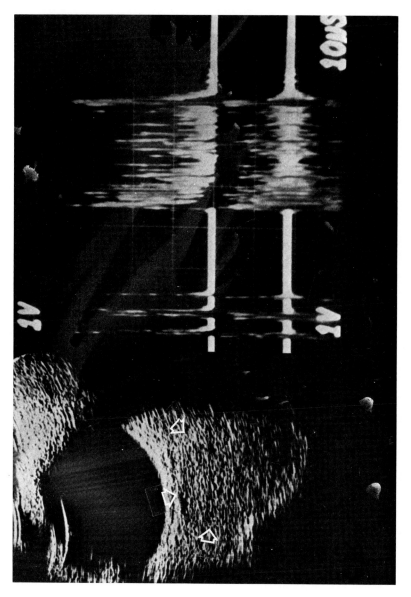

**FIG. 14.** Orbital cavernous hemangioma with the muscle cone (*arrows*), demonstrating a well-circumscribed configuration and moderately strong reflectivity. The echoes are of moderate height and regularly spaced on A-scan.

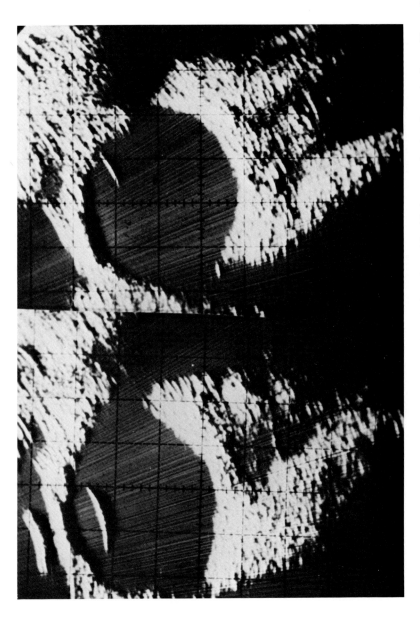

**FIG. 15.** Optic sheath meningioma. The optic nerve shadow is irregularly enlarged in this large optic sheath meningioma. The patient was asymptomatic with visual acuity 20/20.

## REFERENCES

1. Binkhorst, R. D.: Biometric A-scan ultrasonography and intra-ocular lens power calculation. In: *Current Concepts in Cataract Surgery*, edited by J. M. Emery pp. 175–182. C. V. Mosby, St. Louis, 1978.
2. Blumenkranz, M. S., and Byrne, S. F. Standardized echography (ultrasonography) for the detection and characterization of retinal detachment. *Ophthalmology*, 89: 821–831, 1982.
3. Cappaert, W. E., Kipnov, R. V., and Frank, K. E. Sector B-scan ultrasonographic "hemangioma-like" pattern. *Arch. Ophthalmol.*, 101: 74–77, 1983.
4. Coleman, D. J., and Lizzi, F. L. *In vivo* choroidal thickness measurement. *Am. J. Ophthalmol.*, 88: 369–375, 1979.
5. Coleman, D. J., and Lizzi, F. L. Computerized ultrasonic tissue characterization of ocular tumors. *Am. J. Ophthalmol. (in press)*, 1983.
6. Coleman, D. J., Lizzi, F. L., and Jack, R. L. *Ultrasonography of the Eye and Orbit*. Lea and Febiger, Philadelphia, 1977.
7. Coleman, D. J., Lizzi, F. L., Sliverman, R. H., Rondeau, M. J. Smith, M. E., and Torpey, J. H. Acoustic biopsy as a means for characterization of intraocular tumors. *Acta Ophthalmol. (in press)*, 1983.
8. Dallow, R. L. (Ed.) Ophthalmic ultrasonography: comparative techniques. *Int. Ophthalmol. Clin.*, 19(4):1979.
9. Dallow, R. L., and Coleman, D. J. Ultrasound in orbital diagnosis. In: *Ocular and Adnexal Tumors*, edited by F. A. Jakobiec, pp. 311–340. Aesculapins, Birmingham, 1978.
10. Johns, G. E. Clinical evaluation of the DBR A-scan unit. *J. Am. Intraocul. Implant Soc.*, 5:213–217, 1979.
11. Lizzi, F. L., Greenebaum, M., Feleppa, E. J., Elbaum, M., and Coleman, D. J. Theoretical framework for spectrum analysis in ultrasonic tissue characterization. *J. Acoust. Soc. Am. (in press)*, 1983.
12. Maloney, W. F., Kratz, R. P., Mazzocco, T. R., et al. Posterior chamber intraocular lens power calculation in 441 cases. *J. Am. Intraocul. Implant Soc.*, 5:349–350, 1979.
13. Ossoinig, K. C. Standardized echography: basic principles, clinical applications and results. *Int. Ophthalmol. Clin.*, 19(4): 127–210, 1979.
14. Ossoinig, K. Echography of the eye, orbit and periorbital region. In: *Radiology of the Orbit*, edited by P. H. Arger, pp. 229–233. Wiley, New York, 1977.
15. Ossoinig, K. C., Cennamo, G., and Byrne, S. Echographic differential diagnosis of optic nerve lesions. In: *Ultrasonography in Ophthalmology*, edited by J. M. Thijssen, and A. M. Verbeek, pp. 327–332. Proceedings of the 8th SIDUO Congress, Junk, The Hague, 1981.
16. Retzlaff, J. A new intraocular lens calculation formula. *J. Am. Intraocul. Implant Soc.*, 6:148–152, 1980.
17. Reuter, R., Lepper, R. D., and Haigos, W. Comparative measurements in ultrasonic pulse-echo equipment with the echosimulator in ultrasonography in ophthalmology. *Proceedings of the 8th SIDUO Congress, Junk, Hague, 1981*, edited by J. M. Thijssen, and A. M. Verbeek, pp. 463–472.
18. Sanders, D., and Kraff, M. C. Improvement of IOL power calculation using empirical data. *J. Am. Intraocul. Implant Soc.*, 6:263–267, 1980.
19. Schroeder, W., and Guthoff, R. Ultrasonography of the optic nerve. In: *Ultrasonography in Ophthalmology*, edited by J. M. Thijssen, and A. M. Verbeek, pp. 359–362. Proceedings of the 8th SIDUO Congress, Junk, The Hague, 1981.
20. Shammas, H. J. F., Minckler, D. S., and Ogden, C. Ultrasound in early thyroid orbitopathy. *Arch. Ophthalmol.*, 98: 277–279, 1980.
21. Slavin, M. L., and Glaser, J. C. Idiopathic orbital myositis. *Arch. Ophthalmol.*, 100:1261–1265, 1982.
22. Spoor, T. C., Kennerdell, J. S., Dekker, A., Johnson, B. L., and Rickoff, P., Orbital fine needle biopsy with B-scan guidance. *Am. J. Ophthalmol.*, 89: 274–277, 1980.
23. Susal, A. L., Gaynon, M. W., and Walker, J. T. Linear array multiple transducer ultrasonic examination of the eye. *Ophthalmology*, 90: 266–271, 1983.

Ultrasound Annual 1983, edited by R. C. Sanders and M. Hill. Raven Press, New York © 1983.

# Sonography of the Upper Abdominal Venous System

*Michael C. Hill and †Roger C. Sanders

*Department of Radiology, The George Washington University Medical Center, Washington, D.C. 20037; and †Department of Radiology, The Johns Hopkins Hospital, Baltimore, Maryland 21205

In this chapter we will focus on the role of sonography in diagnosing congenital and acquired conditions affecting the inferior vena cava, the central portal venous system, and the hepatic veins.

## INFERIOR VENA CAVA

The inferior vena cava (IVC) carries blood from all of the body below the diaphragm into the right atrium. It is formed to the right of the vertebral body of L5 by the junction of the right and left common iliac veins (101). It runs superiorly, anterior to the spine and to the right of the aorta. After passing through the diaphragm it angles slightly forward and medially to enter the right atrium. As it ascends in the abdomen, it is related posteriorly to the right psoas muscle, right renal artery, right crus of the diaphragm, and the medial portion of the right adrenal gland (Fig. 1). Along its right side, it is related to the right ureter and the medial border of the right kidney, and anteriorly to the posterior parietal peritoneum below the level of the horizontal portion of the duodenum. Above this level, it is directly related to the head of the pancreas and then to the first portion of the duodenum from which it is separated by the portal vein and common bile duct (Fig. 1). Above this, it forms the posterior margin of the epiploic foramen before becoming surrounded to a variable degree by liver parenchyma.

The tributaries of the inferior vena cava include the previously mentioned two common iliac veins, the lumbar veins (four on each side), gonadal veins, renal veins, right suprarenal and inferior phrenic veins, and the hepatic veins (Figs. 2, 3, 31). The gonadal veins drain in at different levels; the one on the right enters laterally below the level of the right renal vein, while the one on the left drains directly into the left renal vein (Fig. 2) (101). The lumbar veins are connected to the ascending lumbar vein which branches off the common iliac vein and ascends posterior to the psoas muscle, lateral to the lumbar vertebral bodies, and anterior to the transverse processes. Having passed

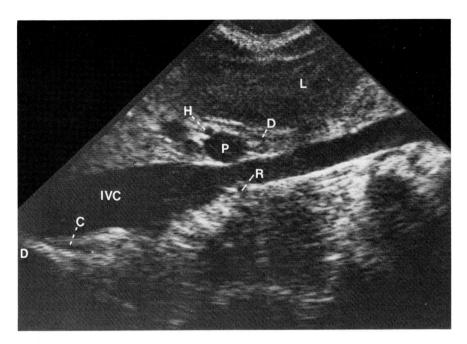

**FIG. 1.** Longitudinal sonogram of a normal inferior vena cava (IVC). The main portal vein (P) is seen anterior to the IVC while the right renal artery (R) and right crus of the diaphragm (C) are seen posterior to the IVC which contains low level echoes. Liver (L). Hepatic artery (H). Common bile duct (D) in the head of the pancreas. Diaphragm (D).

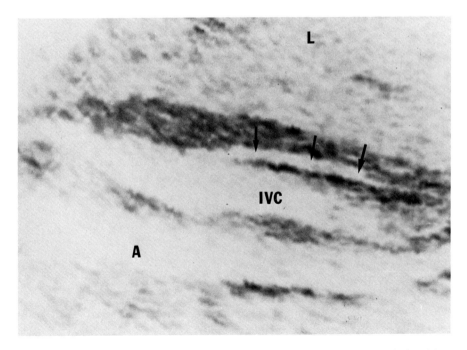

**FIG. 2.** Longitudinal sonogram along the right flank with the patient in the left decubitus position. Using the liver (L) as an acoustic window, the right gonadal vein *(arrows)* can be identified arising from the inferior vena cava (IVC). Aorta (A).

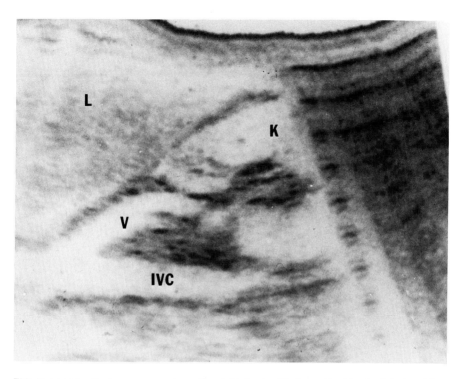

**FIG. 3.** Longitudinal sonogram along the right flank with the patient in the left decubitus position. Using the liver (L) as a sonic window, the right renal vein (V) can be seen arising from the inferior vena cava (IVC) and entering the right kidney (K).

deep to the crus of the diaphragm, these veins ascend in the thorax as the azygous and hemiazygous veins. The importance of these veins lies in the fact that they act as collateral pathways when there is obstruction of the IVC.

Sonographic visualization of the upper IVC is usually possible in most patients, but the lower portion may be obscured by overlying bowel gas. If this is the case, the lower IVC may be visualized by placing the patient in the left decubitus position and by using the liver, right kidney or right psoas muscle as an acoustic window (Figs. 2, 3). The normal IVC can be indented by the caudate lobe of the liver and head of pancreas. Its size increases as it ascends in the abdomen and changes with the cardiac cycle and phase of respiration (Fig. 1). In normal individuals its size can vary greatly; it can be surprisingly large in a thin female while at the same time be small and difficult to see in a well-built muscular male. The greatest distention and, therefore, the optimal sonographic visualization of the IVC is best achieved by simple breath holding or at the end of expiration (44). Although there are conflicting reports on the issue, deep inspiration and the valsalva maneuver usually decrease the size of this vessel making it difficult to visualize. In inspiration, because of the negative intrathoracic pressure, the IVC blood is forced into the right heart. With a valsalva maneuver, the increase in intra-abdominal pressure is sufficient in most people to force the blood out of the IVC into the heart. This is the exact opposite to what happens in the jugular veins in the neck where a valsalva maneuver causes distention since they are not subjected to the high external pressures generated within the abdomen.

The right renal and right gonadal vein are best identified entering the IVC with the patient in the left decubitus position by scanning through the right flank using the right kidney as a sonic window (Figs. 2, 3). The right renal artery can be seen posterior to the IVC, and by angling the transducer more medially one may identify its origin from the aorta (Fig. 1). This technique can be used in patients with abdominal aortic aneurysms to determine whether the aneurysm involves the origins of the renal arteries (54). The left renal vein can be identified both longitudinally and transversely as it crosses between the aorta and the superior mesenteric artery (Fig. 4). The degree of distention of the left renal vein is greater to the left of the midline

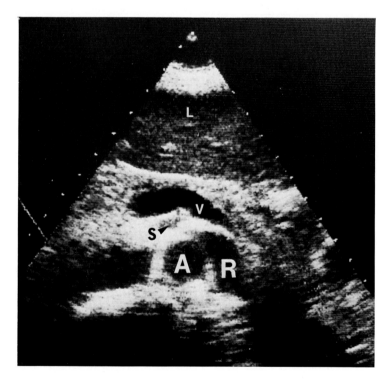

**FIG. 4.** Transverse sonogram through the upper abdomen using the left lobe of the liver (L) as a sonic window. The left renal (R) vein is dilated to the left of the midline prior to where it crosses between the aorta (A) and the superior mesenteric artery (S). Splenic vein (V).

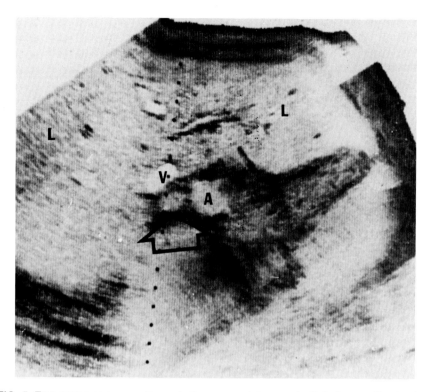

**FIG. 5.** Transverse sonogram through the upper abdomen. A dilated ascending lumbar vein *(arrow)* is seen posterior to the inferior vena cava (V). The patient had congestive cardiac failure. Aorta (A). Liver (L).

where it runs between the superior mesenteric artery and the aorta owing to the pinch cock effect of these two vessels (15). The degree of distention can be 4 times greater to the left of the midline. It is found only when the distance between the superior mesenteric artery and aorta measures 15 mm or less or when the third portion of the duodenum crosses at the same level as the left renal vein (15). The presence of a left varicocele appears to have only a limited relationship to the size of this vein; however, elevated left renal vein pressures have been found (107). The left renal vein may be abnormally dilated and even be varicoid in patients with portal hypertension owing to the development of gastrorenal or splenorenal collaterals (91, 95).

The normal lumbar veins, right adrenal vein, and phrenic veins cannot be sonographically identified. The right ascending lumbar vein can be identified in up to 70% of patients as an anechoic tubular structure running posterior to the IVC (Fig. 5) (62). Its internal diameter typically measures no more than 2 mm. It should not be confused with the anechoic right crus of the diaphragm; however, this mistake can be avoided by scanning transversely and showing that it has a true tubular shape (Fig. 5).

With high resolution real-time scanners, low level echoes can be identified within the IVC (Fig. 1). The exact etiology of these echoes is not known, but it is postulated that they are secondary to turbulent blood flow. They travel in the direction of blood flow and are seen mainly at junction points where there is mixing of blood (22).

### Congenital Anomalies

The IVC is formed by three pairs of cardinal veins in the retroperitoneum that undergo sequential development and regression (Fig. 6) (28, 35, 65, 83). The posterior cardinal veins appear at 6 weeks and form no part of the normal adult IVC, although they play a part in certain adult anomalies. The subcardinal veins appear at 7 weeks and give rise to the prerenal segment of the inferior vena cava (Fig. 6). The supracardinal system appears at 8 weeks and gives rise to the postrenal segment of the IVC below the diaphragm. Above the diaphragm, the supracardinals form the azygous and hemiazygous veins. The anastomoses between the subcardinal and supracardinal systems form the renal veins (Fig. 6). In normal people, the left cardinal system involutes and the right IVC is composed of the posterior infrarenal supracardinal vein, renal segment, anterior suprarenal subcardinal vein, and the confluence of the hepatic veins (Fig. 6).

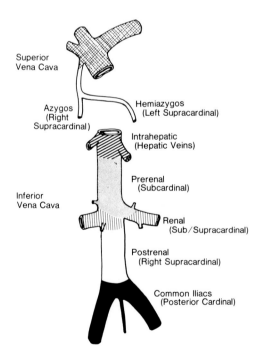

Superior
Vena Cava

Azygos
(Right
Supracardinal)

Hemiazygos
(Left Supracardinal)

Intrahepatic
(Hepatic Veins)

Prerenal
(Subcardinal)

Inferior
Vena Cava

Renal
(Sub/Supracardinal)

Postrenal
(Right Supracardinal)

Common Iliacs
(Posterior Cardinal)

**FIG. 6.** Diagram of the embryological derivation of the different segments of the inferior vena cava.

With a double IVC (incidence 0.3 to 2.8%) the size of the two vessels can be the same or vary depending upon which side is dominant. To the unsuspecting, a left IVC can mimic para-aortic adenopathy on CT. The commonest type is where the left IVC joins the left renal vein which crosses the midline at its normal level to join the right IVC (28, 65, 83). With this anomaly, there is no continuation of the left inferior vena cava above the left renal vein. A less common type of double inferior vena cava occurs when the right IVC joins the azygous and the left IVC joins the hemiazygous system. With a single left IVC (incidence 0.2%), it joins the left renal vein which crosses the midline to join the right renal vein to form a right-sided IVC. The left-sided IVC should not be confused with a left gonadal vein, both of which join the left renal vein. The left IVC can be identified arising from the left common iliac vein while the left gonadal vein exits the abdomen through the inguinal canal (83). The left IVC can persist above the level of the left renal vein whereas the right IVC is not present above this point. In such cases, the left IVC ascends into the thorax by joining the hemiazygous vein (96). Recognition of a caval duplication is important when surgical ligation or umbrella placement is being considered in a patient with thromboembolic disease or when retroperitoneal surgery is necessary, i.e., resection of an abdominal aortic aneurysm (83).

Infrahepatic interruption of the IVC is due to failure of union of the hepatic veins and right subcardinal vein and with it there can be azygous or, less commonly, hemiazygous continuation (Fig. 6) (35). Dilatation of these latter veins can mimic a paravertebral and/or right tracheobronchial angle mass on a chest radiograph. This anomaly is associated with cyanotic and acyanotic congenital heart disease, abnormalities of cardiac position, abdominal situs, and with asplenia and polysplenia. Sonographically, the azygous vein continuation can be identified as a large vessel comparable in size to the normal IVC that passes alongside the aorta medial to the right crus of the diaphragm (35). The hepatic veins do not drain into it, but drain via an independent confluence that passes through the diaphragm to enter into the right atrium in the usual position of the IVC.

The true position of the left renal vein is very important when a splenorenal shunt is being considered in a patient with portal hypertension, and in a prospective renal transplant donor. The incidence of a circumaortic renal vein varies from 1.5 to 8.7% and that of a retroaortic left renal vein from 1.8 to 2.4%; both can be identified sonographically (Fig. 7) (83). The posterior component crosses behind the aorta to join the right-sided inferior vena cava at a level one to two vertebral bodies below that of the preaortic segment (Fig. 7) (65).

Membranous obstruction of the inferior vena cava can simulate infrahepatic interruption of the IVC with azygous continuation (50). In this condition, a web or membrane obstructs the IVC at the level of the diaphragm and leads to chronic congestion of the liver with centrilobular and periportal

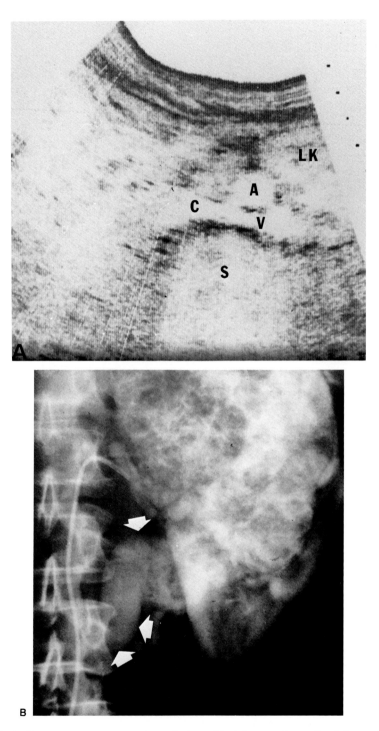

**FIG. 7. A:** Transverse sonogram through the mid-abdomen shows the left renal vein crossing behind the aorta (A) to enter the inferior vena cava (C). A mass is identified arising from the left kidney (LK). Spine (S). **B:** Venous phase of a selective left renal angiogram shows the retroaortic left renal vein *(arrows)* descending from the L2 to the L3 level before crossing behind the abdominal aorta. A vascular hypernephroma is seen involving the left kidney.

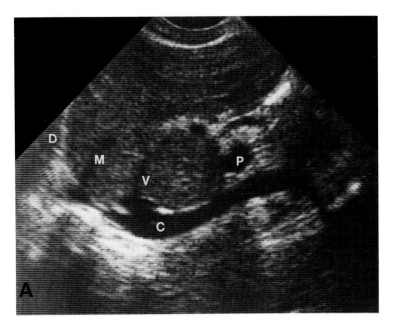

**FIG. 8. A:** Longitudinal sonogram of the hepatic portion of the inferior vena cava (C). The inferior vena cava cannot be demonstrated passing through the diaphragm (D) to enter the right atrium. The middle hepatic vein (M) and a hepatic vein from the caudate lobe (V) can be seen entering the upper portion of the inferior vena cava. Portal vein (P).

fibrosis (Fig. 8). Clinically, these patients present in the third and fourth decade with portal hypertension, and an increased incidence of hepatoma has been described. Sonographically, the obstruction can be identified at the level of the diaphragm along with dilatation of the azygous system (Fig. 8) (50). An inferior vena cavogram will show conical obstruction of the inferior vena cava at the level of the diaphragm with marked collateralization through the azygous and hemiazygous systems. Hepatic venography will show patency of the major intrahepatic veins, which can also be demonstrated sonographically (Fig. 8). The etiology of this condition is unknown and it has been postulated to be either congenital or acquired (injury, thrombosis, infection).

### Thrombosis and Tumor Involvement of the Inferior Vena Cava

The wall of the inferior vena cava is sonographically echogenic, well-defined, and uniformly thin (Fig. 1) (58). As mentioned previously, low level luminal echoes can be identified moving in the direction of blood flow with high resolution, real-time ultrasound equipment. With thrombosis or tumor invasion of the IVC, single or multiple focal echogenic nodules may be seen along the wall and may extend into the lumen for a varying length as

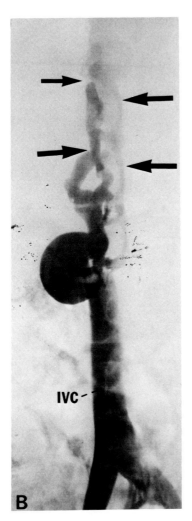

**FIG. 8. B:** Inferior vena cavogram demonstrates azygous continuation of the inferior vena cava *(arrows)*. The hepatic portion of the inferior vena cava is not identified as blood is flowing downward in that portion.

a tail (Fig. 9) (40, 45, 90). In some instances, the IVC itself may be distended and entirely filled with diffuse fine intraluminal echoes (Fig. 10) (40). Tumor thrombus tends to have a fine homogeneous echo pattern whereas blood clot alone has an inhomogeneous coarse echo pattern. By extending the examination to evaluate the remaining portions of the IVC and its tributaries along with the adjacent organs, one can usually confirm the cause of the caval thrombus (Figs. 10, 11).

The most common tumor to invade the IVC is a renal cell carcinoma (9%) which is usually on the right side because of the close proximity of the right renal parenchyma to the caval lumen (Figs. 10, 11) (40, 41, 45, 61). The presence of venous extension is directly related to the size of the renal tumor (41). The tumor may be seen extending along the involved renal vein into the cava and may, in fact, extend all the way superiorly into the right atrium; this is extremely important to know prior to surgery (86). In children, a Wilms tumor can grow into the IVC in a similar fashion (88). It should be remembered that in renal tumors with arteriovenous shunting, the renal vein may be dilated in the absence of venous extension of the tumor itself (95). The IVC above the involved renal vein will be dilated in such cases. Other tumors that may invade the IVC include hepatocellular carcinoma, via the hepatic veins, and adrenal cell carcinoma (27, 88, 94). Other much less common tumors that may do this include retroperitoneal liposarcomas, leiomyosarcomas, osteosarcomas, and rhabdomyosarcomas. Benign tumors such as a renal angiomyolipoma have also been reported to invade the IVC (27, 59). When no cause for an echogenic mass arising from the caval wall can be identified (although extremely rare), one should consider a primary tumor of the IVC, such as a leiomyosarcoma (105).

All of the above mentioned tumors may not only invade the IVC, but may also displace and compress it owing to associated lymphadenopathy and/or direct tumor extension (Fig. 12) (9, 42). The direction and degree of displacement depends upon the origin of the tumor, and its size (58). A hypernephroma of the right kidney could displace the cava anteriorly and medially, and in

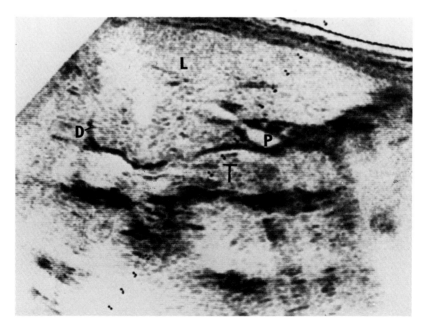

**FIG. 9.** A longitudinal sonogram of the IVC demonstrates echogenic thrombus (T) filling its entire lumen. This thrombus had extended from a deep venous thrombosis in the leg. Liver (L). Main portal vein (P). Diaphragm (D).

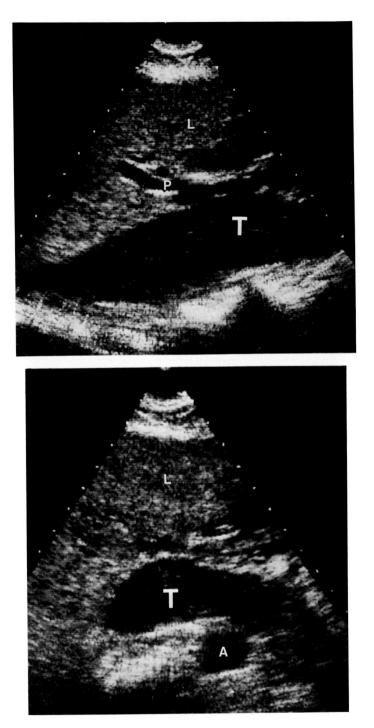

**FIG. 10. A:** Longitudinal sonogram of the inferior vena cava, which is filled with low level echoes secondary to tumor thrombus (T). Liver (L). Main portal vein (P). **B:** Transverse sonogram at the level of a dilated thrombus-filled left renal vein (T). This was secondary to a hypernephroma of the left kidney. Aorta (A). Liver (L).

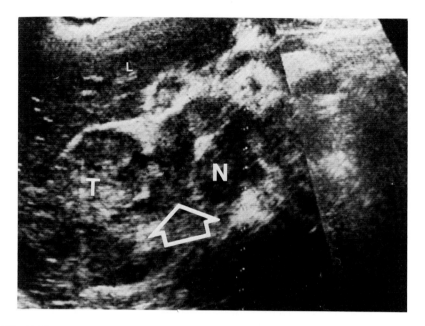

**FIG. 11.** Transverse sonogram through the mid-abdomen showing the inferior vena cava *(arrow)* filled with echogenic thrombus which is secondary to a hypernephroma of the right kidney (T). Adenopathy (N) can be seen surrounding the inferior vena cava. Liver (L).

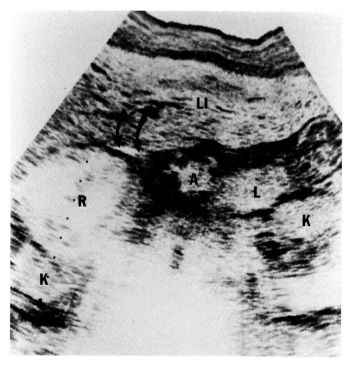

**FIG. 12.** Transverse sonogram through the upper abdomen demonstrates enlargement of the right adrenal gland (R) displacing the inferior vena cava *(arrows)* anteriorly. There is also enlargement of the left adrenal gland (L). This was secondary to metastatic disease. Liver (L1). Aorta (A). Kidneys (K).

fact may envelope it (Fig. 11). A right adrenal gland or neurogenic tumor along with a right renal artery aneurysm can displace an IVC anteriorly, whereas a mass in the head of the pancreas displaces it posteriorly (Fig. 12) (9, 42, 58). Although uncommon, a tortuous abdominal aorta can extend to the right behind the IVC, displacing it anteriorly. A tumor of the liver displaces the IVC posteriorly (9, 58). This is especially true for lesions of the caudate lobe such as enlargement secondary to cirrhosis or the presence of a tumor, cyst, or abscess (Figs. 13, 14). With uniform hepatomegaly, the IVC is compressed rather than being displaced. Adenopathy secondary to metastatic disease or lymphoma can produce diffuse displacement of the inferior vena cava, usually anteriorly (8, 58).

Nontumoral clot in the IVC usually results from extension from the iliac veins or renal veins (21, 80). Extension from the iliac veins can be due to an inflammatory process in the pelvis, or due to a thrombus of the deep venous system of the calf extending along the popliteal, femoral, and iliac veins (Fig. 9). Thrombosis of the renal veins leads to the nephrotic syndrome and is usually idiopathic; however, it can occur secondary to shock, sepsis, and

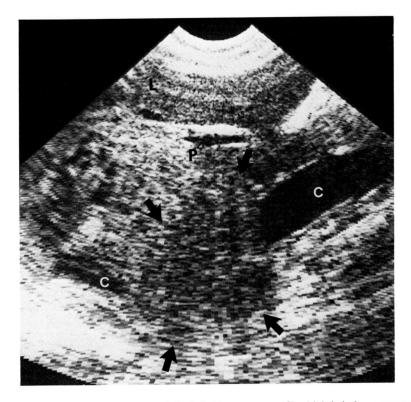

**FIG. 13.** Longitudinal sonogram of the inferior vena cava (C) which is being compressed by a hepatic adenoma (*arrows*) involving the caudate lobe of the liver which has bled. Main portal vein (P). Normal liver (L).

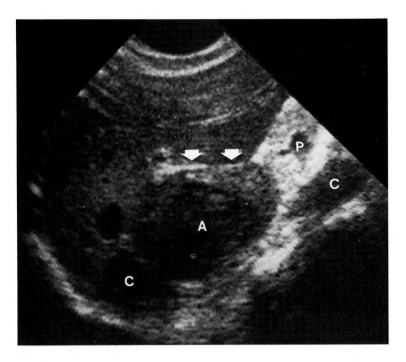

**FIG. 14.** Longitudinal sonogram through the inferior vena cava (C) which is being compressed by an amoebic abscess (A) that is involving the caudate lobe of the liver. Main portal vein (P). Ligamentum venosum *(arrows)*.

trauma, while in neonates it may be due to dehydration or maternal diabetes mellitus (Fig. 15) (13, 21, 80). Sonographically, the involved kidney develops increased cortical echoes with preservation of the corticomedullary junction (81). This finding is present for 1 to 3 weeks, while beyond this stage the size of the involved kidney decreases as the cortical echogenicity increases, and there is a loss of cortico-medullary definition.

Computed tomography and inferior vena cavography are used to stage tumors of the retroperitoneum and to evaluate whether there is caval involvement. On CT and intravenous cavography, a false positive diagnosis of tumor invasion can occur at the level of the renal veins when a pedal injection of contrast is given (5, 36). This is due to the inflow of nonopacified renal blood. A cavogram can also suggest the presence of tumor compression in the area of the caudate lobe of the liver (88). Sonography represents a noninvasive way of determining whether a possible lesion is real or not.

### Abnormal Dilatation of the Inferior Vena Cava

Abnormal dilatation of the IVC in the absence of intrinsic disease can occur with right-sided heart failure (53). An M-mode tracing of the IVC in

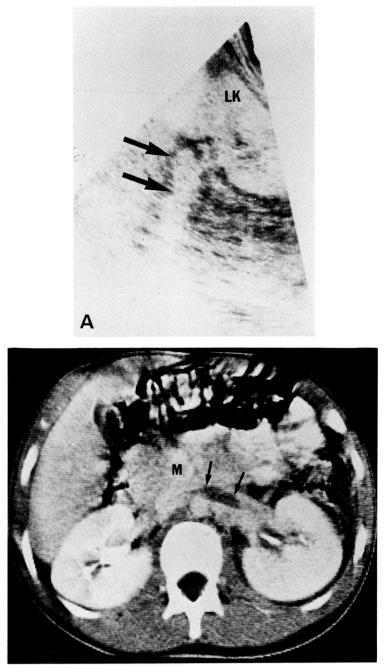

**FIG. 15. A:** Longitudinal sonogram through the left kidney (LK) with the patient in the right decubitus position demonstrates echogenic thrombus in the left renal vein *(arrows)*. **B:** A computed tomogram following the intravenous administration of contrast demonstrates clot in the left renal vein *(arrows)*. There is an ill-defined mass seen involving the retroperitoneal vessels and mesenteric vessels (M). At surgery, this proved to be idiopathic retroperitoneal and mesenteric fibrosis.

normal patients demonstrates a small presystolic A-wave and a smaller systolic V-wave, and there is a 50% decrease in the dimension of the IVC with inspiration (66, 69). Absence of this inspiratory decrease along with a large A-wave implies significant right heart dysfunction which may be due to atherosclerotic heart disease, pulmonary hypertension, pericardial tamponade, constrictive pericarditis, or atrial tumors. If any of these entities is suspected, based upon a sonographic examination of the cava, an echocardiographic study should be performed. With severe tricuspid insufficiency, the M-mode tracing of the IVC has a large V-wave owing to the reversal of blood flow from the right atrium into the IVC with ventricular contraction (66, 69). If saline is injected into an arm vein, and reflux of this "contrast medium" is noted into the upper IVC following a ventricular contraction, then this is a more sensitive sign of tricuspid insufficiency than an M-mode tracing of the IVC (102).

### Inferior Vena Cava Filter Devices

The commonest origin of pulmonary emboli is from venous thrombosis in the lower extremities. This is usually treated with anticoagulants unless their use is contraindicated, i.e., history of a bleeding peptic ulcer. Until recently, the only alternative was surgical ligation or clipping of the IVC, which has a substantial morbidity (4 to 50%) and mortality depending on patient selection and operative techniques. Complications that can occur include shock from a rapid decrease in circulating blood volume, lower extremity edema, and recurrent embolization. In recent years, the transvenous insertion of filter devices into the IVC has been advocated to prevent recurrent embolization in patients who cannot tolerate anticoagulants (7). These devices can be implanted under local anesthesia and are placed in the IVC just proximal to the renal veins.

The true position of these filter devices can be followed sonographically, and some of their complications can be detected (Fig. 16). The filter can migrate either cranially or caudally and can perforate the cava leading to retroperitoneal bleeding. Perforation of the duodenum, aorta, ureter, and hepatic veins has been described along with lower extremity thrombophlebitis, edema, and stasis dermatitis. The filter device itself may become thrombosed and can be a source of recurrent pulmonary emboli (7). The overall morbidity related to these filter devices is stated to be approximately 1% (7). The commonest filter devices used are the Mobin-Uddin (MU) and the Kim-Ray-Greenfield (KG) filters. The KG filter is less thrombogenic, and is less likely to perforate than the MU filter (Fig. 16) (7). Either filter device can migrate caudally and may, in fact, do so all the way down to one of the common iliac vessels, thus defeating the whole purpose of its function.

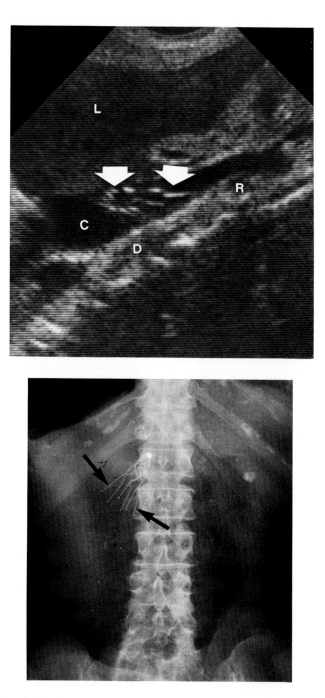

**FIG. 16. A:** Longitudinal sonogram through the inferior vena cava (C). A Kim-Ray-Green-field filter *(arrows)* can be identified in the inferior vena cava superior to the right renal artery (R). Liver (L). Right crus of the diaphragm (D). **B:** Radiograph of the Kim-Ray-Greenfield filter device showing the metallic prongs *(arrows)* by wich it attaches itself to the caval wall.

### Portasystemic Shunts

A portacaval shunt joins the end or side of the main portal vein to the adjoining portion of the IVC (Fig. 17). A mesocaval shunt joins the end or side of the superior mesenteric vein to the IVC, and with a splenorenal shunt the splenic vein is joined to the side of the left renal vein (Warren shunt) (Fig. 18). The site and size of the shunt can be determined sonographically, and with Doppler ultrasound shunt patency can be determined (33). Indirect evidence of shunt patency can be inferred by the absence of visualization of collaterals, which occurs when the shunt is occluded. The easiest shunt to identify sonographically is the portacaval shunt followed by the mesocaval shunt (38). With a portocaval shunt, there is dilatation of the IVC just above the site of the anastomoses and absence of this dilatation could indicate occlusion of the shunt (Fig. 17) (38). This type of caval dilatation is less frequently present with mesocaval shunts; however, there is dilatation of the superior mesenteric vein above the site of a functioning prosthetic side-to-side mesocaval shunt (Fig. 18) (49). It is usually not possible to evaluate the patency of a splenorenal shunt as the anastomotic site is often overlain by adipose tissue and bowel gas despite longitudinal scanning through the spleen with the patient in the right decubitus position (31). Dynamic CT scanning offers a noninvasive way of evaluating the patency of the above mentioned shunts (33).

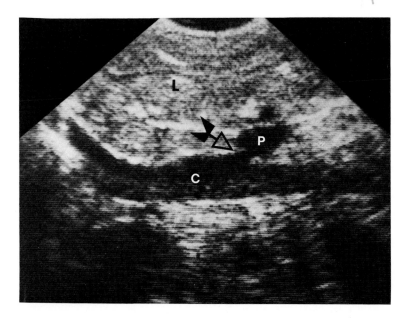

**FIG. 17.** Longitudinal sonogram of the inferior vena cava (C) demonstrating an end-to-side portacaval shunt *(arrow)*. Main portal vein (P). Liver (L).

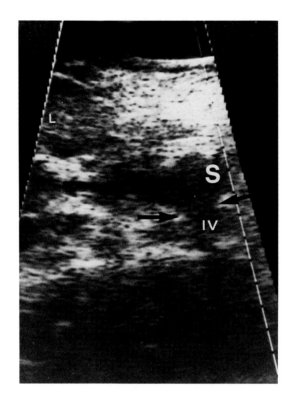

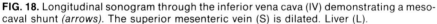

**FIG. 18.** Longitudinal sonogram through the inferior vena cava (IV) demonstrating a meso-caval shunt *(arrows)*. The superior mesenteric vein (S) is dilated. Liver (L).

## CENTRAL PORTAL VENOUS SYSTEM

The normal anatomy of the portal venous system has been well described (4, 16, 25, 30, 101). The main portal vein is formed by the junction of the superior mesenteric and splenic veins behind the neck of the pancreas. Once formed, this vein runs superiorly to the porta hepatis with a varying degree of obliquity in the free edge of the lesser omentum anterior to the inferior vena cava where it divides into right and left branches (Fig. 19) (30). The right portal vein is larger than the left and can be identified in most (96%) patients. It courses horizontally in the right lobe of the liver before dividing into anterior and posterior branches that run in the anterior and posterior segments of the right lobe of the liver (Fig. 19) (63). An echogenic ligament can often be seen running from the right portal vein down to the gallbladder fossa, and this ligament (main lobar fissure) is helpful in locating a small gallbladder (76). The proximal portion of left portal vein runs superiorly, anterior to the caudate lobe, before making an abrupt anterior turn into the left intersegmental fissure where it gives off branches to the medial and lateral segments of the left lobe of the liver (4, 16, 63). The ligamentum teres, which is the remnant of the umbilical vein, arises from the anterior tip of the left portal vein. The umbilical vein runs inferiorly to the umbilicus in the falciform ligament which is a fold of peritoneum that in its upper portion runs in the left intersegmental fissure.

The branches of the portal venous system in the liver are intrasegmental whereas those of the hepatic veins run between the segments (63). These veins are easily identified from each other by tracing out their branching patterns and by noting that the walls of the portal branches are echogenic whereas those of the hepatic veins are usually not echogenic (Figs. 19, 31) (17). Approaching the porta hepatis, the portal vein branches increase in size, as do the hepatic veins, as one moves superiorly to where these veins enter the inferior vena cava just before it passes through the diaphragm to enter into the left atrium.

The degree of visualization of the extrahepatic portal venous system depends upon the patient's body habitus; however, in the majority of patients one can identify the main portal vein, the splenic vein, and the proximal

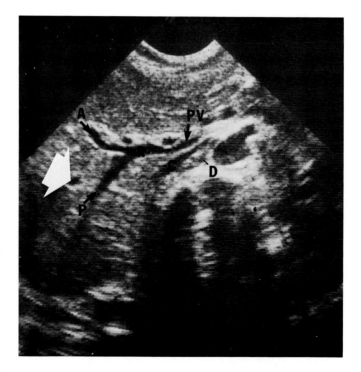

**FIG. 19.** Transverse sonogram through the upper abdomen demonstrating the main portal vein (PV) and the right portal vein (R) with its anterior (A) and posterior (P) divisions. Inferior vena cava (C). Right hepatic vein *(arrow).* Right crus of the diaphragm (D).

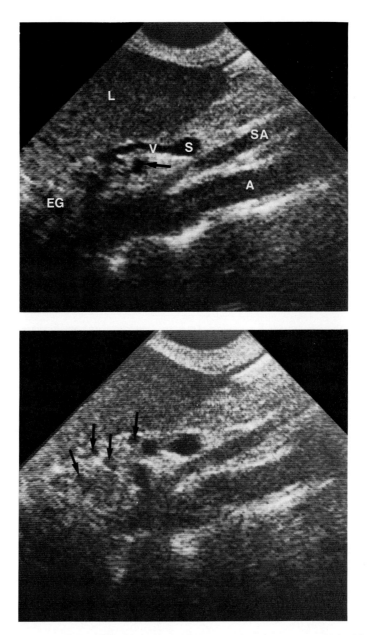

**FIG. 20. A:** Longitudinal midline sonogram demonstrating the coronary vein (V) arising from the superior aspect of the splenic vein (S). The coronary vein can be identified running toward the esophagogastric junction (EG) close to the under surface of the liver (L). Aorta (A). Celiac axis *(arrow)*. Superior mesenteric artery (SA). **B:** Longitudinal sonogram slightly to the left of Fig. 20A demonstrating varices *(arrows)* along the lesser curvature of the stomach at the level of and just below the esophagogastric junction.

portion (4 to 6 cm) of the superior mesenteric vein. The walls of these veins are well defined and echogenic whereas the lumen is echo-free (Fig. 20). With high resolution, real-time ultrasound equipment, low level echoes can be identified in the central portion of the lumen of the larger veins moving in the direction of the flow of blood (22). The exact etiology of these echoes is not known, but they may be due to the turbulent flow of blood. The splenic vein can be traced running along the posterior superior aspect of the body and tail of the pancreas to the splenic hilus (Fig. 27). Along its course, the splenic vein lies posterior and inferior to the splenic artery and anterior to the left crus of the diaphragm, left adrenal gland, and upper portion of the left kidney, where it lies in the splenorenal ligament. Its tributaries include the short gastric, left gastroepiploic, and inferior mesenteric veins along with a varying number of pancreatic veins (25). With the exception of the short gastric veins, these veins are usually not visualized sonographically. This is also true of the tributaries of the superior mesenteric vein from the small bowel and right colon, with the exception of the right gastroepiploic and inferior pancreaticoduodenal veins which can on occasion be identified.

The coronary (left gastric) vein can be seen in 20% of normal patients and its internal diameter should not exceed 4 mm (Figs. 20, 21) (23). It is best identified by scanning longitudinally just lateral to where the splenic vein

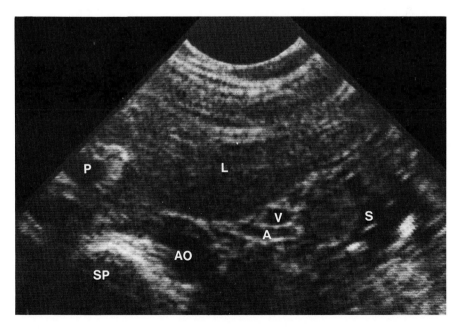

**FIG. 21.** Transverse sonogram through the upper abdomen demonstrating branches of the coronary vein (V) and left gastric artery (A) along the lesser curvature of the stomach (S). Liver (L). Aorta (AO). Spine (SP). Left portal vein (P).

joins the superior mesenteric vein to form the main portal vein. Usually, it joins the superior portion of the main portal vein in this area; however, it can drain more medially into the superior portion of the splenic vein (Fig. 20). It is formed by veins from the stomach and runs superiorly along its lesser curvature to the esophagogastric junction (Figs. 20, 21). Here it makes an abrupt turn inferiorly and posteriorly behind the lesser sac to join the main portal vein. The right gastric vein runs along the pyloric portion of the lesser curvature of the stomach in the lesser omentum and it is joined by the prepyloric vein before draining directly into the main portal vein (25, 101). Sonographically these veins are usually not seen.

The left gastric artery takes a similar course to the left coronary vein, and their branches along the lesser curvature of the stomach can be confused with one another unless traced back to their origins (Fig. 21). This is best done by performing an oblique longitudinal scan along the true axis of the main vessels where they can be identified arising from either the celiac axis or draining into the main portal vein (Fig. 20).

### Portal Hypertension with Porta-Systemic Collaterals

The causes of portal hypertension include (73, 87):

Intrahepatic:   Cirrhosis
                  Hepatic venous obstruction (Budd-Chiari syndrome)
Presinusoidal:  (a)  Extrahepatic—obstructed portal vein
                                 increased splenic blood flow
                (b)  Intrahepatic—sarcoidosis
                    Presinusoidal—congenital fibrosis
                                 schistosomiasis
                                 primary biliary cirrhosis
                                 lymphoma
                                 toxins (polyvinyl chloride)

In the presinusoidal forms of portal hypertension, the hepatocellular function studies and wedge hepatic venous pressure are normal (87). The exact opposite is true of cirrhosis where liver failure is evident and the wedge hepatic venous pressure is elevated. The porta-systemic collaterals associated with portal hypertension have been well described in the angiographic literature (24, 32, 72, 84). They can be identified sonographically, especially with real-time ultrasound equipment. Doppler ultrasound can determine the direction of blood flow, and can be used to grade the severity of the portal hypertension (33, 46, 89). When ultrasound is not successful in visualizing the portal system, which may be due to the size of the patient or the presence of massive ascites, then CT represents a noninvasive way of identifying porta-systemic collaterals (20, 52).

The easiest porta-systemic collateral to identify is the coronary vein with its associated gastroesophageal varices (Fig. 20) (23, 26, 56, 57, 92). The involved coronary vein usually has an internal diameter greater than 4 or 5 mm (23). Having identified its origin from the cephalic aspect of the main portal vein or adjoining splenic vein, the varices can be identified by longitudinal oblique scanning of the gastroesophageal junction and lesser curvature of the stomach (Fig. 20). The esophageal varices can be seen by scanning transversely with the transducer angled cranially through the left lobe of the liver. In some individuals, a dilated inferior mesenteric vein may be identified joining the splenic vein along its caudal aspect just to the left of the midline (23). Gastrorenal and splenorenal veins along with dilated short gastric branches are best identified by scanning longitudinally through the spleen with the patient in the right decubitus position (Fig. 22) (23, 57). The proximal splenic vein can be identified, being formed in the splenic hilus by a varying number (2 to 5) of splenic branches. The short gastric veins are seen along the wall of the stomach medial to the spleen above the splenic hilus while the gastrorenal and splenorenal collaterals are best seen longitudinally

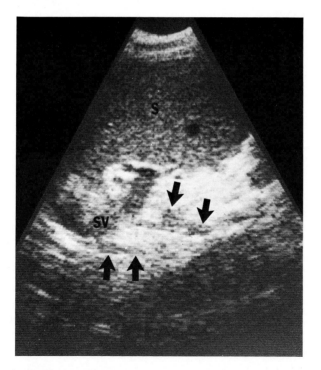

**FIG. 22.** Longitudinal sonogram through the spleen (S) with the patient in the right decubitus position. Splenorenal collaterals can be identified *(arrows)* running inferiorly from the splenic vein (SV) to the left renal vein.

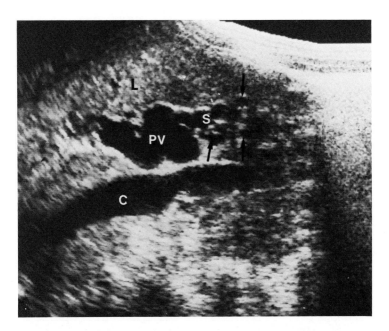

**FIG. 23.** Longitudinal sonogram along a dilated main portal vein (PV). A large number of collateral vessels *(arrows)* can be identified around the superior mesenteric vein (S) in the area of the distal antrum of the stomach and proximal duodenum. Inferior vena cava (C). Liver (L).

through the lower portion of the spleen and the upper pole of the left kidney (Fig. 22) (23, 26, 56, 57).

Varices can also be identified along the greater curvature of the stomach and in the adjacent mesentery (gastroepiploic veins) (Fig. 23) (92). The varices in this area can be large and drainage into the superior mesenteric vein via the right gastroepiploic vein may be seen. Other veins that can be sonographically identified include paraduodenal, periportal, and pelvic collaterals (Figs. 23–25) (6, 92).

The umbilical vein runs from the umbilicus to the left portal vein in the falciform ligament. Normally, it is only the fat surrounding the vein that is seen since the vein itself is usually not patent. In portal hypertension, the vein acts as a collateral channel carrying blood from the portal to the systemic venous system via anterior abdominal wall veins (epigastric veins) (Fig. 26) (1, 23, 37, 57, 92). This is called the Cruvalhier Baumgarten syndrome and when these veins are clinically apparent they can be seen radiating from the umbilicus; this is called a caput medusa (56, 75). The presence of a dilated umbilical vein indicates that the cause of the portal hypertension is within the liver itself (e.g. cirrhosis) and may not be identified angiographically owing to hepatofugal flow. Sonographically the umbilical vein is best identified by scanning transversely across the left intersegmental

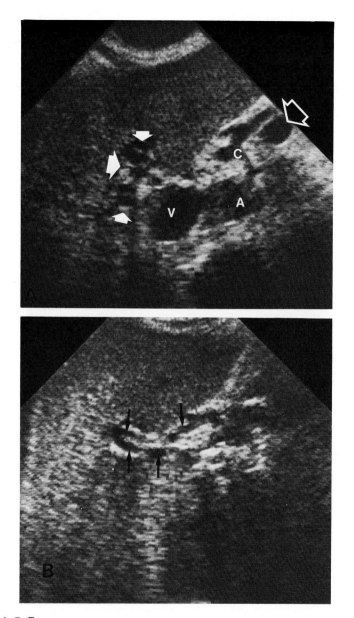

**FIG. 24. A, B:** Transverse sonogram through the upper abdomen reveals numerous small branches in the area of the porta hepatis *(arrows);* however, no main portal vein can be identified. Aorta (A). Inferior vena cava (V). Celiac axis (C). Splenic vein *(open arrow).*

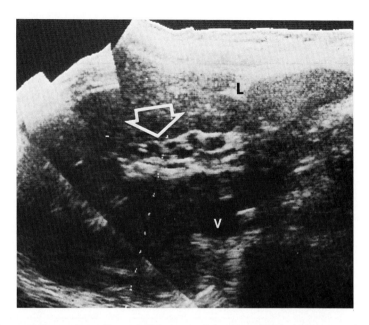

**FIG. 25.** Transverse sonogram through the upper abdomen reveals numerous periportal collaterals *(arrow)* in the area of the porta hepatis. Liver (L). Inferior vena cava (V).

fissure where it has a "bull's eye" appearance as the dilated vein is surrounded by the echogenic fat in the falciform ligament (Fig. 26) (85). On longitudinal scanning, it can be seen arising from the anterior tip of the left portal vein and running inferiorly to the umbilicus (Fig. 26) (23, 34, 37, 56). If too much scanning pressure is used, the vein may be rendered nonvisible due to compression.

The portal venous system distends with deep inspiration. This is due to descent of the diaphragm with compression of the liver and its hepatic veins. Portal venous outflow is slowed while inflow continues, thus distending the central portal venous system. No dilatation occurs in portal hypertension as the veins are already maximally distended (12).

The size of the central portal venous system cannot be used to indicate the presence of porta-systemic collaterals (2, 98, 100). In some patients with cirrhosis, the development of porta-systemic collaterals can be so effective at shunting blood that the central portal venous system does not dilate and would be considered normal by a size criterion alone (48). Dilatation of the central portal venous system occurs with splenomegaly in the absence of porta-systemic collaterals and is in response to increased blood flow (Fig. 27) (87).

The mapping out of the porta-systemic collaterals is important in patients who are candidates for shunt surgery. The effective collateral pathways

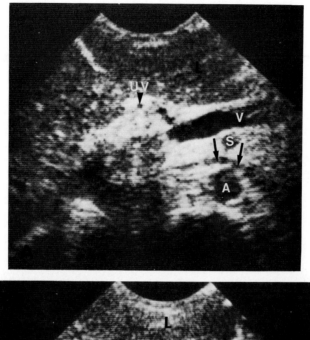

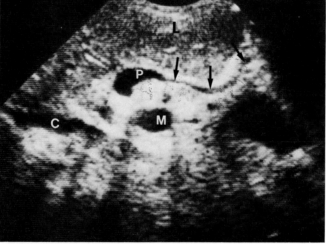

**FIG. 26. A:** A recanalized umbilical vein (UV) is present in the left intersegmental fissure surrounded by echogenic fat. Note the abnormal echo texture of the liver (L). Splenic vein (V). Superior mesenteric artery (S). Left renal vein *(arrows)*. Aorta (A). **B:** Longitudinal sonogram along the axis of the recanalized umbilical vein *(arrows)*. It can be seen arising from the tip of the left portal vein (P). Main portal vein (M). Inferior vena cava (C). Liver (L).

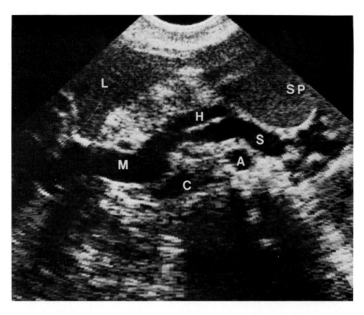

**FIG. 27.** Transverse sonogram through the upper abdomen shows dilatation of the main portal vein (M) and splenic vein (S) associated with marked splenomegaly (SP) secondary to Gaucher disease. Liver (L). Common hepatic artery (H). Aorta (A). Inferior vena cava (C).

should be preserved and one should make sure that the left renal vein is not retroaortic when a splenorenal shunt is contemplated (Fig. 7). One also has to be careful when performing upper abdominal aspiration biopsies in patients with portal hypertension as a varix can be inadvertently punctured, leading to a hemoperitoneum (74). Hopefully, this can be avoided by identifying the varices in advance of an aspiration procedure.

In patients with portal hypertension of unknown etiology, one should look for obstruction of the hepatic veins and central portal system and for signs of parenchymal liver disease (11, 43, 67). The sonographic findings of parenchymal disease depend upon its cause, severity, and length of time it has been present. There is an increase in fine parenchymal echoes associated with increased attenuation of the sound beam with or without hepatomegaly (Fig. 26). In advanced cirrhosis there is shrinkage of the liver, especially of the right lobe, with compensatory enlargement of the caudate lobe and in some instances the left lobe (10). The liver outline becomes lobulated and prominent fat deposits may be seen in the left intersegmental fissure, porta hepatis, gallbladder fossa, and hepatorenal fossa. Focal areas of regeneration (regenerating nodules) may be seen causing marked lobulation of the liver outline and they can simulate a hepatic mass. These regenerating nodules can be differentiated from a hepatoma in that the serum alpha fetal protein will be normal and they may take up the technetium sulfur colloid on a liver spleen scan, but do not take up gallium (60).

## Thrombosis of the Portal Venous System

Thrombosis of the portal venous system has many causes. It may be due to (a) tumors—hepatoma, pancreatic and gastric carcinoma, or lymphoma, (b) inflammation—intraabdominal or pelvic infections, e.g., appendicitis or diverticulitis, inflammatory bowel disease, omphalitis, sepsis, (c) cirrhosis, (d) trauma, (e) blood dyscrasias, and (f) idiopathic (3, 19, 51, 67, 68, 77, 78, 99). The portal venous thrombosis can be intra- or extrahepatic and may cause partial or complete obstruction of the involved vein (Figs. 28, 29). Sonographically, obstruction can be identified only in the large branches of the central portal venous system as the smaller branches cannot be sonographically identified (67, 77). In such cases, venous thrombosis may be identified on a contrast enhanced CT scan (97, 106).

If there is only partial obstruction of the involved vein, echogenic thrombus will be identified along the wall (Figs. 29, 30). If the vein is entirely filled with echogenic clot, one may have difficulty identifying the vein and collaterals may be present (Fig. 28) (3, 67). If there is complete obstruction of the main portal vein, numerous periportal collaterals may be seen (cavernous transformation) (Figs. 24, 25) (64, 67). On occasion, if the tumor causing portal vein thrombosis is intrahepatic, such as a hepatoma, there may be invasion of the umbilical vein (29).

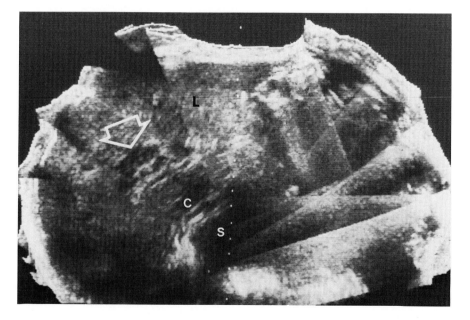

**FIG. 28.** Transverse sonogram through the upper abdomen shows the right portal vein to be filled with echogenic material *(arrow).* This represented thrombus in a patient on birth control pills. Liver (L). Inferior vena cava (C). Spine (S).

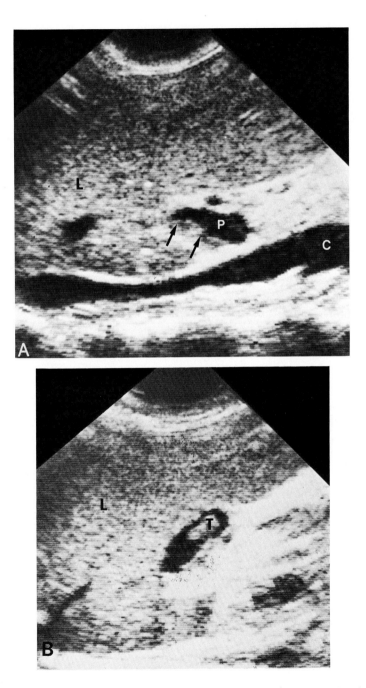

**FIG. 29. A:** Longitudinal sonogram along the main portal vein (P) demonstrating thrombus *(arrows)* along its posterior wall. Inferior vena cava (C). Liver (L). **B:** Longitudinal sono-gram slightly to the left of **A** demonstrates tumor thrombus (T) partially filling the left portal vein. These thrombi were due to portal pyelophlebitis secondary to acute diver-ticulitis. Liver (L).

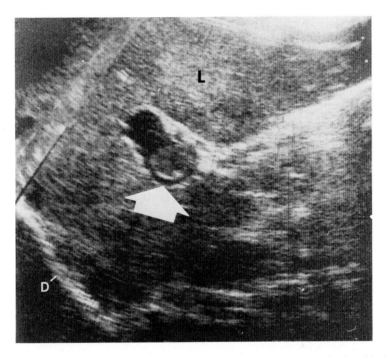

**FIG. 30.** Longitudinal sonogram through the junction of the main portal vein with the left portal vein demonstrating a thrombus *(arrow)* almost completely occluding the vein lumen. The etiology of this thrombus was unknown. Liver (L). Diaphragm (D).

Occlusion of the splenic vein is usually secondary to an inflammatory or neoplastic process of the pancreas (19, 39, 70, 79, 93, 99, 103). This is associated with fundal varices in the absence of esophageal varices, and they may be so prominent as to simulate a gastric neoplasm. Collaterals can be identified along the walls of the stomach draining via the coronary vein into the main portal vein and along the greater curvature of the stomach into the superior mesenteric vein via the gastroepiploic veins (39, 70). There may be associated splenomegaly (55). When there is obstruction of the superior mesenteric vein proximal to its junction with the splenic vein, collaterals develop around the duodenum (pancreatic, duodenal and prepyloric veins) and drain into the main portal vein via the right gastric vein (Fig. 23) (92).

## HEPATIC VEINS

The hepatic veins are not as easily visualized sonographically as the portal veins unless a specific effort is made. They are best identified by scanning both longitudinally and transversely with the patient's breath held in inspiration so that the lower portion of the liver descends beneath the costal margin and can thus be used as a sonic window. Instead of scanning directly

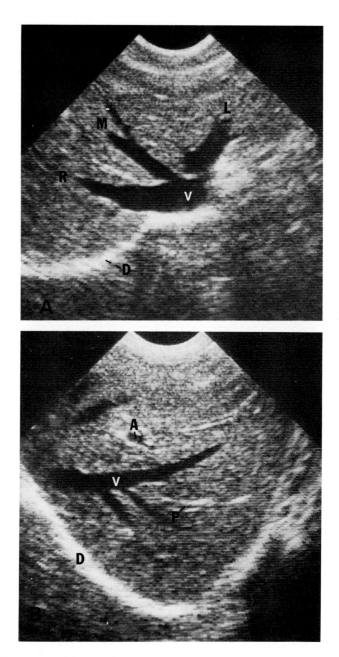

**FIG. 31. A:** Transverse oblique subcostal scan in deep inspiration demonstrating the right (R), middle (M), and left (L) hepatic veins draining into the inferior vena cava (V). Diaphragm (D). **B:** Oblique longitudinal sonogram along the axis of the right hepatic vein (V). It can be seen coursing between the anterior (A) and posterior (P) branches of the right portal vein. Diaphragm (D).

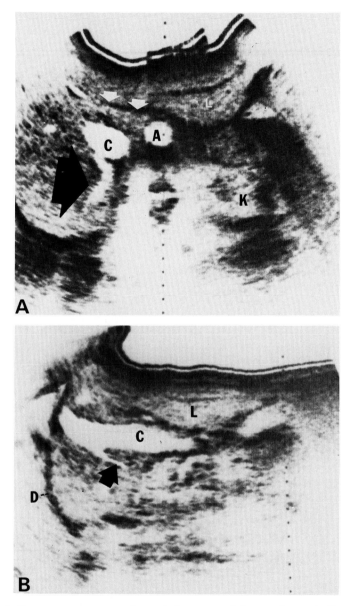

**FIG. 32. A:** Transverse sonogram through the upper abdomen demonstrating a variant right hepatic vein *(arrow)* draining into the posterior aspect of the inferior vena cava (C). The caudate lobe can be identified lying between the inferior vena cava and the ligamentum venosum *(white arrows)*. Aorta (A). Liver (L). Left kidney (K). **B:** Longitudinal sonogram along the inferior vena cava (C) showing the aberrant right hepatic vein *(arrow)* entering its posterior aspect. Liver (L). Diaphragm (D).

transversely, it is better to scan obliquely along the axis of the subcostal margin as it is in this plane that all three veins can be best identified entering the IVC (Fig. 31). The hepatic veins course between the hepatic lobes and segments unlike the branches of the portal veins which course within the segments (Fig. 31) (63). The branching pattern of the hepatic veins is such that their junctions point toward the diaphragm and their caliber increases as one approaches the IVC (63). The walls of the portal veins are more echogenic than those of the hepatic venous system when the beam strikes them at right angles (Figs. 19, 31) (17). This distinguishing feature, however, should never be used alone in differentiating between these veins.

The right hepatic vein is the largest and can be identified emptying into the right lateral aspect of the IVC just beneath the right hemidiaphragm (Fig. 31). It runs an oblique course in the intersegmental fissure between the anterior and posterior segments of the right lobe, where it separates the anterior and posterior branches of the right portal vein (Figs. 19, 31) (63). The middle hepatic vein enters the anterior or right anterior surface of the IVC at the same level. It marks the junction between the true right and left lobes of the liver, and so is an important landmark when surgical resection of a solitary mass in the liver is contemplated. The left hepatic vein drains into the IVC along its anterior or left anterolateral margin. It runs in the left

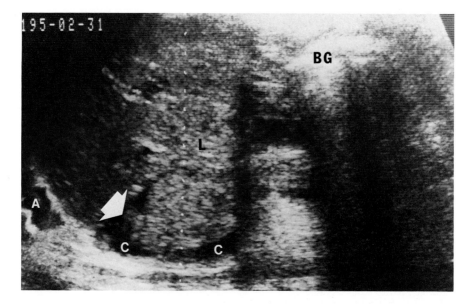

**FIG. 33.** Longitudinal sonogram along the axis of the inferior vena cava (C). Thrombus can be identified *(arrow)* in the middle hepatic vein at its confluence with the inferior vena cava. In this patient with Budd-Chiari syndrome no cause could be found. Liver (L). Right atrium (A). Bowel gas (BG).

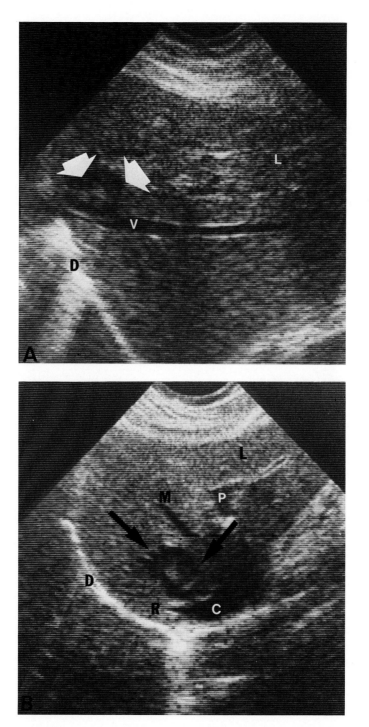

**FIG. 34. A:** Longitudinal oblique sonogram through the right lobe of the liver (L). The right hepatic vein (V) can be seen being compressed by a metastatic lesion *(arrows)*. Diaphragm (D). **B:** Transverse sonogram through the liver (L). The metastatic lesion *(arrows)* is seen compressing the right hepatic vein (R) and middle hepatic vein (M) near their junction with the inferior vena cava (C). Left portal vein (P). Diaphragm (D).

intersegmental fissure between the medial and lateral segments of the left lobe (Fig. 31) (63). The caudate lobe lies between the ligamentum venosum and portal vein anteriorly, and the IVC posteriorly (Fig. 32) (14). Its venous drainage is separate from that of the rest of the liver, being drained by one or two veins that enter directly into the anterior aspect of the adjacent IVC (Fig. 8). On occasion, a separate right hepatic vein can be seen draining into the posterior aspect of the IVC (Fig. 32).

Hepatic venous thrombosis (Budd-Chiari syndrome) is a rare condition that is characterized by upper abdominal pain, hepatomegaly, and ascites. It is caused by hypercoagulable states (polycythemia rubra vera, oral contraceptives), trauma, congenital webs and bands, and also by direct compression and invasion by tumors such as hepatomas, renal cell carcinoma, and pancreatic carcinomas (11, 47, 104). In the majority (50 to 70%) of cases, however, no cause can be found.

Sonographically the caudate lobe is enlarged and has reduced echoes. Echogenic clot may be identified in the hepatic veins or they may be reduced in size or not be visualized due to compression (Fig. 33) (11, 47, 104). There may also be narrowing of the intrahepatic portion of the IVC with ascites (104). The findings on hepatic scintigraphy are classic and include enlargement of the caudate lobe with increased uptake of the technetium sulfur colloid in comparison to the rest of the liver (71, 104). The reason for this may be the preservation of function of the caudate lobe due to its separate venous drainage (18, 104). On CT, the caudate lobe is also enlarged and there is patchy enhancement of the rest of the liver with lack of visualization of the hepatic veins (47, 82, 104). Other reports have described marked homogenous enhancement of the caudate lobe which may be due to preferential flow away from the obstructed segments of liver to the unobstructed veins of the caudate lobe (18, 104). These abnormal collateral channels can be identified sonographically (47). With the partial Budd-Chiari syndrome, where a single vein is obstructed, the involved segment of the liver on CT has a low density which can simulate a neoplasm (71, 82). Mass lesions in the liver can compress a hepatic vein without producing obstruction or invasion (Fig. 34).

## REFERENCES

1. Aagaard, J., Jenson, L. I., Sorensen, T. I. A., Christensen, U., and Burcharth, F. Recanalized umbilical vein in portal hypertension. *AJR*, 139:1107–1109, 1982.
2. Abdel-Latif, Z., Abdel-Wahab, F., and El-Kady, N. M. Evaluation of portal hypertension in cases of hepatosplenic schistosomiasis using ultrasound. *J. Clin. Ultrasound,* 9:409–412, 1981.
3. Babcock, D. S. Ultrasound diagnosis of portal vein thrombosis as a complication of appendicitis. *AJR,* 133:317–319, 1979.
4. Bandai, Y., Makuuchi, M., Watanabe, G., Ito, T., Sugiura, M., and Wada, T.

Sonographic differentiation between the umbilical portion of the left portal vein and intrahepatic bile ducts. *J. Clin. Ultrasound*, 8:207–211, 1980.

5. Barnes, P. A., Bernardino, M. E., and Thomas, J. L. Flow phenomenon mimicking thrombus: A possible pitfall of the pedal infusion technique. *J. Comput. Assist. Tomogr.*, 6(2):304–306, 1982.

6. Berger, R. B., Taylor, K. J. W., and Rosenfield, A. T. Pelvic varices simulating cystic ovaries: Differentiation by pulse Doppler. *J. Clin. Ultrasound*, 10:186–189, 1982.

7. Berland, L. L., Maddison, F. E., and Bernhard, V. M. Radiologic follow-up of vena cava filter devices. *AJR*, 134:1047–1052, 1980.

8. Bernardino, M. E., Green, B., and Goldstein, H. M. Ultrasonography in the evaluation of post-nephrectomy renal cancer patients. *Radiology*, 128:455–458, 1978.

9. Bernardino, M. E., Libshitz, H. I., Green, B., and Goldstein, H. M. Ultrasonic demonstration of inferior vena caval involvement with right adrenal gland masses. *J. Clin. Ultrasound*, 6:167–169, 1978.

10. Birnholz, J. C. Ultrasound evaluation of diffuse liver disease. In: *Clinics in Diagnostic Ultrasound—Diagnostic Ultrasound in Gastrointestinal Disease*, Vol. 1, edited by K. J. W. Taylor, pp. 23–33. Churchill Livingstone, New York, 1979.

11. Blickman, J. G., and McArdle, C. R. Budd-Chiari syndrome. *J. Comput. Assist. Tomogr.*, 5(3):409–410, 1981.

12. Bolondi, L., Gandolfi, L., Arienti, V., et al. Ultrasonography in the diagnosis of portal hypertension: Diminished response of portal vessels to respiration. *Radiology*, 142:167–172, 1982.

13. Braun, B., Weilemann, L. S., and Weigand, W. Ultrasonographic demonstration of renal vein thrombosis. *Radiology*, 138:157–158, 1981.

14. Brown, B. M., Filly, R. A., and Callen, P. W. Ultrasonographic anatomy of the caudate lobe. *J. Ultrasound Med.*, 1:189–192, 1982.

15. Buschi, A. J., Harrison, R. B., Brenbridge, A. N. A. G., Williams, B. R. J., Gentry, R. R., and Cole, R. Distended left renal vein: CT/sonographic normal variant. *AJR*, 135:339–342, 1980.

16. Callen, P. W., Filly, R. A., and DeMartini, W. J. The left portal vein: A possible source of confusion on ultrasonograms. *Radiology*, 130:205–206, 1979.

17. Chafetz, N., and Filly, R. A. Portal and hepatic veins: Accuracy of margin echoes for distinguishing intrahepatic vessels. *Radiology*, 130:725–728, 1979.

18. Cho, K. J., Geisinger, K. R., Shields, J. J., and Forrest, M. E. Collateral channels and histopathology in hepatic vein occlusion. *AJR*, 139:703–709, 1982.

19. Cho, K. J., and Martel, W. Recognition of splenic vein occlusion. *AJR*, 131:439–443, 1978.

20. Clark, K. E., Foley, W. D., Lawson, T. L., Berland, L. L., and Maddison, F. E. CT evaluation of esophageal and upper abdominal varices. *J. Comput. Assist. Tomogr.*, 4(4):510–515, 1980.

21. Coleman, C. C., Saxena, K. M., and Johnson, K. W. Renal vein thrombosis in a child with the nephrotic syndrome: CT diagnosis. *AJR*, 135:1285–1286, 1980.

22. Cosgrove, D. O., and Arger, P. H. Intravenous echoes due to laminar flow: Experimental observations. *AJR*, 139:953–956, 1982.

23. Dach, J. L., Hill, M. C., Pelaez, J. C., LePage, J. R., and Russell, E. Sonography of hypertensive portal venous system: Correlation with arterial portography. *AJR*, 137:511–517, 1981.

24. Doehner, G. A., Ruzicka, F. F., Rousselot, L. M., and Hoffman, G. The portal venous system: On its pathological roentgen anatomy. *Radiology*, 66:206–217, 1956.

25. Douglass, B. E., Baggenstoss, A. H., and Hollinshead, W. H. The anatomy of the portal vein and its tributaries. *Surg. Gynecol. Obstet.*, 91:562–576, 1950.

26. Dökmeci, A. K., Kimura, K., Matsutani, S., et al. Collateral veins in portal hypertension: Demonstration by sonography. *AJR*, 137:1173–1177, 1981.

27. Dunnick, N. R., Doppman, J. L., and Geelhoed, G. W. Intravenous extension of endocrine tumors. *AJR*, 135:471–476, 1980.

28. Faer, M. J., Lynch, R. D., Evans, H. O., and Chin, F. K. Inferior vena cava duplication: Demonstration by computed tomography. *Radiology*, 130:707–709, 1979.

29. Fakhry, J., Gosink, B. B., and Leopold, G. R. Recanalized umbilical vein due to portal vein occlusion: Documentation by sonography. *AJR*, 137:410–412, 1981.
30. Filly, R. A., and Laing, F. C. Anatomic variation of portal venous anatomy in the porta hepatis: Ultrasonographic evaluation. *J. Clin. Ultrasound*, 6:83–89, 1978.
31. Foley, W. D., Gleysteen, J. J., Lawson, T. L., et al. Dynamic computed tomography and pulsed Doppler ultrasonography in the evaluation of splenorenal shunt patency. *J. Comput. Assist. Tomogr.*, 7(1):106–112, 1983.
32. Foley, W. D., Stewart, E. T., Milbrath, J. R., SanDretto, M., and Milde, M. Digital subtraction angiography of the portal venous system. *AJR*, 140:497–499, 1983.
33. Foley, W. D., Varma, R. R., Lawson, T. L., Berland, L. L., Smith, D. F., and Thorsen, K. Dynamic computed tomography and duplex ultrasonography: Adjuncts to arterial portography. *J. Comput. Assist. Tomogr.*, 7(1):77–82, 1983.
34. Funston, M. R., Goudie, E., Richter, I. A., Butterworth, A. M., and Allan, J. C. Ultrasound diagnosis of the recanalized umbilical vein in portal hypertension. *J. Clin. Ultrasound*, 8:244–246, 1980.
35. Garris, J. B., Kangarloo, H., and Sample, W. F. Ultrasonic diagnosis of infrahepatic interruption of the inferior vena cava with azygous (hemiazygous) continuation. *Radiology*, 134:179–183, 1980.
36. Glazer, G. M., Callen, P. W., and Parker, J. J. CT diagnosis of tumor thrombus in the inferior vena cava: Avoiding the false-positive diagnosis. *AJR*, 137:1265–1267, 1981.
37. Glazer, G. M., Laing, F. C., Brown, T. W., and Gooding, G. A. W. Sonographic demonstration of portal hypertension: The patent umbilical vein. *Radiology*, 136:161–163, 1980.
38. Goldberg, B. B., and Patel, J. Ultrasonic evaluation of portacaval shunts. *J. Clin. Ultrasound*, 5(5):304–306, 1977.
39. Goldstein, G. B. Splenic vein thrombosis causing gastric varices and bleeding. *Am. J. Gastroenterol.*, 58:319–325, 1972.
40. Goldstein, H. M., Green, B., and Weaver, R. M. Ultrasonic detection of renal tumor extension into the inferior vena cava. *AJR*, 130:1083–1085, 1978.
41. Goncharenko, V., Gerlock, A. J., Kadir, S., and Turner, B. Incidence and distribution of venous extension in 70 hypernephromas. *AJR*, 133:263–265, 1979.
42. Gosink, B. B. The inferior vena cava: Mass effects. *AJR*, 130:533–536, 1978.
43. Gosink, B. B., Lemon, S. K., and Scheible, W. Accuracy of ultrasonography in diagnosis of hepatocellular disease. *AJR*, 53:440–444, 1979.
44. Grant, E., Rendano, F., Sevinc, E., Gammelgaard, J., Holm, H. H., and Gronvall, S. Normal inferior vena cava: Caliber changes observed by dynamic ultrasound. *AJR*, 135:335–338, 1980.
45. Green, B., Goldstein, H. M., and Weaver, R. M. Abdominal pansonography in the evaluation of renal cancer. *Radiology*, 132:421–424, 1979.
46. Greene, E. R., Volpicelli, N., and French, F. B. Noninvasive estimation of normal and abnormal portal vein blood flow variables. Paper No. 706, Presented at the 26th Annual Meeting of the American Institute of Ultrasound in Medicine. San Francisco, California, August 1981.
47. Harter, L. P., Gross, B. H., St. Hilaire, J., Filly, R. A., and Goldberg, H. I. CT and sonographic appearance of hepatic vein obstruction. *AJR*, 139:176–178, 1982.
48. Hill, M. C., Druy, E. M., Dach, J. L., and Steinberg, W. M. The abnormal portal venous system. Paper No. 231, Presented at the World Federation for Ultrasound in Medicine and Biology, Brighton, England, July 1982.
49. Holmin, T., Alwamark, A., and Forsberg, L. The ultrasonic demonstration of portacaval and interposition mesocaval shunts. *Br. J. Surg.*, 69:673–675, 1982.
50. Huberman, R. P., and Gomes, A. S. Membranous obstruction of the inferior vena cava. *AJR*, 139:1215–1216, 1982.
51. Inamoto, K., Sugiki, K., Yamasaki, H., and Miura, T. CT of hepatoma: Effects of portal vein obstruction. *AJR*, 136:349–353, 1981.
52. Ishikawa, T., Tsukune, Y., Ohyama, Y., Fujikawa, M., Sakuyama, K., and Fujii, M. Venous abnormalities in portal hypertension demonstrated by CT. *AJR*, 134:271–276, 1980.
53. Isikoff, M. B., Hill, M. C., Sinner, W. N., and Diaconis, J. N. Ultrasonic diagnosis of a

mega cava presenting as a retroperitoneal mass (German). (Progress in Radiology and Nuclear Medicine), 130:608–610, 1979.

54. Isikoff, M. B., and Hill, M. C. Sonography of the renal arteries: Left lateral decubitus position. *AJR*, 134:1177–1179, 1980.

55. Itzchak, Y., and Glickman, M. G. Splenic vein thrombosis in patients with a normal size spleen. *Invest. Radiol.*, 12:158–163, 1977.

56. Jüttner, H. U., Jenney, J. M., Ralls, P. W., Goldstein, L. I., and Reynolds, T. B. Ultrasound demonstration of portosystemic collaterals in cirrhosis and portal hypertension. *Radiology*, 142:459–463, 1982.

57. Kane, R. A., and Katz, S. G. The spectrum of sonographic findings in portal hypertension: A subject review and new observations. *Radiology*, 142:453–458, 1982.

58. Kurtz, A. B., Rubin, C., and Goldberg, B. B. Ultrasound diagnosis of masses elevating the inferior vena cava. *AJR*, 132:401–406, 1979.

59. Kutcher, R., Rosenblatt, R., Mitsudo, F. M., Goldman, M., and Kogan, S. Renal angiomyolipoma with sonographic demonstration of extension into the inferior vena cava. *Radiology*, 143:755–756, 1982.

60. Laing, F. C., Jeffrey, R. B., Federle, M. P., and Cello, J. P. Noninvasive imaging of unusual regenerating nodules in the cirrhotic liver. *Gastrointest. Radiol.*, 7:245–249, 1982.

61. Madayag, M. A., Ambos, M. A., Lefleur, R. S., and Bosniak, M. A. Involvement of the inferior vena cava in patients with renal cell carcinoma. *Radiology*, 133:321–326, 1979.

62. Manor, A., Itzchak, Y., Strauss, S., and Graif, M. Sonographic demonstration of the right ascending lumbar vein. *AJR*, 138:339–341, 1982.

63. Marks, W. M., Filly, R. A., and Callen, P. W. Ultrasonic anatomy of the liver: A review with new applications. *J. Clin. Ultrasound*, 7:137–146, 1979.

64. Marx, M., and Scheible, W. Cavernous transformation of the portal vein. *J. Ultrasound Med.*, 1:167–169, 1982.

65. Mayo, J., Gray, R., St. Louis, E., Grossman, H., McLoughlin, M., and Wise, D. Anomalies of the inferior vena cava. *AJR*, 140:339–345, 1983.

66. Meltzer, R. S., McGhie, J., and Roelandt, J. Inferior vena cava echocardiography. *J. Clin. Ultrasound*, 10:47–51, 1982.

67. Merritt, C. R. B. Ultrasonographic demonstration of portal vein thrombosis. *Radiology*, 133:425–427, 1979.

68. Miller, E. I., and Thomas, R. H. Portal vein invasion demonstrated by ultrasound. *J. Clin. Ultrasound*, 7:57–59, 1979.

69. Mintz, G. S., Kotler, M. N., Wayne, R. P., Abdulmassih, S. I., and Kane, S. A. Real time inferior vena caval ultrasonography: Normal and abnormal findings and its use in assessing right heart function. *Circulation*, 64:1018–1025, 1981.

70. Muhletaler, C., Gerlock, A. J., Goncharenko, V., Avant, G. R., and Flexner, J. M. Gastric varices secondary to splenic vein occlusion: Radiographic diagnosis and clinical significance. *Radiology*, 132:593–598, 1979.

71. Nakamura, H., Tanaka, T., Hori, S., Yoshioka, H., and Kuroda, C. Partial Budd-Chiari syndrome. *J. Comput. Assist. Tomogr.*, 6(4):833–835, 1982.

72. Nunez, D., Russell, E., Yrizarry, J., Pereiras, R., and Viamonte, M. Portosystemic communications studied by transhepatic portography. *Radiology*, 127:75–79, 1978.

73. O'Brien, M. J., and Gottlieb, L. S. Portal hypertension. In: *Pathological Basis of Disease*, 2nd ed., edited by S. L. Robbins and R. S. Cotran, pp. 1047–1062, W. B. Saunders, Philadelphia, 1979.

74. Palaez, J. C., Hill, M. C., Dach, J. L., and Isikoff, M. B. Abdominal aspiration biopsies—Sonographic versus CT guidance. Paper No. 77, Presented at the American Roentgen Ray Society Meeting. New Orleans, Louisiana, May 1982.

75. Park, S. C., Glanz, S., Gordon, D. H., and Johnson, M. Computed tomography and angiography in the Cruveilhier-Baumgarten syndrome. *J. Comput. Assist. Tomogr.*, 5(1):19–21, 1981.

76. Parulekar, S. Ligaments and fissures of the liver: Sonographic anatomy. *Radiology*, 130:409–411, 1979.

77. Pauls, C. H. Ultrasound and computed tomographic demonstration of portal vein thrombosis in hepatocellular carcinoma. *Gastrointest. Radiol.*, 6:281–283, 1981.
78. Reh, T. E., Srivisal, S., and Schmidt, E. H. Portal venous thrombosis in ulcerative colitis: CT diagnosis with angiographic correlation. *J. Comput. Assist. Tomogr.*, 4(4):545–547, 1980.
79. Rice, R. P., Thompson, W. M., Kelvin, F. M., Kriner, A. F., and Garbutt, J. T. Gastric varices without esophageal varices. *JAMA*, 237(18):1976–1979, 1977.
80. Rosenberg, E. R., Trought, W. S., Kirks, D. R., Sumner, T. E., and Grossman, H. Ultrasonic diagnosis of renal vein thrombosis in neonates. *AJR*, 134:35–38, 1980.
81. Rosenfield, A. T., Zeman, R. K., Cronan, J. J., and Taylor, K. J. W. Ultrasound in experimental and clinical renal vein thrombosis. *Radiology*, 137:735–741, 1980.
82. Rossi, P., Sposito, M., Simonetti, G., Sposato, S., and Cusumano, G. CT diagnosis of Budd-Chiari syndrome. *J. Comput. Assist. Tomogr.*, 5(3):366–369, 1981.
83. Royal, S. A., and Callen, P. W. CT evaluation of anomalies of the inferior cava and left renal vein. *AJR*, 132:759–763, 1979.
84. Ruzicka, F. F., and Rossi, P. Arterial portography: Patterns of venous flow. *Radiology*, 92:777–787, 1969.
85. Schabel, S. I., Rittenberg, G. M., Javid, L. H., Cunningham, J., and Ross, P. The "bull's-eye" falciform ligament: A sonographic finding of portal hypertension. *Radiology*, 136:157–159, 1980.
86. Shenoy, S. S., and Rowland, D. M. Ultrasound demonstration of right atrial invasion by hypernephroma. *J. Clin. Ultrasound*, 8:52–54, 1980.
87. Sherlock, S. The portal venous system and portal hypertension. In: *Diseases of the Liver and Biliary Tract*, 6th ed., edited by S. Sherlock, pp. 134–176, Blackwell Scientific Publications, London, 1981.
88. Slovis, T. L., Philippart, A. I., Cushing, B., et al. Evaluation of the inferior vena cava by sonography and venography in children with renal and hepatic tumors. *Radiology*, 140:767–772, 1981.
89. Smith, D. F., Lawson, T. L., Berland, L. L., Foley, W. D., and Thorsen, M. K. Pulsed Doppler evaluation of porto-systemic collaterals in portal hypertension. Paper No. 313, Presented at the 27th Annual Meeting of the American Institute of Ultrasound in Medicine. San Francisco, California, August 1981.
90. Sonnenfeld, M., and Finberg, H. J. Ultrasonographic diagnosis of incomplete inferior vena caval thrombosis secondary to periphlebitis: The importance of a complete survey examination. *Radiology*, 137:743–744, 1980.
91. Spira, R., Kwan, E., Gerzof, S. G., and Widrich, W. C. Left renal vein varix simulating a pancreatic pseudocyst by sonography. *AJR*, 138:149–150, 1982.
92. Subramanyam, B. R., Balthazar, E. J., Madamba, M. R., Raghavendra, B. N., Horii, S. C., and Lefleur, R. S. Sonography of portosystemic venous collaterals in portal hypertension. *Radiology*, 146:161–166, 1983.
93. Sutton, J. P., Yarborough, D. Y., and Richards, J. T. Isolated splenic vein occlusion. *Arch. Surg.*, 100:623–626, 1970.
94. Teng, S. S., and Laing, F. C. Ultrasonographic demonstration of inferior vena caval invasion. *J. Clin. Ultrasound*, 6:424–426, 1978.
95. Thomas, J. L., and Bernardino, M. E. Neoplastic-induced renal vein enlargement: Sonographic detection. *AJR*, 136:75–79, 1981.
96. Train, J. S., Henderson, M. R., and Smith, A. P. Sonographic demonstration of left-sided inferior vena cava with hemiazygous continuation. *AJR*, 134:1057–1059, 1980.
97. Vigo, M., De Faveri, D., Biondetti, P. R., and Benedetti, L. CT demonstration of portal and superior mesenteric vein thrombosis in hepatocellular carcinoma. *J. Comput. Assist. Tomogr.*, 4(5):627–629, 1980.
98. Webb, L. J., Berger, L. A., Sherlock, S. Grey-scale ultrasonography of portal vein. *Lancet*, October 1, 1977.
99. Weinberger, G., Mitra, S. K., and Yoeli, G. Ultrasound diagnosis of splenic vein thrombosis. *J. Clin. Ultrasound*, 10:345–346, 1982.
100. Weinreb, J., Kumari, S., Phillips, G., and Pochaczevsky, R. Portal vein measurements by real-time sonography. *AJR*, 139:497–499, 1982.

101. Williams, P. L., and Warwick, R. The inferior vena cava. In: *Gray's Anatomy*. 36th ed., pp. 761–763. W. B. Saunders, Philadelphia, 1980.
102. Wise, N. K., Myers, S., Fraker, T. D., Stewart, J. A., and Kisslo, J. A. Contrast M mode ultrasonography of the inferior vena cava. *Circulation*, 63:1100–1103, 1981.
103. Yale, C. E., and Crummy, A. B. Splenic vein thrombosis and bleeding esophageal varices. *JAMA*, 217(3):317–320, 1971.
104. Yang, P. J., Glazer, G. M., and Bowerman, R. A. Budd-Chiari syndrome: Computed tomographic and ultrasonographic findings. *J. Comput. Assist. Tomogr.*, 7(1):148–150, 1983.
105. Young, R., Friedman, A. C., Hartman, D. S. Computed tomography of leiomyosarcoma of the inferior vena cava. *Radiology*, 145:99–103, 1982.
106. Zerhouni, E. A., Barth, K. H., and Siegelman, S. S. Demonstration of venous thrombosis by computed tomography. *AJR*, 134:753–758, 1980.
107. Zerhouni, E. A., Siegelman, S. S., Walsh, P. C., and White, R. I. Elevated pressure in the left renal vein in patients with varicocele. *J. Urol.*, 123:512–513, 1980.

*Subject Index*

# Subject Index